Classics in Movement Science

Mark L. Latash, PhD
Vladimir M. Zatsiorsky, PhD
The Pennsylvania State University

Editors

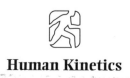

Human Kinetics

Library of Congress Cataloging-in-Publication Data

Latash, Mark L., 1953-
    Classics in movement science / Mark L. Latash, Vladimir M. Zatsiorsky
      p. cm.
    Includes bibliographical references and index.
    ISBN 0-7360-0028-3
      1. Human mechanics. 2. Human locomotion. I. Zatsiorsky, Vladimir M., 1932- II.
Title.

    QP301 .L358 2001
    612.7'6--dc21

                                00-053857

ISBN: 0-7360-0028-3

Acquisitions Editor: Judy Patterson Wright, PhD; **Managing Editor:** Amy Stahl; **Assistant Editors:** Derek Campbell, Amanda S. Ewing; **Copyeditor:** Joyce Sexton; **Proofreader:** Erin T. Cler; **Indexer:** Marie Rizzo; **Permission Managers:** Courtney Astle, Dalene Reeder; **Graphic Designer:** Stuart Cartwright; **Graphic Artist:** Tara Welsch; **Photo Manager:** Clark Brooks; **Cover Designer:** Nancy Rasmus; **Art Manager:** Craig Newsom; **Illustrator:** Chuck Nivens; **Printer:** Edwards Bros.

Printed in the United States of America   10 9 8 7 6 5 4 3 2 1

Human Kinetics
Web site: www.humankinetics.com

United States: Human Kinetics, P.O. Box 5076, Champaign, IL 61825-5076
800-747-4457
e-mail: humank@hkusa.com

Canada: Human Kinetics, 475 Devonshire Road Unit 100, Windsor, ON N8Y 2L5
800-465-7301 (in Canada only)
e-mail: orders@hkcanada.com

Europe: Human Kinetics, Units C2/C3 Wira Business Park, West Park Ring Road, Leeds LS16 6EB, United Kingdom
+44 (0) 113 278 1708
e-mail: humank@hkeurope.com

Australia: Human Kinetics, 57A Price Avenue, Lower Mitcham, South Australia 5062
08 8277 1555
e-mail: liahka@senet.com.au

New Zealand: Human Kinetics, P.O. Box 105-231, Auckland Central
09-523-3462
e-mail: hkp@ihug.co.nz

Contents

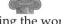

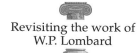

Preface

In his classical book *On Dexterity and Its Development*, N.A. Bernstein wrote: "No natural phenomenon can be understood without carefully considering how it emerged" (1996, p. 45). This statement can be equally applied to a particular phenomenon (for example, dexterity) or to an area of science. Many theories can be truly understood and appreciated only when considered within their particular historical context, including the prevailing trends in philosophy, the state of other areas of science, technology, and even politics (Bongaardt, 1996; Flesher, 1997). Recently, more and more scholars working in movement science have started to appreciate the necessity of understanding the history of this discipline. Papers and book chapters on the history of movement science have been published (Meijer et al., 1988; Cappozzo et al., 1992; Latash & Latash, 1994; Bongaardt, 1996; Flesher, 1997; Bongaardt & Meijer, 1998), and a special historical section, "Bernstein's Heritage," has been established in one of the journals in the area, *Motor Control* (Latash, 1998). This trend does not show signs of running out of steam.

So a major purpose of the present volume is to put together influential papers from the past, or sections from them, and to present these works together with commentaries, both historical and scientific, written by contemporary authorities in movement science. History cannot be separated from its interpretation. Therefore, subjective views of the contributors to this volume have certainly affected the way they present the "classic papers" and their authors. This subjectivity need not be viewed as bad. Actually, it provides two things for the price of one: an understanding of the thinking of a famous scientist of the past and that of his or her contemporary counterpart!

The names of Bernstein, Denny-Brown, Fenn, Hill, Hughlings Jackson, Woodworth, Sherrington, von Helmholtz, and other great scientists who worked in areas that are now associated with biomechanics, neurophysiology of movements, and motor control are frequently cited in textbooks and research papers. However, very rarely students or even researchers have an opportunity to read the original publications. This is due partly to the poor accessibility of some of the original sources, partly to the fact that some of these papers have never been translated into English, and partly to the style of the original papers—which may seem wordy and difficult to extract important facts and ideas from. However, in many cases, ideas expressed by great scientists of the past are anything but obsolete, while citations of these classic papers commonly contain direct misrepresentations of what the authors actually tried to say. Such misrepresentations travel from paper to paper and from textbook to textbook. One of the most glaring examples is the frequent reference to a paper by Sir A.V. Hill (1938) within the context of joint or muscle viscosity: In this paper, Hill actually wrote that the notion of viscosity was inapplicable to muscles and joints!

We strongly believe that students and researchers in biomechanics and motor control need to read at least some of the greatest works of the past. The purpose of this volume is to present, under one cover, a selection of classic papers with commentaries that will hopefully make these papers more understandable for contemporary students and will also put their studies into an appropriate historical and contemporary scientific context.

It is probably impossible to define universally acceptable criteria for selecting particular papers and their authors into the group of "classics." We started this project by posting an Internet message and asking our colleagues to nominate up to three great scientists of the past whose works should be included into this volume. We are very much grateful to all those who responded to our posting and helped us make the final decision. Two more criteria were used in the selection process, mostly to avoid unnecessary uneasy feelings among competing influential directions in movement science. First, the original publications should have appeared at least 50 years ago. Second, only publications by late authors were accepted. We also wanted to have different areas of movement science represented in the volume including physics (von Helmholtz), behavioral research (Woodworth), clinical studies (Hughlings Jackson), and certainly biomechanics and neurophysiology.

We are indebted to Onno Meijer for his fantastic introductory chapter, which covers movement science from ancient Greece and Rome to the 19th century. This chapter is an excellent example of Onno's brilliantly provocative style, including his unique ability to use simple examples to illustrate complex notions and ideas. This chapter is a tremendous piece of work that will certainly be appreciated by future readers.

Some of the "classics" are presented in their entirety, while others have been shortened. In certain cases, only quotations from a "classic" are presented. Decisions on how exactly to present a piece of these classics were left to the authors of the chapters, with only soft guidelines provided by the editors. We are very much grateful to Dagmar Sternad who not only wrote a commentary on works by Wachholder but also translated his original papers. A translation of the famous 1935 paper by Bernstein was available (Bernstein, 1967). However, meticulous reading showed its inadequacy. Therefore, a new translation was prepared by one of the editors (Mark Latash).

We are very much grateful to all the contributors to this volume, to Human Kinetics Publishers for their patience and high professionalism, and to the copyright holders of the original publications for allowing us to reproduce the "classics."

References

Bernstein NA (1967) *The co-ordination and regulation of movements*. Oxford: Pergamon Press.

Bernstein NA (1996) On dexterity and its development. In: Latash ML & Turvey MT (Eds.), *Dexterity and its development*, pp. 3-246. Mahwah, NJ: Erlbaum.

Bongaardt R (1996) *Shifting focus: The Bernstein tradition in movement science*. Doctoral Dissertation. Free University, Amsterdam.

Bongaardt R & Meijer OG (1998) Bernstein's theory of movement behavior: Historical development and contemporary relevance. *J Mot Behav*, 32 (1): 57-71.

Cappozzo A, Marchetti M, & Tosi V (1992) (Eds.) *Biolocomotion: A century of research using moving pictures*. Rome: Promograph.

Flesher MM (1997) Repetitive order and the human walking apparatus: Prussian military science versus the Webers' locomotion research. *Ann Sci*, 54: 463-487.

Hill AV (1938) The heat of shortening and the dynamic constants of muscle. *Proc Roy Soc London Ser B*, 126: 136-195.

Latash LP & Latash ML (1994) A new book by N.A. Bernstein: "On Dexterity and Its Development." *J Mot Behav*, 26: 56-62.

Latash ML (1998) Bernstein's papers in "Motor Control." *Mot Control*, 2: 1.

Meijer OG, Wagenaar RC, & Blankendaal FCM (1988) The hierarchy debate: Tema con variazioni. In: Meijer OG & Roth K (Eds.), *Complex movement behavior: "The motor-action controversy,"* pp. 489-561. Amsterdam: North-Holland.

Credits

Figure 1.1 Reprinted, by permission, from J.A. García-Diego, 1986, *Juanelo Turriano Charles V's Clockmaker: The man and his legend.* (Madrid: Editorial Castalia), xxxviii; by kind permission of the Fondación Juanelo Turriano.

Figure 1.3 Reprinted by kind permission of Fray Francisco de Andrés, Prior of the monastery.

Figure 1.5 Reprinted, by permission, from E. Wickersheimer, 1926, *Anatomies de Mondino dei Luzzi et de Guido de Vigevano.* (Paris: Droz), page not numbered.

Figure 1.9 Reprinted, by permission, from J.A. García-Diego, 1986, *Juanelo Turriano Charles V's Clockmaker: The man and his legend.* (Madrid: Editorial Castalia), lxxiii; by kind permission of the Fondación Juanelo Turriano.

Figure 1.10 Reprinted, by permission, from K.E. Rotschuh, Ed., 1969, *René Descartes.* (Heidelberg: Lambert Schneider), 68; with the kind help of the *Institut für Theorie und Geschichte der Medizin*, Münster.

Figure 1.11 Reprinted, by permission, from G.A. Borelli, 1989, *On the movement of animals* (original work published 1680-1681, trans. from Latin by P. Maquet). (Berlin: Springer), Table III, Figures 4 & 5; by kind permission of Springer-Verlag, Heidelberg.

Figure 1.13 Adapted, by permission, from P.N. Kugler and M.T. Turvey, 1987, *Information, natural law, and the self-assembly of rhythmic movement.* (Hillsdale, NJ: Lawrence Erlbaum), 117.

Chapter 4 Reprinted, by permission, from D. Denny-Brown and J. B. Pennybacker, 1938, "Fibrillation and fasciculation in voluntary muscle," *Brain* 61: 311-334.

Fenn photo, chapter 5 Reprinted, by permission, from W.O. Fenn, 1963, *History of the American Physiological Society: The third quarter century.* (Bethesda, MD: The American Physiological Society), 14.

Chapter 5 Reprinted, by permission, from W. O. Fenn, 1930, "Frictional and kinetic factors in the work of sprint running," *American Journal of Physiology* 92: 583-611. Reprinted, by permission, from H. Elftman, 1939, "Forces and energy changes in the leg during walking," *American Journal of Physiology* 125: 339-356.

Figures 5.1–5.5 Reprinted, by permission, from W. O. Fenn, 1930, "Frictional and kinetic factors in the work of sprint running," *American Journal of Physiology* 92: 583-611.

Figures 5.6–5.14 Reprinted, by permission, from H. Elftman, 1939, "Forces and energy changes in the leg during walking," *American Journal of Physiology* 125: 339-356.

Figure 5.15 Reprinted, by permission, from V.M. Zatsiorsky and R.J. Gregor, 2000, Mechanical power and work in human movement. In *Energetics of human activity,* edited by W.A. Sparrow (Champaign, IL: Human Kinetics), 196.

Tables 5.1-5.4 Reprinted, by permission, from W. O. Fenn, 1930, "Frictional and kinetic factors in the work of sprint running," *American Journal of Physiology* 92: 583-611.

Tables 5.5 and 5.6 Reprinted, by permission, from H. Elftman, 1939, "Forces and energy changes in the leg during walking," *American Journal of Physiology* 125: 339-356.

Granit photo, chapter 6 Reprinted from R. Granit, 1972, "Discovery and understanding," *Annual Review of Physiology* 34.

Chapter 6 Reprinted, by permission, from R. Granit, 1950, "Reflex self-regulation of muscle contraction and autogenic inhibition," *American Journal of Neurophysiology* 13: 351-372.

Figures 6.1–6.17 Reprinted, by permission, from R. Granit, 1950, "Reflex self-regulation of muscle contraction and autogenic inhibition," *American Journal of Neurophysiology* 13: 351-372.

Jackson photo, chapter 9 Reprinted from M. Critchley and E.A. Critchley, 1998, *John Hughlings Jackson: Father of English neurology.* (New York: Oxford University Press.)

Lombard photo, chapter 10 Reprinted, by permission, from W.O. Fenn, 1968, *History of the International Congresses of Physiological Sciences 1889-1968.* (Bethesda, MD: The American Physiological Society), plate XX.

Chapter 11 Reprinted, by permission, from C.S. Sherrington, 1932, "Inhibition as a coordinative factor," Nobel Lecture, December 12, 1932. In *Les Prix Nobel* (Stockholm: Nobel Foundation), 278-289. © The Nobel Foundation 1932.

Figure 11.1a Reprinted, by permission, from C.S. Sherrington, 1913, "Reflex inhibition as a factor in the co-ordination of movements and postures," *Quarterly Journal of Experimental Physiology* 6: 251.

Figure 11.1b Reprinted, by permission, from R. Granit, 1966, *Charles Scott Sherrington: An appraisal* (Surrey, United Kingdom: Thomas Nelson and Sons, Ltd.), 55.

Figure 11.2 Reprinted, by permission, from E.G.T. Liddell and C. S. Sherrington, 1924, "Reflexes in response to stretch (myotatic reflexes)," *Proceedings of the Royal Society of London Series B: Biological Science* 96: 212.

Wachholder photo, chapter 12 Reprinted, by permission, from M. Weisendanger, 1997, Paths of discovery in human motor control. A short historical perspective. In *Perspectives of motor behavior and its neural basis,* edited by M.-C. Hepp-Reymond and G. Marini (Basel, Switzerland: S. Karger AG), 109. Photograph from the Institute of Physiology.

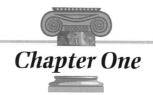

Chapter One

Making Things Happen: An Introduction to the History of Movement Science

Onno G. Meijer

Faculty of Human Movement Sciences, Vrije Universiteit, Amsterdam, The Netherlands

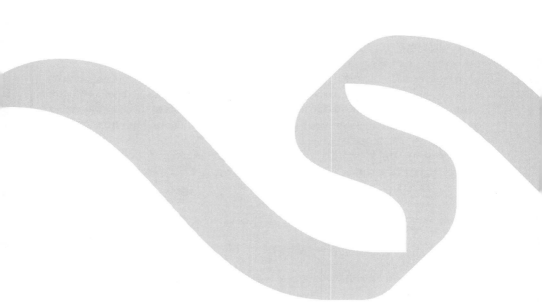

Abstract

This introductory chapter focuses on the problem of understanding coordination and control in a mechanical world. Charles V is presented as exemplar of the difficulties that arose as soon as mechanical metaphors were accepted. Charles was obsessed with his collection of clocks, trying to have them sound together on the hour. He couldn't.

In the world view preceding the era of Charles V, the world was intrinsically goal directed (Plato, Aristotle, Galen as he would be known by posterity, and Muslim culture). In such a goal-directed world, control and coordination are not much of a problem. But at the time of Charles V, mechanical metaphors were on the rise, and it became difficult to properly understand coordination and control. This is taken to define "Charles' problem."

Descartes and Borelli claimed control from outside the world, that is, by an immaterial soul. But it is impossible to reconnect such a soul with the material world. In the alchemically inspired views of Harvey and Newton, matter has surprising properties, and the problem of reconnection did not present itself. Nevertheless, Harvey and Newton failed to couch their views of matter within a scientifically acceptable framework. When observing synchronization between clocks, Christiaan Huygens stumbled upon a technical solution to Charles' problem, but the importance of the phenomenon was not recognized. Had Charles known of Huygens' finding, he would have been able to make his clocks strike together; but he could never have predicted exactly when they would do so.

In the 18th and 19th centuries, the dominance of mechanicism was not seriously threatened. To the contrary, it was the soul that suffered—by first becoming passive and then disappearing altogether. Thus, it was through the end of the 19th century that we failed to understand the need to change the world view that had led to Charles' problem.

With the 20th century came vastly different metaphors, and maybe we are now able to solve Charles' problem. Still, old habits die hard, and the reader of this book is invited to wonder, with every chapter, how far the views of the author in question would do the job. It is irrelevant how the author thinks about the soul; it is the understanding of the world that matters. In view of biological flexibility, the to-be-coordinated/controlled needs some "Speelruimte" *(Spielraum)* for itself (slack, space to play, freedom to negotiate). At least, that's how I see it.

The Clocks of Charles V (1500-1558)

On August 12, 1550, Juanelo Turriano had to go to Augsburg. To bring the clock.[1]

There is no doubt that the clock was a masterpiece. It has not survived to our present time, but contemporary descriptions allow us to envisage what it looked like (figure 1.1). Of course, the clock indicated time, as had sundials from time immemorial, Chinese water clocks,[2] or Muslim candle clocks.[3] Turriano's clock was mechanical, with a spring that could be wound. The clock was small enough to be put on a table. It had eight faces, probably with separate displays of the motions of the firmament, the sun and the moon, the time of sunrise and sunset, the phases of the moon, and the date of Easter Sunday, for instance, in any particular year. The clock also depicted the trajectories of the planets, large circles with smaller ones protruding from their surface ("epicycles"), sometimes arching backward in a way too complicated to understand and thus certainly the work of God.[4] Bishop Vida, just like Turriano born in Cremona, wrote that the clock was

> a clock of admirable, unusual and incredible artifice which not only measures daily the course of the sun as it goes from rising to setting and divides the day into 24 hours of equal duration by means of mechanisms and hidden energy, either from propelling weights or from a steel spring strongly rolled up and wound round an axis. . . , but figures out the order of the heavens and the constitution and form of the world by means of its continuous motion. . . . I believe . . . its egregious artificer, with his eminent talent and goaded eagerness for investigation, has emulated the divine, . . . inimitable activity of God himself in the construction of the Universal World and Nature entire. . . . *This is, in fact, transferring what is divine to men and like contending with Nature herself and—if it is lawful to say so—emulating the Eternal Craftsman.*[5]

It was, in other words, a clock worthy of an emperor.

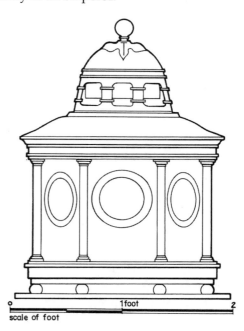

Figure 1.1
Turriano's clock (reprinted from García-Diego 1986).

Augsburg, in southern Germany, was a prosperous town, famous center of clock making. It also was the residence of Jacob Fugger, the banker, who had helped Charles V to buy his election to become Emperor of the Holy Roman Empire.[6] From August 8, 1550, to November 3, 1551, Charles resides in Augsburg—to educate his son, to meet with the Imperial Council (the Diet), and to discuss some family problems. His son Philip is doing well. He finds the Germans a bit uncivilized, but he "is doing his best. . . . He often goes out to join in their sports. . . ."[7] In the Diet, relations with the Protestants are strained. Maurice of Saxony and the Princess Palatine have asked Philip to intercede with Charles to release the prisoners from the battle of Mühlberg, but Charles is angry and refuses. Things do not go any better in Charles's family. Ferdinand, his brother, cannot accept Philip as future emperor and is campaigning for his own son, Maximilian.

So it was in the eye of the storm—with the greatest power in Christendom on the verge of collapse—that Juanelo Turriano must[8] have arrived. To date, Turriano, the engineer-clockmaker-astrologist, is best known in the Spanish-speaking world. "In Mexico the saying is 'like Juanelo's egg'."[9] This fame derived from a later period, when Turriano built the waterworks in Toledo for King Philip II, raising the water by 90 meters from the Tajo to the Alcázar.[10] Turriano was born around 1511 in a village near Cremona, in Northern Italy. He trained himself to be a mechanical engineer. "His face and figure are very rough, ugly and coarse. He does not show any dignity, any character, any sign of ability. It is . . . repulsive to see him always with his face, hair and beard covered . . . with plenty of ash and . . . tar. His hands and . . . fingers are always coated with rust. He is dirty, badly and excentrically dressed. . . ."[11] Juanelo Turriano was to be the closest friend of Emperor Charles V.

Charles had quite a collection of clocks already, but Turriano's clock was to be the jewel in his crown. The clock was not finished yet, and Juanelo had to bring it back to Milan. They met again in Innsbruck, in Tyrol, where Charles was hiding from the troops of Maurice of Saxony. Isolated from his own army, in actual danger of losing everything, Charles was delighted to see the clock. On March 7, 1552, he decreed from Innsbruck:

> We, Charles V, by the Grace of Divine Mercy, August Emperor of the Romans and King of Germany, the Spains, the two Sicilies, Jerusalem, Hungary, Dalmatia, Croatia, etc., Archduke of Austria, Duke of Burgundy and Milan, Count of Habsburg, Flanders, Tyrol, etc.,[12] recognize . . . the praiseworthy artistic and practical work which . . . has been executed by Our dear Janellus Turrianis [sic], a mathematician of Cremona . . . in constructing for Us . . . an exceptional Clock . . . never seen anywhere else up to the present time, which shows not only all the hours of the Sun and of the Moon, but also all the other signs of the planets . . . in a true, exact and visible order with consummate ability and to Our greatest satisfaction. We have conceded . . . to Janellus

himself . . . an annual pension of one hundred gold escudos . . . by the testimony of these letters signed by Our hand and provided with Our seal.[13]

Charles asked Juanelo Turriano to remain in his service.[14]

Two months later, they had to run. Maurice of Saxony had taken Augsburg and now his troops were entering Innsbruck. Charles V escaped on foot, the small group carrying a litter because his gout prohibited him from negotiating the Brenner Pass. It is hard to resist the mythologies that were written later, such as the raging snowstorm,[15] and I cannot stop imagining how Juanelo saved the clock by carrying it on his back. The group arrived safely in Lienz, where the duke of Alba joined the emperor with his troops. Once more, the candle was allowed to flicker, and Charles attempted to recapture Metz from the French. In December, 1552, he gave up the siege.

Charles was severely depressed. In a confidential report from the Low Countries, Francisco Duarte wrote to Philip:

> His Majesty does not have a Nobleman in his court nor does he want to, and he has not talked to anybody who deserves respect; nor does he want to hear about business, or to sign the few [documents] that are presented; day and night he is attending to his clocks, occupying himself with adjusting them and bringing them in concert; these are his principal concern, together with another new clock, which he invented and ordered to be placed in a window sill. At night, as he is not able to sleep when he wants to, he makes his attendants and others get up often, and candles and torches are lighted, so that he can take his clocks apart and put them back together to bring them in concert [desbaratar y tornar a conçertar].[16]

Because of his gout, three fingers were amputated, but he "amused himself with putting clocks together with the other two."[17] When he complained of tasteless food, his cook mocked: "I do not know . . . what more I can do to please your Majesty, unless I . . . make your Majesty a new dish, a broth of clocks. . . . For there is nothing in the world . . . which His Majesty likes so much as standing to look at clocks."[18] In October, 1555, Charles abdicated, ceding Spain and the Low Countries to his son. He retired to the monastery of Yuste, in the Extremadura, meeting Juanelo daily and trying to have his clocks sound together. He died in Yuste on September 21, 1558.

Intermezzo 1: Holiday in Spain

For me, this whole story began in June, 1998, on a holiday in Spain with Yang Tit Man. In the Museum of the University of Salamanca, we saw an anatomical model, with ball-and-socket joints for the articulations (figure 1.2). The model was made in 1570, about a century earlier than I would have deemed possible. Mark Latash had already asked me to write a chapter on the early history of movement science, and I felt that this model could help me unravel the early mechanization of the world view in the West. In the cathedral of Santiago de Compostella I bought a book, written by Mark Williams (1996), on the history of Spain. According to Williams, Charles V once exclaimed:

How could I possibly have hoped to unite all my dominions when I cannot make these clocks strike the hour together?[19]

I decided that I wanted to know more of Charles V. About a year later, Professor José Ramón-Nieto, conservator of the Museum of the University of Salamanca, informed us that the ball-and-socket joints in the model had not been added in later reconstructions.[20] We obtained a copy of Francisco Duarte's report[21] in the *Archivo General de Simancas*. In the monastery of Yuste, the *Padre Prior* Fray Francisco de Andrés, gave us a picture of Charles's wheelchair (figure 1.3), showed us a

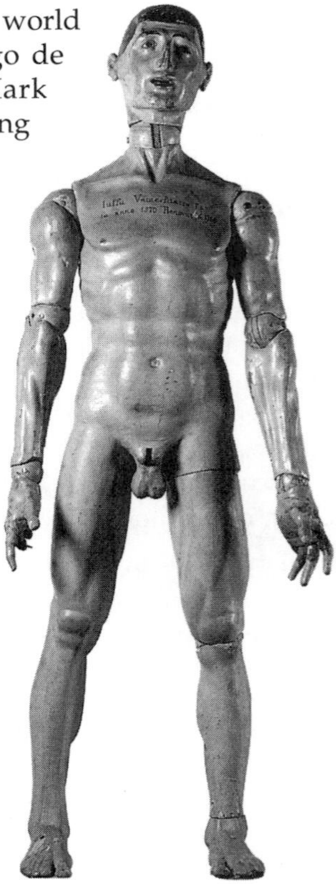

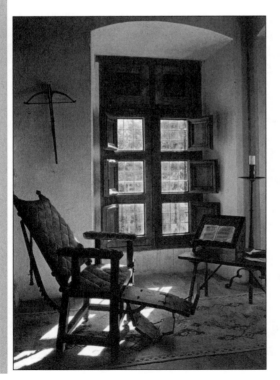

Figure 1.2
Anatomical model at the University of Salamanca, 1570 (Universitas Studii Salamantini, p. 19; by kind permission of Professor José Ramón-Nieto).

Figure 1.3
The wheelchair of Charles V in Yuste (by kind permission of Fray Francisco de Andrés, prior of the monastery).

book by José García-Diego on Juanelo Turriano,[22] and gave us the telephone number of the author. Monasteries are a wee bit timeless, and it turned out that García-Diego had died several years before. From his inheritance, the *Fondación Juanelo Turriano* was created. The next day, we had lunch with the technical director of that foundation, Professor Ignacio González-Tascón,[23] and his wife, Beatriz Presmanes-Arizmendi. For the four of us, it was friendship at first sight. It is to them that I dedicate this chapter.

For the present chapter, I have two questions: Why was Charles V so obsessed with his clocks? And: What can we learn from that?

When García-Diego tells us that Charles was obsessed with clocks "because" they were his hobby,[24] or when González-Tascón informs us that mechanical engineering was popular in 16th-century Spain "because" it had no religious implications,[25] we can see that they belong to that generation of Spanish intellectuals who explicitly refrain from conceptual analysis, while alluding to conceptual developments all the time. Granted that conceptual analysis easily leads us astray, it is nevertheless what we have to try to do.

People have been fascinated with clocks at all times and in all cultures. Wrote Needham and Wang in *Science and Civilisation in China*:

> The clock is the earliest and most important of complex scientific machines. Its influence upon the world-outlook of developing modern science was incalculable. . . . "The fundamental solution . . . of the problem of securing steady motion by intersecting the progress (of a . . . powered train) into intervals of equal duration, must be considered as the work of a . . . genius." The essential engineering task was to devise means of slowing down the rotation of a wheel so that it would keep a constant speed continuously . . . in time with the . . . diurnal revolution of the heavens. The essential invention was the escapement [cf. figure 1.13].[26]

So, clocks are special devices, but why was Charles obsessed with them?

Europe was holding its breath in the year 1500, when Charles was born in the city of Ghent, in Flanders. An unprecedented inheritance was awaiting him: the house of Habsburg, that of Burgundy, and the two Spains.[27] All over Europe, the dream of Empire was revived.[28] Eight years before Charles' birth, Spain had removed the last trace of Muslim power (Granada), and in the same year Columbus had reached America. These were times of tremendous change. How could young Charles learn to do what was expected of him? There certainly was no shortage of tutors. In the North, Desiderius Erasmus of Rotterdam wrote a book, in 1516, *The Education of a Christian Prince*,[29] telling Charles about virtue, generosity, justness, and the love of peace. The South followed suit, with Bishop Antonio de Guevara, "court preacher and historiographer to the emperor,"[30] who wrote, in 1529, *Libro del Emperador Marco Aurelio con el Relox de Principes [Book of the*

Emperor Marcus Aurelius, with the Clock of Princes].[31] De Guevara takes the clock as the symbol of virtue[32] and orderliness. For him, time is

> the inventor of all noveltyes and a Regestre certayne of antiquities, which seeth of it selfe the beginning, the middelst, and the end of all thinges. And finally, time is he that endeth al. . . . By this, all men shall see . . . that it was . . . my minde . . . to make a diall [clock] for princes, whereby all christen people may be governed and ruled.[33]

God is eternal, our world temporal, and nobody can escape time;[34] but the wise prince uses his understanding of time to govern and rule. Clearly, De Guevara's book shows that the image of the clock was unusually popular in 16th-century Spain.[35]

Still, García-Diego's description of how Turriano's clock was received, and Bishop Vida's statement that the clock emulated "the eternal Crafts-man,"[36] reveal that the meaning of Turriano's clock was much more specific. Turriano successfully captured the movements of the planets, thereby allowing humans to have, so to speak, "a look into God's kitchen." Thus, the clock became a mechanical metaphor for the universe. God is an engineer, and the clock revealed how he did it. What could Charles learn from that? He had a collection of clocks, and one sees him tightening or loosening the springs, putting some oil here and there, or adjusting screws, then waiting to see whether all his clocks will sound together. So, *Charles attempted to coordinate*[37] *his devices by separately controlling each and every one of them.* He couldn't. In this way he confronted his impotence[38] as emperor. Surely the clocks were a metaphor for his realms. In my mind, this metaphor is too exact and to the point to be a coincidence.[39] Replace "devices" with "realms" in the italicized statement, and it will be equally accurate.

Apart from the Catholic faith, under threat since Luther (1517), Charles himself was the only unifying force of his empire. He tried to take each country seriously, visiting the realms, listening to the councils, and even apologizing for his mistakes.[40] But the separate realms continued to have their own agendas.[41] Sometimes he would "take them apart and put them back together," as in the battle of Mühlberg (1547),[42] but still they wouldn't sound in concert. Nor would his clocks. In a mechanical universe, *desbaratar y tornar a conçertar*[43] does not work. God may be a clockmaker, but does he bring the clocks into harmony by separately controlling each and every one? Nobody knew. Charles V, God's representative on earth, failed to bring about the harmony that was expected of him because, he must have thought, he had failed to properly control his separate realms. I propose to conclude that he was obsessed with his clocks because they confronted him with the problem of coordination in a mechanical universe.

What can we learn from that?

The Challenge of Movement Science

From the dawn of human history, men and women have wondered how things come about. Some things we cannot influence, such as earthquakes or floods; we invented the gods to attribute causal responsibility to them. Some things we ought to control but cannot, such as our feeling sick in the course of an unhappy love affair; traditionally, such sickness has been attributed to sorcery. And then, there are the things that we can control, directly so. When you want to raise your arm, you raise your arm. As long as you are not paralyzed, it is you who are in control over your arms and legs.

Ideas on motor control and coordination, therefore, reveal how we think about ourselves. In this chapter on the early history of movement science, I refrain from summing up who discovered what, when, and where. Instead, I present history in the guise of a theoretical debate, pinpointing some of the metaphors that shaped movement science in the past and still influence the present. The first time when "movement science" could be recognized as a more or less separate enterprise was during the scientific revolution, at the peak of what Dijksterhuis called the "mechanization" of the world view,[44] in which "the physical universe is seen as a large machine that, once it is set in motion, will do, because of its construction, the work for which it was called into life."[45] The first major metaphors of mechanicism arose during the reign of Charles V.

From Goal-Directedness to Mechanical Metaphors

Of course, Charles was no scientist, let alone a movement scientist. Still, I have focused on his obsession with clocks as an example of the difficulties one may encounter when trying to solve the central problem of movement science, that is, understanding coordination and control.[46] In the following section, I sketch the prehistory of movement science, starting with the "discovery of rationality" in Greece. When we arrive at the 16th century for the second time, I will suggest that Charles also understood the body as a mechanical device. Next, I generalize his inability to understand coordination and control by defining "Charles' problem." Important developments in the 17th century are then presented as if they aimed at solving Charles' problem. In that respect they failed, as did others until deep into the 19th century. In closing my argument, I will point to the intellectual challenges that are the hallmark of movement science, and will hint at what I regard as prerequisites to understanding the coordination and control of movement.

The Charioteer: Plato (±428-348 B.C.)

In Plato's *Phaedrus,* we find the first major metaphor for Western conceptions of control and coordination. Since Plato was Christianized for many centuries and the context of his analysis sounds unusual, I will present his argument in some detail. The young Phaedrus meets Socrates and tells him about a speech that questioned whether a young man should give in to an older suitor who is in love with him or to one who just desires him. The answer is clear: the suitor who just desires, because then the young man has more choice.

Having captivated his audience with this surprising start, Plato introduces the soul as that which moves but is not moved by something else.

> Now that we have seen that that which is moved by itself is immortal, we shall feel no scruple in affirming that precisely that is the essence and definition of soul, to wit self-motion. Any body that has an external source of motion is soulless; but a body deriving its motion from a source within itself is animate or *besouled*. . . .[47]

For Plato, the soul is in control. So he comes back to the problems of love and presents his now-famous metaphor of wanting to let go and wanting to restrain yourself at the same time:

> Let [the soul] be likened to the union of powers in a team of . . . steeds [horses] and their . . . charioteer. . . . It is a pair of steeds that the charioteer controls; moreover, one of them is noble and good . . . , while the other has the opposite character. . . . Hence the task of our charioteer is difficult and troublesome.
>
> Now when the driver beholds the person of the beloved . . . the obedient steed, constrained . . . by modesty, refrains from leaping upon the beloved; but his fellow, heeding no more to the driver's goad or whip, leaps and dashes on, sorely troubling his companion and his driver and forcing them to approach the loved one. . . .[48]

Sure, it is the driver who pulls the reins, but it is not always easy to control the horses:

> . . . when they lie side by side, the wanton horse of the lover's soul would have a word with the charioteer, claiming a little guerdon [reward] for all his trouble. The like steed in the soul of the beloved has no word to say, but swelling with desire . . . he kisses the lover. . . . When they lie by one another, he is minded not to refuse to do his part in gratifying his lover's entreaties; yet his yoke-fellow in turn, being moved by reverence and heedfulness, joins with the driver in resisting.[49]

In Plato's philosophy, it is the soul that moves; more importantly, the good soul constrains. And at the end, they don't do it.

Until the scientific revolution, Plato's metaphor of the charioteer was quintessential Western philosophy of control and coordination. The horses are controlled and coordinated from the outside (by the driver, i.e., the soul). Charles V also tried to control and coordinate his clocks as an outside entity. But there is one conspicuous difference.

For Charles V, the clocks are passive, while for a charioteer, the horses are active—they all have "their own agendas." In my mind, mechanism[50] implies that the to-be-coordinated/controlled is passive and stupid, fully deriving its intelligence from an external, superior authority (figure 1.4). There is no doubt that for Plato's charioteer, control and coordination are hard work. But if the to-be-coordinated/controlled were to become completely passive, as in mechanism, wouldn't then there be even more work to do—in fact, more than humanly possible?

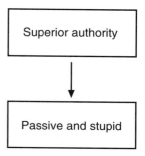

Figure 1.4
Definition of mechanism.

Intrinsic Goal-Directedness: Aristotle (384-322 B.C.)

While Plato thought that this-world-here is but a shadow of the perfect world of ideas, his student Aristotle did not share this "otherworldliness."[51] Aristotle liked to go at things, sit down, and stare at them.

I invite the reader to have an imaginary walk with a medieval teacher who is trying to explain the Aristotelian world view. Behold, I take this stone in my hand and then let it go: It falls back to Earth. But didn't we take it from Earth in the first place? So, we see the first truth: Earth returns to Earth, finding its own place.[52] Now I take a vessel of Water and pour it out over the Earth. A puddle will form and the Water will stay at its natural place, just above Earth. When it is heated by the Sun and becomes Air, it will collect itself in clouds, higher than both Earth and Water. Or when you breathe on a cold night, will not the Air climb up a little? Certainly, not as much as Fire—you can see that when I light a torch and hold it down, the Fire will still strive upward. So, Fire, as we can observe in the Sun and the Stars, has the highest place in our Universe. This should be sufficient: Our world consists of Earth, Water, Air, and Fire, and each has its proper place.

Because everything has its own place, the world of Aristotle is *intrinsically goal-directed* (as are the horses of Plato's charioteer, but not the clocks of Charles V). In such a world, harmony (coordination) comes naturally, as is clear from Aristotle's famous metaphor of the city-state:

> The constitution of an animal can be considered as that of a well-governed city-state. For when order is once established in a city there is no need of a special ruler with arbitrary powers to be present at every activity, but each individual performs his own task. . . . And in the animals the same process goes on . . . because each part of them . . . is naturally suited to perform its own function; so that there is no need of soul in each part, but since it is situated in a central origin of authority over the body [the heart[53]], the other parts live by their structural attachment to it and perform their own functions in the course of nature.[54]

Thus, between the views of Aristotle and Plato there is a difference in emphasis: For the Aristotelian soul, coordination comes almost for free and not much control is needed.

According to Aristotle, "Nature never does anything without a purpose."[55] For example: "The business of the hands is to take hold and to keep hold of things, and this is done by means of that part of the hand which bends; therefore the fingers must be long."[56] Aristotle wrote separate books on the *Movement of Animals* and the *Locomotion of Animals*,[57] very much in agreement with his overall philosophy of nature. Essential to our understanding of what it was that Turriano's clock came to replace is Aristotle's argument that animal movements are not those of marionettes:

> The movement of animals resembles that of marionettes which move as the result of a small movement, when the strings are released . . . or a toy-carriage which the child that is riding upon it himself sets in motion in a straight direction, and which afterwards moves in a circle because its wheels are unequal, for the smaller wheel acts as a centre. . . . Animals have similar parts in their organs, namely, the growth of their sinews and bones. . . . In the marionettes and the toy-carriages no alteration takes place, though if the inner wheels were to become smaller and then again larger, the same circular movement would take place. In the animal, however, the same part can become both greater and smaller and change its form, the members increasing through heat and contracting again through cold and thus altering.[58]

The movement organs of animals alter by themselves. In mechanicism, such alteration would become very hard to understand. One may assume that Charles V did not expect (parts of) his clocks to grow or wane since machines do not do that.[59] In classical antiquity the central metaphors were derived from the living, while in fact inanimate nature was not "invented" before the arrival of the mechanical metaphors of the 16th century.

The Mechanics of Control: Galen (129-201 A.D.)

Almost 500 years elapsed between classical Greece and the peak of the Roman Empire. Galen (Galenus) wrote his most important books around 165 A.D., during the reign of Marcus Aurelius, the "last of the good emperors." In the works of Galen we recognize that knowledge of the body had gained remarkable precision since Plato and Aristotle. In the old days, muscles had been "flesh" (σαρξ, *sarx*), "foam rubber" to protect the bones and to regulate temperature, while movement was caused by the contraction of the tendons, all stemming from the "beginning"[60] (αρχη, *archè*), that is, the heart. In the view of Galen, "The rational soul is lodged in the encephalon" (ενκεφαλον[61])—nerves departing from it, or from the spinal cord, to control the muscles, "the instruments of voluntary movement."[62] Galen decided to write on the usefulness of bodily organs since "all the parts of the body are in sympathy with one another, all cooperate in producing one effect."[63] Thus, we find Aristotle's "intrinsic goal-directedness" back in Galen's work, a "hymn of praise to our Architect."[64] It is because of their use that things are what they are:

> . . . man is the most intelligent of the animals and so, also, hands are the instruments most suitable for an intelligent animal. For it is not because he has hands that he is the most intelligent, as Anaxagoras says, but because he is the most intelligent that he has hands, as Aristotle says, judging most correctly. Indeed, not by his hands, but by his reason has man been instructed in the arts. Hands are an instrument,[65] as the lyre is the instrument of the musician, and tongs of the smith.[66]

Galen wrote a special book called "On the Movement of Muscle."[67] Each muscle contracts with its own particular movement and will stretch because of antagonistic activity. In some movements, however, there is no muscular contraction, such as in falling as opposed to lying down; but then the muscles do not act "as living beings, but as inanimate bodies."[68] Even involuntary movements are due to the soul: "The body of muscles was not created with the faculty to contract themselves, because the soul accomplishes that operation more completely and better."[69] Sleepwalking reveals that the soul is never at rest, always telling the muscles what to do through the appropriate nerves.

> All muscles . . . need to receive from the brain or the spinal cord a nerve which is small to the eye but with a force that is far from small. This you recognize from nerve lesions. In fact, incision, compression, contusion, ligature, or *squirrus* [putrefaction] of the nerve, removes all movement and sentiment from the muscle. . . . Thus, within the nerves there exists a considerable force, flowing down from above, from the great beginning (αρχη, archè). . . . The nerves therefore play the role of conductors, bringing to the muscles the forces they tap from the brain as from a spring. . . . The ligaments, on the other hand, serving to connect and unify the muscles with the bones, give rise to the membranes that surround it, and enter certain internal separations of the flesh of the muscles itself. You can imagine this flesh as a place that is irrigated with several canals . . . , one of which brings hot, thin and steamy blood, and the other cold, thicker blood; the first of these canals we call artery and the second vein.[70]

In Galen's view, muscles receive three different kinds of *pneuma* (spirit).

Nourishment ("natural pneuma") is made in the liver and transported through the body as the thick, cold blood of the veins. When combined with air from the lungs and the heat of the heart, it forms inspiring "vital pneuma" (vital spirit), a thin, hot blood that is injected on every heartbeat by the arteries. And then there is "psychic pneuma" (*spiritus animalis*, animal spirit), the power to cause movement, residing in the ventricles of the brain and from there transported by the nerves to the muscles. This animal spirit is concocted in the arteries of the *rete mirabile* (retiform plexus) in the brain:

> Well, what is this wonderful thing, and for what purpose has it been made by Nature who does nothing in vain? . . . [Wherever] Nature wishes material to be completely elaborated, she arranges for it to spend a long time in the organs concocting it. . . . *Vital pneuma passing up through the arteries is used as the proper material for the generation of psychic pneuma [animal spirit] in the encephalon.* . . . For the whole encephalon is interwoven with these intricately divided arteries. . . . Shall we not, then, marvel at the foresight of the Architect who conducted . . . the arteries from the heart . . . as far as the head itself and then conducted the arteries to the retiform plexus . . . ?[71]

There is no doubt about the mechanical abilities of the Romans, and surely Galen ascribes a mechanical function to muscles, that is, moving bones. The point is that he understands the body so well that now he needs something to be transported from the soul to the muscles, through the nerves. And he gets in trouble. His argument is very convoluted when he presents his animal spirits, and he praises Nature and its Architect more often than normal—as if he knew that the transport of force through thin tubes (nerves) was difficult to imagine. Moreover, this whole *rete mirabile* (retiform plexus) doesn't exist in humans—it was an artifact of Galen's use of animals for his research. In the 16th century, Andreas Vesalius would attack Galen on this very point.

One wonders whether there is a relationship between empire building (with its concomitant upsurge in mechanics) and having problems in understanding control and coordination (Galen, Charles V). In my mind, having an empire combines naturally with thinking about the nature of control.[72] The trouble appears to be that the better one understands control, the more it seems to escape. We know that the Romans had aqueducts and that the transport of nutrition (*pneuma naturalis,* in the veins) was not difficult to imagine. And they had central heating, often with pipes under the floor, so that also the transport of hot blood (*pneuma vitalis,* in the arteries) offered no problem. But the transport of willpower? Through thin pipes? Mechanically, no sense could be made of that.[73] After Galen, the Roman Empire slowly started to collapse, and Galen's problem of the mechanics of control disappeared from sight. The Galen whose views were inherited by Islam and Christendom was the Galen of intrinsic goal-directedness. It was that view that would be challenged by the men Charles V attracted to his court.

The Discovery of Seeing: Andreas Vesalius (1514-1564)

Galen's view remained undisputed from 165 A.D. to 1543, that is, almost one and a half millennia. After the Roman Empire turned Christian, Saint Augustine (354-430) convinced the West that Plato belonged to Christendom—and a long period of otherworldliness ensued. The Roman Empire collapsed, its Eastern counterpart, Byzantium (Istanbul), not even able to preserve a Latin original of Galen's writing. When Mohammed (±570-632) started to preach, Muslims created their own empire. In Baghdad, there was a frantic explosion of translating and comparing manuscripts from the West, from Persia, India, China. During the Mongol Empire, scientific information started to pour back into China. Similarly, Western science, altered and improved, filtered back to the West through Muslim Spain.

In 12th-century Europe, towns were built everywhere, and proud burghers were no longer satisfied with Plato's otherworldliness. Aquinas (Thomas of Aquino, 1225-1274) revealed that Aristotle had been a more Christian heathen than Plato since God had written both the Bible and the Book of Nature, so the good Christian should know them both. The world of Plato, Aristotle, and Galen had been more symbolic than visible. In that respect, they agreed well with Muslim civilization since Islam was hesitant to depict (and venerate) the living. In Christian Europe, pictures had been supposed to illustrate the Bible rather than to tell anything about nature. But Aquinas opened the door to visible nature, and slowly, Europe started to celebrate *seeing*—first in Northern Italy,[74] then with the Flemish Primitives,[75] and in Germany. I invite the reader to visit the Albertina in Vienna, to see how Dürer (1471-1528) made a painting of grass (!) and to realize how Europe was "poised on the threshold of time, waiting for the new era to reveal itself."[76]

In my mind, it is from this tradition of celebrating seeing that one has to understand Andreas Vesalius, the 16th-century anatomist who was to challenge the authority of Galen.

Andreas Vesalius was born in Brussels, in the same Flanders where Charles V spent his youth.[77] Vesalius studied medicine in Paris and Louvain, to obtain his doctorate in Venice in 1537. He was appointed lecturer in surgery in Padua, also giving anatomical demonstrations in Bologna. There, he strongly disagreed with the famous Curtius on the anatomical rationale for bloodletting:

> When the lecture of Curtius was finished, Vesalius . . . asked Curtius to accompany him to the anatomy. For he wanted to show him that his theory was quite true. . . . Now, he said, excellentissime Domine, here we have our bodies. We shall see whether I have made an error. . . . Curtius answered smiling . . . No . . . Domine, we must not leave Galen, because he always well understood everything. . . . Oh, Vesalius said, you want to talk about things not visible and concealed. I, again, talk about what is visible. Curtius answered: Indeed, I always deal with what is most obvious. Domine, you do not well understand . . . Galen. . . . Vesalius replied: It is quite true, because I am not so old a man as you are. . . . I have said that Galen has erred in this, and this is evident here in these bodies, as also many other mistakes of his.[78]

Until Vesalius, anatomy had been symbolic, with nothing "visible" as we would understand that notion today (figure 1.5). When, in 1543, Vesalius published his anatomical atlas in Basel, *De Humani Corporis Fabrica* (*On the Construction of the Human Body*), the body could finally be "seen" (figure 1.6). The *Fabrica* hit like a bomb, people realizing, as with Turriano's clock, that they were looking into "God's kitchen." God is an engineer, and Vesalius revealed how he did it—the human body was no longer a mystery.

The story of the *rete mirabile*[79] (retiform plexus) is both amusing and typical. In the same course in which he had quarreled with Curtius, Vesalius demonstrated the brain. Normally, he used freshly killed criminals for this purpose, but now he also brought a sheep (which has a *rete mirabile*, whereas humans do not).

> At last he showed us the rete mirabile . . . in the middle of the cranium . . . forming the plexus in which the spiritus animales [animal spirits] are produced. . . . It was a reddish, fine, netlike web of arteries lying above the bones, which I afterwards touched with my hands. . . .[80]

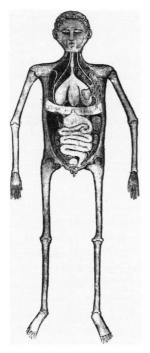

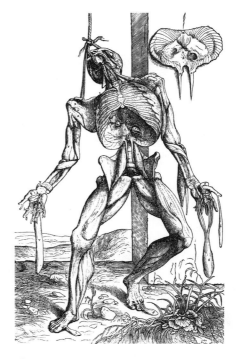

Figure 1.5
Anatomical drawing from the 1345 atlas of Guido de Vigevano (reprinted from Wickersheimer 1926).

Figure 1.6
Anatomical drawing from the 1543 atlas of Andreas Vesalius (1543, p. 190).

One cannot help wondering how Vesalius' students must have felt, touching the "origin of the soul," unaware that it does not exist in humans. In the *Fabrica* (1543), however, Vesalius boldly states the facts:

> As to Galen's retiform plexus, I really cannot tell otherwise than what is already established beyond doubt if one carefully looks at my series [of pictures] of the vessels of the brain, . . . that we found that Galenus was deluded by his dissecting a cow, and that he hasn't reported on the human brain and its vessels, but on the cow.[81]

Vesalius includes a picture of the difference between cow and man (figure 1.7), and even shows the seat of the soul, the ventricles. But then, if the basic facts are wrong, how can one trust the conclusions? Nevertheless, Vesalius himself did not replace the theory of animal spirits by a theory of his own. That had to wait until 1664, when Thomas Willis concluded that psychological functions relate to the substance of the brain rather than its fluids.[82]

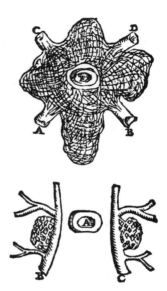

Figure 1.7
The *rete mirabile* (retiform plexus) in the cow (top), compared to the situation in the human preparation (bottom) (Vesalius, 1543, p. 621).

Much of the *Fabrica* is about the locomotor apparatus, which can easily be understood because the other parts of the body stink too much.[83] For us, this circumstance has the advantage that we can clearly see how Vesalius thought about movement. As with Galen, his view was that "the muscle . . . is the instrument of voluntary movement."[84] In explaining the function of ligaments, Vesalius shows that the muscles that bring your toes in the direction of your nose are at risk of removing themselves from the ankle joint unless ligaments keep them close to the bones (figure 1.8). The mechanics is sound. But in the picture, the "owner" of the muscles

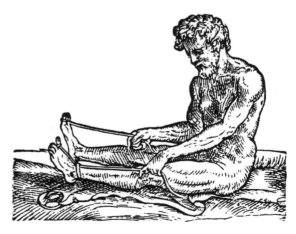

Figure 1.8
Who pulls the ropes? (Vesalius, 1543, p. 215)

controls them with his/her own hands, and one wonders who pulls the ropes. Have human movements, contrary to Aristotle,[85] become like the movements of marionettes? Yes.

Charles' Problem

García-Diego, the biographer of Juanelo Turriano,[86] discusses the popularity of automata in the 16th century. Technically, automata are close to clocks, with a spring that can be wound. Historically, they are connected with churches—the little men coming out of the tower on the hour to strike the bell. Venice has some beautiful examples of them.[87] They are easy to build separately. Leonardo da Vinci (1452-1519), whose anatomical drawings preceded those of Vesalius, made a spectacular robot. Similar machines, all over Europe, were the talk of the day. The Smithsonian Institution in Washington has a friar on display ("the Washington automaton"), who moves not only his arms and his legs but also his eyes and his mouth (figure 1.9).

Juanelo Turriano, the clockmaker, was rumored to have made such automata, but García-Diego is unsure:

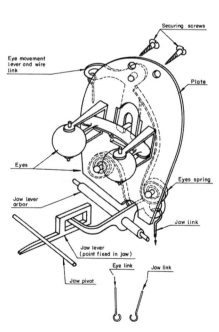

I cannot really imagine the Emperor in Yuste amusing himself with these little figures. Charles V used to discuss Natural History during his meals. Sometimes the works of Pliny had to be fetched in order to decide a discussion. . . . There is another hypothesis . . . that, instead of automatons, the silent Juanelo had fabricated some marionettes. . . . In that age educated people were more interested in marionettes than they are now . . . there were performances by them in churches until this was forbidden—I don't know why—by the Council of Trent.[88]

The evidence is more scant than that for the clock as mechanical metaphor for the universe. Still, given the popularity of marionettes[89] and automata, I venture to conclude that Vesalius saw bodily movements as those of marionettes. In my opinion, his work was taken to strengthen a second mechanical metaphor in Re-

Figure 1.9
The Washington automaton: mechanism of the head (reprinted from García-Diego 1986).

naissance Europe, that is: Living movements are like those of an automaton. Wrote Mark Williams about Charles V:

> The overworked king [Charles] had several lifelike statues of himself made, some with moveable limbs. These would be hauled out whenever a crowd or foreign delegation was deemed unworthy of his attention and propped up at a safe distance from the throngs, who never suspected that they were cheering a dummy.[90]

Apparently, mechanicism ran in the family (of the Spanish Habsburgs). Charles II (1665-1700), the son of Philip IV, was physically so weak that "he had to be presented to the nobles at court held up by strings which his nurse worked like a puppeteer."[91]

As was politically correct, Andreas Vesalius dedicated his *De Humani Corporis Fabrica* (Basel, 1543) "to the divine Charles V, the great, the most invincible, who is the Emperor."[92] In 1544, he was offered a professorship at the faculty of medicine in Pisa. At the same time, the emperor invited him to become physician to the court. Pisa requested of Charles that Vesalius still be allowed to be professor of anatomy, but this "aroused the displeasure of the emperor,"[93] and Vesalius left to join Charles' court.

> The pro-Galen physicians employed at the court brought gravely defamatory accusations against him [Vesalius], but the success of his book kept him in the monarch's favour. As second in rank among the court physicians, it was his duty to attend upon the emperor. . . .[94]

Vesalius was with the court in Augsburg when Juanelo Turriano arrived to bring the clock. We know nothing about their probable meeting.

In 1551, while Vesalius continued to attend the emperor, a chair for Vesalian anatomy was created at the University of Salamanca.[95] It was in that department that the 1570 anatomical model was made with the ball-and-socket joints (figure 1.2) that amazed me so at the beginning of this adventure. When the model was made, both Charles and Vesalius[96] were already dead.

What was it that Charles had seen in Vesalius? Sure, Charles' gout required surgery, and anatomists made excellent surgeons.[97] But was there not also a confluence of the story of the clock and that of the anatomical atlas?

With the evidence at hand, I cannot know for sure that the clock of Juanelo Turriano also reminded Charles of his inability to control his crippled body. He could not coordinate his clocks "because" he couldn't control them well enough. He must have had similar experiences with his body:

> Because the gout that bothers him is often in all the limbs, joints and nerves of his body, it is so bad that it never stops. And the cold is molesting him so much that it brings him to the end . . . he cannot speak, and when he speaks

he cannot be heard or is hardly understood by his attendants. His haemorrhoids have swollen and hurt him so much that he cannot move around without great pain and tears.[98]

This was an emperor who was no longer in control of his own body and who attracted an anatomist to attend upon it day and night.

I propose to define as *Charles' problem:* How on earth can a person or a culture that derives from mechanics the central metaphors for understanding the world (Turriano's clock) and the body (Vesalius' atlas) come to properly understand coordination and control?

Early Attempts at Solving Charles' Problem (17th Century)

Of course, this notion of "Charles' problem" is mine, inspired by his obsession with clocks. In terms of 20th-century science, Charles' problem cuts through very different disciplines. There is a social science aspect to it in that he wanted to bring his realms into agreement. The actual problem he was obsessed with, of course, is of a technical, physical nature: wanting clocks to strike in synchrony on the hour. Finally, the fact that he attracted an anatomist to attend to his body suggests, at least to me, that there was also a "biological"[99] aspect to his obsession. It is in this latter aspect that I best recognize the problems of coordination and control that modern movement science is facing. To date, we know that control and coordination are typically biological phenomena.[100] Thus, it is only with hindsight that I regard the biological aspect of Charles' problem as the most important one.

Having said all this, I can now characterize the history of *movement science* as the systematic attempt to solve Charles' problem.[101]

The Extraterrestrials: Descartes, Borelli

The story so far appears to be fairly simple. Combine proud burghers, who trust no authority but their own, with the discovery of seeing, then invent the mechanical spring—and, lo and behold, the world is no longer intrinsically goal-directed but becomes mechanical.

Of course, the real story is far more complicated and mysterious than that. For Descartes and Borelli, however, I will stick to the simple version, with the world becoming mechanical. Since mechanics cannot control or coordinate itself, it was "concluded" that control and coordination must come from outside the world. This conclusion is known under a variety of terms (dualism, rationalism, mechanicism, etc.). To emphasize the Platonic otherworldliness of the idea, I call its defenders the "extraterrestrials."

René Descartes (1596-1650)

René Descartes failed to find any certainty in the reports of others, in poetry, theology, or philosophy. No, the first rule is "never to accept anything as true that I didn't know to be evidently so. . . ."[102] To Descartes, the hallmark of the scientific method is to put your trust in true ideas, as you recognize them within yourself. "I think, therefore I am."[103] So, now we see self-conscious burghers starting to wrestle the Truth out of the hands of the church. Scared by Galileo's troubles,[104] Descartes hastens to add that the two things he is most certain of are the existence of God and that of the soul.[105]

For Descartes, existence falls apart into two separate realms: "Men are composed . . . of a Soul and a Body."[106] The rational soul consists of that-which-thinks ("res cogitans"), while the body belongs to that-which-is-extended ("res extensa"), passively obeying "laws of nature," which are best understood in terms of geometry. Thus, the living body has become a clock (or automaton):

> . . . those who know what large variety of *automata,* or moving machines, human industry has been able to make, using only a small number of parts when compared to the large number of bones, muscles, nerves, arteries, veins, and all other parts that are in the body of every animal, will conceive this body as a machine which, having been made by the hands of God . . . has movements of itself that are much more admirable than those of anything that could be invented by man.[107]

Descartes even gives a kind of "Turing test":[108] If it looks like a monkey, if it moves like a monkey, we will think it *is* a monkey.

Without the soul, a human being is dead: "Let us conclude that the body of a living man differs as much from that of a dead man as . . . [an intact] clock[109] . . . [differs] from the same clock when it is broken."[110] The moving principle, the soul, controls and coordinates all individual movements for Descartes, as for Galen, through the animal spirits. Descartes mechanized the nervous system (figure 1.10) and thought, contrary to Galen, in terms of "reflexes":

> It is even the case that the mind is not always the determining factor because among the movements that occur in

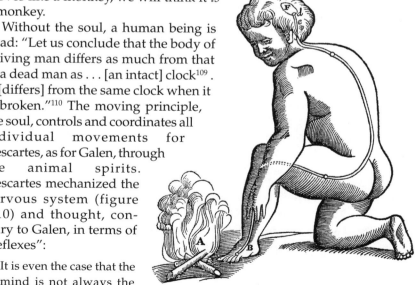

Figure 1.10
Descartes' mechanization of the nervous system (reprinted from Rotschuh 1969).

us, there are several that are completely independent from the mind, like the beating of the heart. . . . And while people who fall from a height put their hands first, to save their head, it is not by the advice of reason that they do this, but only because their senses, touched by the present danger, cause some change in their brain, determining that the animal spirits will enter the nerves in the way that is required to produce this movement, just like in a machine, the mind being unable to stop it.[111]

Note that this is not a "reflex" as a set of particular connections in the nervous system. Descartes does not even use the word "reflex." It was Willis who would introduce the term "reflex motion" ("motus reflexus") in his 1670 book *On Muscular Movement*.[112]

Since the Cartesian soul is responsible for every movement, it is not enough that it is "lodged in the human body, like the navigator in his ship, if only for moving the limbs, but it is necessary that they [the body and the soul] have a much stronger connection."[113] While remaining close to Galen in accepting animal spirits, Descartes is apparently no longer satisfied with the ventricles and the *rete mirabile;* and he starts to look for a localization of this "much stronger connection" between body and soul. In 1649, he announces that he has found the spot:

> . . . investigating this carefully, it . . . appeared to me to be evident that it is not the heart, and also not the whole brain, but only the most interior of its parts, a certain very small gland, in the middle of its substance . . . , [the pineal gland, because] the smallest changes in the spirits . . . have considerable power to change the movements of that gland.[114]

Descartes must have realized the arbitrary nature of his choice for the pineal gland, and Leibniz (1646-1716) subtly concluded that he "gave up the struggle over this problem."[115]

Descartes spent most of his working life in the Dutch Republic, where lectures had been given about his work at the University of Utrecht, where subsequently his work had been forbidden and where a national fight had broken out over the question whether Descartes could be accepted by Christian religion. Public lectures would end in stark turmoil; fistfights between students and professors happened frequently, and a prohibition against carrying arms into the lecture hall was announced. Descartes gave up and left in 1649. He was received into the protection of Protestant Queen Christina of Sweden.[116] In Sweden, Descartes died in 1650, never really having found the place where the soul meets the body.

Giovanni Alfonso Borelli (1608-1679)

With hindsight, one can say that it was bad luck for Giovanni Borelli that he wrote his *On the Movement of Animals* (1680-1681)[117] just before the appearance of Newton's *Mathematical Principles of Natural Philosophy* (1687), that is, just before mechanics could be captured in a simple set of consistent laws.

Borelli, half Spanish and half Italian, dedicates his work to Queen Christina, who also had protected Descartes (by now she had become Catholic). In his dedication, Borelli reminds her that "the language which the Creator speaks in His works is geometry. This was expressed most clearly by the divine Plato."[118] Borelli announces that he will "enlist Anatomy into Physics and Mathematics not less than Astronomy."[119] So, it is in Borelli's work that the ideas of Andreas Vesalius and Juanelo Turriano really meet.

According to Borelli, there is no doubt that movements are caused by the soul:

> . . . everybody agrees that the principle and the effective cause of movement of animals is the soul. . . . The active instrument of the soul is called will . . . and is supposed to reside in the animal spirits. . . . It is known that muscle by itself is a dead and inert machine in the absence of an external motive faculty. . . . But what is actually transmitted to the muscle by the nerves? Is it an immaterial faculty or a gas or some liquid or some movement or an impulse or anything else?[120]

In his book, Borelli attempts to work bottom-up, from the mechanics of muscle function to the nature of the animal spirits—where he has to stop because the nature of the soul itself escapes him.

Because of lever action, it turns out that the human muscles have a remarkable "motive power":

> . . . the motive power exerted by the four muscles flexing the lower leg . . . is thirty times greater than the suspended weight and is more than 949 pounds . . . [when the] trunk, thigh and lower leg are horizontal, the subject lying face down [figure 1.11, left. But] less weight is raised by the same muscles when the trunk and thigh are

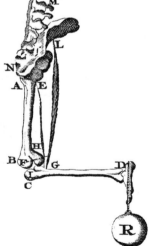
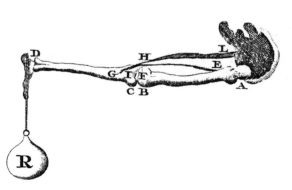

Figure 1.11
Borelli's biomechanics of muscle (reprinted from Borelli 1989).

upright and the lower leg horizontal. . . . Actually, the flexor muscles EG [figure 1.11, right] exert less force than previously because they are somewhat loosened since the distance EG is shortened by flexion of the knee joint.[121]

This statement is just one example that shows how biomechanics began with Borelli.[122] We learn why "going down a slope is somewhat more fatiguing than walking over a horizontal plane,"[123] that "the force of the pectoralis muscles in man is much smaller than what is required for flying,"[124] and that "swimming is a kind of flying."[125]

Muscle contraction is not like the contraction of a tight spring because springs contract only "after they have been stretched and the stretching force has stopped acting."[126] Neither is it a drying "similar to that which occurs in burning hair[127] . . . [because] hardening nerves by roasting or boiling requires much heat which modifies their structure and character so that they cannot resume their previous softness and looseness. This is not true for muscles of animals since they contract and then suddenly loosen."[128] Muscle contraction also "does not occur by puckering [wrinkling] of the fibres as . . . in earthworms. . . ."[129] No, "muscles contract with considerable force because their fibres are swollen by an additional substance as if it were by wedges."[130] Thus:

> Something else must be added [to what] is found in the muscles themselves. . . . Mixing of these substances results in something which, like a fermentation . . . produces this instantaneous contraction of the muscles. . . . Such an operation is possible as appears from countless experiments . . . in chemistry: concentrated spirit of vitriol poured into oil of tartar, all acid spirits mixed with fixed salts suddenly boil by fermentation. Consequently, in muscles some similar thing may occur.[131]

Well, then, "It remains to investigate what is sent through the nerves, with what force and how it is pushed, and through which canals."[132]

> It seems necessary that the spirits be activated in the brain by some motion as is required by their mobile character. . . . It is possible that the cerebral juices . . . shake the origins of the fibres of some nerves by a movement of concussion. . . . They thus irritate and titillate the nerve. The structure and temper of the nerves are very delicate and sensitive, as experience shows. When touching the inside of the nostrils . . . with a light straw, the nerves are shaking so violently along their whole length that they provoke convulsive sneezing[133] and coughing. Therefore, it is not surprising that a slight commotion or irritation of the nerves in the brain provokes some convulsive shaking through their whole length, resulting in the secretion of some droplets of . . . juice which swells the canals of the nervous fibres.[134]

Nerves are shaken by the soul. At their distal ends, droplets of nerve juice then enter the muscle where explosive chemical reactions take place. The muscle swells and contracts, and bones are moved.

To date, we could say that Borelli's shaking is not so very different from "action potentials"; but still, his soul "sneezing" commands into the nervous system leads to insurmountable problems. Borelli confesses "not to understand the mechanism by which the movements . . . in the brain . . . direct [the animal] spirits to titillate certain well-determined muscles. . . . I think that . . . there are as many movements of the spirits in the brain as there are acts of the will."[135] The real problem, however, is who shakes the shaker. Had Borelli invented a meta-shaker, there still would have been the question of who shakes the meta-shaker. If movement is natural and the soul is immaterial, then movement is movement, the soul is the soul, and never the twain shall meet.

This impossibility of reconnecting the soul with the world in mechanicism was recognized by Leibniz,[136] who came to the surprising conclusion that God had created the body and the soul separately, ensuring that they would run in parallel for ever: *harmonia praestabilisata*.[137]

In terms of Charles' problem, the extraterrestrials failed. Granted that one cannot coordinate or control mechanics from within, claiming an outside immaterial soul cannot do the job because of the impossibility of reconnecting it with the material world.[138] If you want to understand control as a form of being active, you may have to assume that also the world is active, as with the horses of Plato's charioteer.[139] Charles saw his clocks as passive and himself as active, wanting to tell his clocks exactly what to do. You cannot, ever.

Given the problem of mechanicism (reconnecting the soul to the world), 17th-century science was aware that alchemy, with its active view of matter, offered a real alternative. Of course, this is not to say that now we all should turn alchemical. In fact, 17th-century alchemy was badly organized and hardly consistent. Still, it contained attractive ideas.

The Alchemists: Harvey and Newton

If we look back at the Arabs and what we inherited from them, we may think of "algebra"—the word stemming from an Arabian root. Or of hospitals. Visit an old town in Germany and look at the front wall of the pharmacy; chances are that it will be the faces of Muslim doctors that stare back at you. Still more important, Muslim culture excelled in alchemy—again, the term has an Arab root. The origin of alchemy is Chinese, but the Arabs liked sweets.[140] If you heat sugar in a dry pan, you get caramel, and so we owe the Arabs toffees and pudding. Boil fruit and let the water escape, you get a syrup to which you later can add water (lemonade) or snow (a sorbet),[141] preferably combined with whipped egg white, as long as you make sure that not a drop of the yellow yolk is added. The Arabs were also great distillers of *al-kohl* (alcohol). If you dissolve sugar in it and add syrup, you get liqueur. Even today, Spanish cuisine is very conscious of its Arabian roots.[142]

Who doesn't know that milk gets sour by itself or that cream turns into butter when you whip it too much? But we do not care much for the modern scientific explanation of these phenomena. Need I go on to show that alchemy is rooted in everyday experience, at least in the eyes of 17th-century Europe? Originally, alchemy had been connected with the melting of ore (the making of "gold"); but now there was gunpowder, and even Borelli the mechanicist saw muscular contraction as a chemical explosion.[143]

In alchemy, matter is active, just like the soul. So, the problems of mechanicism could not arise. During the "scientific revolution" in the 17th century, alchemy was the major competitor of mechanics. The English were very good at it.

William Harvey (1578-1657)

To date, many see Harvey as the one who discovered that the heart is a pump. He never did. Harvey's 1628 De Motu Cordis (On the Movement of the Heart)[144] begins with a dedication to King Charles of "Great Britain, France and Ireland, Defender of the Faith":

> The heart of all creatures is the foundation of their life, the Prince of all their parts, the sun of their microcosm, that . . . from whence all strength and vigour flows. In like manner, the King is the foundation of his kingdom, the sun of his microcosm, the heart of his commonwealth, from whom all power flows and all mercy proceeds.[145]

This may have been just "politically correct," but, anyhow, in Harvey's dedication the heart doesn't appear to be a mechanical device.

Still, Harvey uses mechanical arguments to prove that the blood in the veins streams to rather than from the heart (as Galen would have had it). There are valves in the veins that show this. Moreover, we do not eat enough to produce all the blood that would be needed for Galen's theory. Harvey concludes that blood "circulates":

> When I had perceived that the juice of the food . . . could not suffice to supply the amount of the blood . . . I began to bethink myself whether it might not have a kind of movement as it were in a circle. And this I . . . found to be true . . . that the blood is thrust forth and driven out of the heart through the arteries into the whole structure of the body . . . and that it flows back again through the veins. . . . We may call this motion circular in the same way in which Aristotle says that the air and the rain imitate the circular motion of the heavens. For the earth being wet evaporates by the heat of the sun; the vapours being drawn upwards condense and . . . descend again in raindrops and wet the earth.[146]

It is the heat of the heart that drives the blood out of the arteries (as in boiling over), and when the blood cools down in the periphery, it streams back in the veins. In Harvey's time, such "circulation" (water → vapour →

water) was an alchemical concept, referring to the transmutation of elements.[147]

The metaphor of the pump was added by mechanical philosophers a couple of years after the publication of Harvey's book.[148]

In *De Motu Cordis,* Harvey announces a book on "the motive organs of animals and the structure of the muscles."[149] He never came to finish it, but his notes have survived and were published.[150] For Harvey, "the special action of muscle is contraction."[151] And we see him wrestling with a problem:

> And how, by means of what instruments. . . . NB as in the case of automata. . . . And the first instrument of movement is spirit. . . . And the natural causes of movement are heat and cold . . . the semen goes forth as if itself a living creature and hence too the movement of the heart. . . .
>
> As the magnet attracts iron while it itself remains motionless, so nerve draws muscle towards itself . . . and imparts motive power to . . . the muscle, compare Δ[152] the electric ray, and . . . as . . . the sun illumines the hemisphere, so nerve transmits the command from the brain. . . .
>
> Mechanics should be considered as that which overcomes . . . things [through levers]. . . . In the same way in muscles, Nature nowhere fails to assist in difficulties of this kind. . . . And herein . . . things are to be marvelled at, as how the power of a muscle can cause bones to move and the weights that are tied up to them, as may be seen in elephants with castles on their backs and in the camels of Aleppo. . . .[153]

At the end of his notes, we clearly see that Harvey wrestled with control and coordination. Dealing with "harmony and rhythm," he refers to Aristotle's metaphor of the city-state:[154]

> Nature performs her works in animals by the power of the muscles and attains her end by means of rhythm and harmony. . . . And thus it is with human good in the State . . . nothing is more excellent than the union of the citizens in friendship, nothing better than order. . . . *If through male and female . . . living creatures are perpetuated, their nurturing is effected through diverse concoctions. . . . So things done and things suffered arise from orderliness, from sympathy and antipathy. . . .*[155]

Now, wait a minute! Why is the mixing of male and female concoctions to generate a child, or why are "sympathy and antipathy," relevant to understanding the coordination of movements? This is pure Hermetism.

Intermezzo 2: Hermetism

A major problem in the modern historiography of science is that we don't understand the 17th century, because we don't understand what preceded it, that is, the Renaissance.

When Marsilio Ficino (1433-1499) was translating Plato in Florence, in 1463, word came "that he must translate Hermes first, at once."[156] Here was a work, one assumed, that was even older than Plato, that of the Messenger (Hermes, Mercurius) who had given God's laws to Moses and who had passed God's wisdom on to Plato. In the 16th century, the popularity of Hermes was second only to that of the Bible. Later, in 1614, it was discovered that the Corpus Hermeticum had actually been composed by a collective of Hellenistic authors of the second and third centuries *after* Christ. Still, in the 17th century, the fame of Hermetism was to fade only very, very slowly.

Up to now the trouble we have had is that we have no frame of reference through which to understand Hermetism. To get some feeling for the mystical tone of the Corpus Hermeticum, it is probably best to read the Bible book of Revelation. Then, maybe, one will be able to grasp: "From the Light a certain Holy Word descended upon Nature, and a pure Fire sprang from the moist nature upwards on high. It was light and sharp and drastic also, and the air being light followed The Spirit; it ascended up to the fire from land and water, so that it seemed to be suspended from it."[157] This was the literature that inspired both Harvey and Newton.

Hermetism is the celebration of mystique and magic. It is what shows the simple tale of the uncontested arrival of mechanicism (as told for Descartes and Borelli) to be wrong. Hermetism venerated the sun, which then was placed, by Copernicus (in 1543, the same year as the publication of Vesalius's *Fabrica*), in the middle of the universe. Hermetism thought the earth to be perfect and thus round—a possible influence on Columbus. And by focusing on the oneness of nature, Hermetism very much stimulated alchemical research. "We have said, my child, that there is a body which envelops the whole ensemble of the world; you should represent it to yourself as a circular figure, for thus is the All."[158]

Alas, so often the Oneness is lost, as when you try to mix water and oil. How to restore harmony? You may need a mediator to arrive at "sympathy" again. Experimental research on "sympathy" and "antipathy" was to be an important characteristic of 17th-century alchemy. Both Harvey and Newton derived their ideas on animal motion from this search for "sympathy."

Two substances that are "unsociable," as Newton would say, or in "antipathy," as Harvey had it, can be brought into harmony by introducing a third. Let me say this again, quoting Newton on animal motion:

> . . . knowing how the Spirit [animal spirits] may be used for Animal motion, you may consider, how some things unsociable are made Sociable by the Mediation of a Third. Water, wch[159] will not dissolve copper, will do if the copper be melted with Sulphur. . . .[160]

When Harvey refers to the mixing of male and female concoctions, and to sympathy and antipathy, he is in search of a mechanism to explain the harmony of animal motion. By doing so, he may have been the first premodern scientist to recognize the importance of movement coordination:

> So it happens in the great and nearly all the actions of the body that many muscles work together and X in each action we should look for the muscles involved as in coition. . . . Truly these muscles work together: . . . synergists work with the same regulated movement and follow one another. . . . In great and perfected movements . . . nearly all the muscles work together, D walking and talking, more than 400. . . .

> The muscles, therefore, are moved according to an order and in rhythm at the direction of the soul . . . as playing of the lute, dancing, speaking. It is first, in part, the movement of one finger, one foot, one letter, then the movements connect up and are commanded as on whole and, moreover, as with a given signal. . . .

> Nature sets in motion by signs and watchwords, which are made with little momentum. . . . Just as in the army the soldiers are set in motion by one word as if by a given signal and continue to move until they receive another signal to stop, so the muscles move in order and harmony from established custom.[161]

The least one can say is that William Harvey recognizes that coordination is an important property of animal movement. And he doesn't understand it.

Although Harvey uses a fair amount of mechanical reasoning in all his works, he appears to be convinced that the metaphor of the automaton will not work for understanding coordination. Thus, it is in search of another metaphor that his notes on animal movement end:

> Is the brain the general? The nerves carry the commands, sergeant major. The spinal medulla the lieutenant-cornet. The branches of the nerves which give the signal to the muscles, the captains. The muscles, the soldiers.

> Or is the brain the ruler of the senate for the purpose of deciding what useful things are present? The nerves, the magistrates. The branches of the nerves, the officials. The muscles, the citizens, the populace.

> Or again, is the brain the choir-master? The nerves the time-keepers and prompters, dancers. The muscles, the actors, singers, dancers.

> Or is the brain the architect? The nerves the overseers, surveyors. The branches of the nerves, the clerk of every work. The muscles, the workman.

> Or is the brain the master? The spinal medulla his mate. The nerves, boatswains. The muscles, sailors.

> Or is the brain the prime mover? The nerves, the intelligences. The muscles, the spheres?[162]

All these are social metaphors, as if Harvey had fallen back to the world view of the Middle Ages. In a way, that is true, but in the 17th century, alchemy worked as a progressive program. Whatever we think of alchemy, one has to sympathize with its attempts to retain an active view of matter, if only to avoid the dead end of mechanicism.

Isaac Newton (1642-1727)

The year 1687 marks a watershed with the publication of Newton's *Principia Mathematica Philisophiae Naturalis (Mathematical Principles of Natural Philosophy)*. By claiming universal gravity, working at a distance, Newton could show that the motions of the planets depend on simple, mathematical principles.

Nothing had quite prepared the world when, in 1936, Newton's manuscripts were auctioned and John Maynard Keynes got hold of Newton's alchemical studies.[163] All of a sudden, statements could be read in the public domain that did not sound like the Newton we had imagined:

> . . . two mercuries[164] are the masculine and feminine semens . . . fixed and volatile, the Serpents around the caduceus,[165] the Dragons of Flammel.[166] Nothing is produced from masculine or feminine semen alone. For generation and for the first matter the two must be joined.

> Perhaps the whole frame of Nature may be nothing but various Contextures of some certaine aethereall Spirits or vapours condens'd as it were by precipitation. . . . For Nature is a perpetuall circulatory worker, generating fluids out of solids, and solids out of fluids. . . .[167]

Newton was an ardent anti-Cartesian. He regarded Descartes' ungodly theory of independent matter as "absurd . . . confused and incongruous with reason."[168] For Newton, matter must be part of the All, allowed to carry forces, with God being continuously present in His world. So Newton was an anomaly in 17th-century science in that he was neither a pure mechanicist (with passive matter) nor a pure alchemist (with active matter), but tried to combine the two.[169] Newton realized that passive matter and active spirits cannot be reconciled by themselves, and he needed a "mediator"—which he found in the "ether," the primordial matter of the alchemists, the medium for the spirits.

The first time Newton wrote on animal motion was in a letter to Oldenburg, on December 7, 1675, trying to understand the mechanics of ether:

> Yea & that puzzling Problem: By what means the Muscles are contracted & dilated to cause Animal motion. . . . If there be any power in man to condense & dilate at will the aether that pervades the muscle; that condensation or dilatation must vary the compression of the Muscle, made by the Ambient aether. . . . If both aethers were equally dense, the muscle would be at liberty

as if prest by neither. If there were no aether within, the Ambient would compresse it with the whole force of its Spring.

Now for the changing the consistence of the aether . . . the soule may have an immediate power over the whole aether in any part of the body to Swell or Shrink at will: but then how depends the Muscular motion on the nerves. Others . . . may . . . think it done by some aethereall Spirit included in the *Dura Mater* . . . but still theres a difficulty . . . it should susteyne more or less the force of the Outward Aether. A third supposition may be that the Soul has a power to inspire any muscle with this Spirit by impelling it thither through the Nerves, but this too has its difficulties; for . . . it is hard to conceive, how so great force can be exercised amidst so tender matter as the braine is and besides, why does not this aethereall Spirit . . . go away through the *Dura Mater.* . . .[170]

The pressure of ether in the muscle is different from that of the ambient ether. Muscle is not controlled directly by the soul but via the nerves, which cannot just bring ambient ether because then nothing would happen. Nor can they directly transport the force because it would leak away.

Newton tells Oldenburg how he thinks "it may be done," introducing "sociableness" and his "Mediation of a Third":

First then, I suppose, there is such a Spirit . . . the Animal Spirits[171] . . . Subtile enough to pervade the Animal juices as freely as the Electric or perhaps Magnetic effluvia do glass. . . . So some fluids (as Oyle and water) though their pores are in freedome enough to mix with one another, yet by some secret principle of unsociableness they keep asunder, & some that are Sociable may become unsociable by adding a third thing to one of them. . . . And in like manner the aethereall Animal Spirit in a man may be a mediator between the common aether & the muscular juices to make them mix more freely; & so by sending a little of the Spirit into any muscle . . . it may cause . . . the Swelling or Shrinking of the Muscle & consequently the Animal motion depending thereon. . . . Thus may therefore the Soul . . . cause all the motions we see in Animals. . . .[172]

Between the letter to Oldenburg and the *Principia*, Newton realized that ponderable ether would be problematic,[173] if only for the same infinite regress that was already troubling mechanicism: If particles of ether are moved by other particles of ether, then how are the latter moved? In the *Principia*, Newton refrained from using ether altogether, replacing direct interaction between "particles" with force-at-a-distance, a concept his peers would find occult, if not impossible to accept.

In his years at Trinity College in Cambridge, Newton worked very much in isolation. Apart from the odd letter to Oldenburg, secretary of the Royal Society, not much from his hand was known to his contemporaries. He needed the encouragement of Halley to publish his calculus and the theory of universal gravitation.[174] When the *Principia* appeared, in 1687, there was instantaneous fame; but Newton collapsed, probably because his relationship with the young mathematician Fatio de Duillier came to an end.[175] After that, there was a complete turnaround in Newton's life. He decided to become a civil servant and was appointed, in 1696, as warden of the Mint,[176] and reorganizing the Mint would take the bulk of his energies. Once in a while he would still occupy himself with science, and he even became president of the Royal Society, but he would avoid outspoken views as much as possible—after all, by now he was a civil servant.

Seventeen years after the *Principia*, in 1704, Newton published his *Opticks*,[177] mostly based on earlier studies. He regarded his research as unfinished and added personal speculations as "Queries" at the end. The book went through several reprints, the number of Queries increasing all the time. I quote Query 31 from the fourth edition (1730):

> Have not the small Particles of Bodies certain Powers, Virtues, or Forces, by which they act at a distance . . . ? For it's well known, that Bodies act one upon another by the Attractions of Gravity, Magnetism, and Electricity. . . .

> When Spirit of Vitriol poured upon common Salt or Salt-petre makes an Ebullition with the Salt, and unites with it . . . does not this argue that the fix'd Alcaly of the Salt attracts the acid Spirit of the Vitriol more strongly than its own Spirit, and not being able to hold them both, lets go its own?

> The *Vis inertiae* is a passive Principle by which Bodies persist in their Motion or Rest. . . . By this Principle alone there never could have been any Motion in the World.[178]

Once more, we see Newton reject the world of Descartes: The passivity of mechanicism would preclude motion, while ours is an active world, full of attraction and repulsion. Again, in Newton's mind we need an "Aetherall Medium" to connect active principles with passive matter. By now the ether has become imponderable, but still, it obeys mechanical principles—as we can see in Query 24 on animal motion:

> Is not Animal Motion perform'd by the Vibrations of this Medium, excited by the Brain by the power of the Will, and propagated from thence through the . . . Capillamenta of the Nerves into the Muscles, for contracting and dilating them? I suppose that the Capillamenta of the Nerves are . . . solid and uniform, that the vibrating Motion of the Aethereall Medium may be propagated along them from one end to the other uniformly, and without interruption: For Obstructions in the Nerves create Palsies.[179]

So, the "mediator" has become a "medium," with "vibrations" that are strongly reminiscent of Borelli's "sneezing" commands into the nerves.[180] Had Newton given up his synthesis between alchemy and mechanics? I don't think so. But then, neither had he been successful, and the Queries show that he was fully aware of his failure.

Intermezzo 3: Mechanicism, Coordination, and Definitions

The 1973 *Shorter Oxford English Dictionary* offers the following definition of "mechanics": "a. Orig. (and still in pop. use): That body of theoretical and practical knowledge which is concerned with the invention and construction of machines, the explanation of their operation, and the calculation of their efficiency. b. That department of applied mathematics which treats of motion and tendencies to motion: comprising *kinematics,* the science of abstract motion, and *dynamics* (including *statics* and *kinetics*), the science of the action of forces in producing motion or equilibrium."

The first definition may be of all times; the second is not. In Newton's day, "mechanical philosophy" assumed that mechanical interaction depends on direct contact between bodies. In that sense, Newton's forces-that-act-at-a-distance falsified mechanical philosophy. To date, we know of contraptions with suspended metal balls that continue to move in a magnetic field, but such was not the kind of "machine" known to 17th-century science. It was thus a leap of "faith in science" to continue to see the universe as a machine after Newton's *Principia.* But this is exactly what happened. Hence, Newton's *Principia* not only falsified mechanical philosophy, but also allowed for its resurrection from the ashes. Mechanicism is dead, long live mechanicism.

In the new form of mechanicism (with action at a distance), the problems of Descartes and Borelli were not solved; but neither was Newton's "mediator" accepted (or "medium," in its alchemical sense), nor was Harvey's "harmony" understood. If one is to understand "coordination," however one defines it, it will have to entail the notion that separate processes have something in common. When thinking on the nature of harmony in animal motion, Harvey ended with a long series of questions. And also Newton published his hunches about the ethereal medium in the form of a query. His "mediation by a third" would be forgotten by posterity until the 20th century. In my mind, late 17th-century science was farther away from understanding coordination than ever.

In terms of Charles' problem, we cannot but be ambivalent about alchemy. It did give rise to alternative metaphors, such as that of an army (Harvey), or of "mediation by a third" (Newton); but however attractive these metaphors may have been, at least in principle, Harvey and Newton failed to couch their dissident thoughts in a scientific framework that had the same rigor as mechanical philosophy (or the new laws of mechanics). While Descartes and Borelli had created a conceptual problem that could not be solved, Harvey and Newton, although maybe on the right track, failed to find an acceptable solution to Charles' problem. In fact, about a century later, alchemy would disappear from science without a trace.

Hang Them Together: Christiaan Huygens

On February 22, 1664, Christiaan Huygens (1629-1695), the "doyen of European science,"[181] stumbled upon a technical solution to Charles' problem.[182] Clocks that were together suspended from metal bars (figure 1.12), put on top of wooden chairs, turned out to tick in concert. On February 26, Huygens wrote to his father:

> Pain in the side. winds.... Observation of the sympathy of clocks, admirable phenomenon, witness to the precision of clocks because so little is needed to bring them in perpetual agreement.... While I had been obliged to guard the room for some days . . . I have perceived an admirable effect, & of which nobody else could have thought before. That is to say . . . two clocks, suspended besides each other, with a distance of one or two feet, kept such exact mutual precision, that the two clocks always ticked together, without ever varying. I have admired this for some time; I finally found that this happened because of a kind of sympathy.... I removed them from each other, hanging one in a corner of the room & the other fifteen feet away: & then I saw that in one day there was a difference of 5 seconds so that their agreement didn't present itself but in a little bit of sympathy, which in my mind can have no other cause than the imperceptible agitation of the air as produced by the movement of the clocks.[183]

To date, we find the synchronization of Huygens' clocks highly significant.[184] But that is because we are looking for principles of biological organization, interpreting such ticking-in-concert in terms of the theory of dynamical systems. Contrary to the theories of the 17th and 18th centuries, dynamical systems are nonlinear,[185] complex,[186] and often unpredictable.[187]

On March 16, 1664, Huygens published his finding in the *Journal des Sçavans [Journal of Learned Men]*. But it failed to cause a stir. Later, Huygens himself did not pay much attention to the synchronization

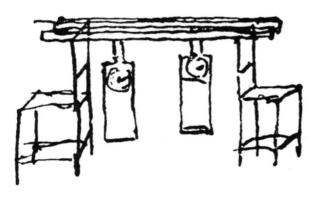

Figure 1.12
Technical solution to Charles' problem (Huygens, 1932, p. 185).

of his clocks. Why did he fail to get enthusiastic?[188] The simplest and most trivial explanation of Huygens' inability to see a new major metaphor in the "sympathy" of his clocks is that nonlinear[189] differential equations just weren't there. Calculus was on its way (Leibniz, Newton, Huygens himself), and it would have been a bit early to recognize that two stable states are possible when clocks are coupled (in-phase and anti-phase).[190] In fact, 17th-century calculus attempted to capture movement by excluding it, that is, by focusing on the snapshot in which Δtime (time elapsed) becomes zero.[191]

Huygens' own biography[192] also leaves little room for imagining him as enthusiastic about the "sympathy" between clocks: For Huygens, sympathy belonged to alchemy. In his youth, Descartes had been a family friend. What Huygens admired most in Descartes was that he had succeeded in removing mystical concepts such as "sympathy" and "antipathy" from science. In 1657, Huygens invented "a clock which is so regular that there is a considerable probability that we can measure longitude at sea if it can be transported."[193] This pendular clock would give him world fame. Even today, we know it as a "grandfather clock" and use it to illustrate the notion of "escapement" (figure 1.13). The thing is, for Huygens, that the clock meant *precision*; and in the letter to his father it was the precision[194] of clocks in sympathy he so much admired, while detesting the notion of "sympathy" itself.

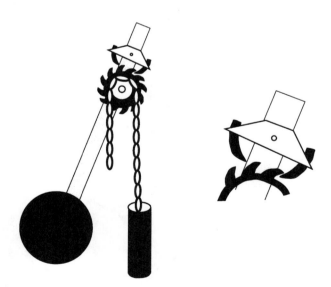

Figure 1.13
Escapement (right), illustrated on a grandfather clock (left) (adapted from Kugler & Turvey 1987).

At the time, theoretical debates within the Dutch Republic were fierce: Religious fundamentalism, mechanicism, alchemy, and a host of "superstitious" beliefs were competing for hegemony.[195] Still, to the outside world, the Dutch formed one united front, dedicated to mechanicism. In 1607, De Gheyn depicted the sequence of postures for musketeers who had to shoot— by doing so, De Gheyn turned his musketeers into automata (figure 1.14).[196] When Descartes entered the Dutch Republic, his theories were well received,[197] and so was Harvey's idea of the circulation of blood.[198] When Galileo was forbidden to publish, he still wrote a book and had it published in Leyden.[199] After the peace of Münster (1648),[200] the Dutch Republic busied itself with exporting[201] its own mix of Calvinism and mechanical philosophy, rather than bothering about the fine points. How could they ever have debased the quality of one of their best products? The Dutch never do such a thing.[202]

Poor Charles! More than a century after his obsession, a technical solution to his problem was found, but it was not recognized as such. There was no mathematics to make it very interesting; Huygens saw a kind of alchemy in it; and the Dutch were just engaged in exporting mechanicism, without bothering too much about the small print.

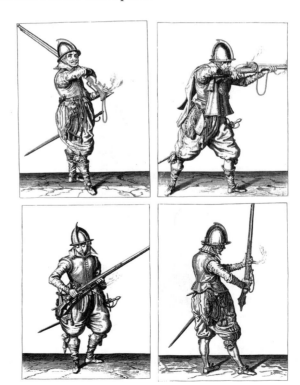

Figure 1.14
Musketeers or automata? Positions 2 (upper left), 11 (upper right), 18 (lower left), and 20 (lower right) of the first series (Roers), with 42 positions (De Gheyn, J., 1607, Wapenhandelinghe van Roers, Musquetten ende Spiessen, 's Gravenhage).

Where Have We Arrived?

We started off with an ailing emperor who failed to have his clocks sound together on the hour. Charles V may have thought that the problem of his clocks was a problem of precision, but to date we have quartz clocks and we know that it is impossible to give them other than finite precision. If you have them right for n decimals, decimal $n + 1$ will soon start to bother you. So it is impossible to individually control clocks in such a way that they acquire absolute predictability.

In the works of Descartes and Borelli, it was recognized that one cannot control a mechanism from within, so these "extraterrestrials" speculated that control came from without. But it turned out to be impossible to reconnect the immaterial soul with the material world. Still, the view of Descartes and Borelli is close to how we personally experience our ability to make things happen, and society at large did not bother too much about the conceptual problems. Sure, Harvey and Newton avoided these problems; but they failed to reach a scientifically acceptable understanding of the causes of "harmony" or the mechanisms of "mediation by a third." Alchemy may have appeared attractive to 17th-century science; but in the end, it failed.

Conceptually, Newton's "mediation" was close to what happened with Huygens' clocks. Huygens offered his clocks something in common (the rhythm of the metal bar over the chairs). What could Charles have learned from that fact? We saw how he focused on the individual clocks, that is, on the parts—as when you bring your car to the garage and do not expect the mechanic to say that all parts are in order, while it is only the whole that fails. But coordination has to do with relationships, with a whole as opposed to its parts. Coordination is when separate processes acquire something in common.

So, if Charles wanted to coordinate his realms, he ought to have ensured that they had enough in common—as in the Roman Empire, the system of justice, together with the economic connectedness of the Mediterranean harbors. No such commonality was reached in the empire of Charles V. Similarly with his clocks—they remained standing on their own. He could have connected them with soft springs,[203] and they would probably have sounded together. Still, there would have been a price to pay: With such a loosely connected system of clocks, you never know exactly when it will sound, let alone being able to predict that the clocks will strike "on the hour." Such self-organizing systems tend to have an agenda of their own.[204]

Continued Failure (18th and 19th Centuries)

Of course, I could continue my story with other attempts to solve Charles' problem in the 18th and the 19th centuries, but I won't. The principles should be clear by now. They remained valid at least until the 20th century, notwithstanding the fantastic discoveries that were being made, such as the steam engine as a new metaphor for the world (replacing the clock), electricity as the secret of the nervous system, quantitative chemistry without the mystique of alchemy, or Darwin's statistical theory of the origin of biological goal-directedness.

With hindsight, one might have expected scientists in the 18th and 19th centuries to have developed more exalted views of matter. After all, with the passive stupidity of mechanicism, they now could know that the demands on the soul were impossibly large. Most scientists, however, continued to adhere to mechanicism. Instead, it was the soul that suffered, going passive in the 18th century and disappearing altogether in the 19th. Without a soul, the problem of Descartes and Borelli disappears; but if you continue to stick to mechanicism, it becomes logically impossible to make things happen.

I will wrap up my story by summarizing what happened to the soul in the 18th and 19th centuries. To avoid possible misunderstanding, let me say beforehand that I personally do not think the soul can solve any problems of movement science. Nor is it harmful per se—Islamic science, for instance, goes on to have an active soul and there is no problem with that. What is essential is your image of the world itself. The passive stupidity of mechanicism should be replaced with a somewhat more respectful image of matter—so that coordination and control can become natural phenomena and "activity" becomes possible *within* the world. For the arrival of such images, we had to wait until the 20th century. Historically (but not logically), this happened because the soul went away: It was only after discarding the soul that science started to realize that matter must be more surprising than we had thought.

The Soul Goes Passive

In the year following the publication of Newton's *Principia,* the troops of William III, stadtholder of the Dutch Republic, and Mary, daughter of Catholic King James II, landed in Torbay, on November 15, on their way to the British throne.[205] On February 23, 1689, they received the crown and proclaimed the Declaration of Rights in which, maybe for the first time in Europe, basic rights of the citizens were guaranteed. England had become a modern, democratic nation: the Glorious Revolution.[206]

As a matter of course, Christiaan Huygens followed in the wake of his stadtholder, and on July 8 he met with King William at Hampton Court, asking the king if he would accept Newton as regent of a Cambridge college.[207] The king would not.[208] Some weeks later, Huygens visited Robert Boyle (1627-1691), the famous physicist-chemist, who failed to convert him to alchemy.[209] "He [Boyle] did an experiment for us with two cold liquids which when combined give a flame. With the one, smelling almost like anise, he drenched linen in a silver spoon. The other one, that he poured over it, was in a small bottle; when it was opened smoke came out. . . . Boyle promised to give me the recipe to make ice without ice or snow."[210]

A feeling of unprecedented satisfaction entered Protestant England. When Boyle died, in 1691, he left a sum to be used for sermons on "The proof of the Christian religion against notorious infidels, namely Atheists, Theists, Pagans, Jews and Mohammedans, not descending lower to any controversies that are among the Christians themselves."[211] A series of such sermons was given by William Derham (1657-1735), author of a book with a rather lengthy title:

> *The Artificial Clockmaker, A Treatise of Watch and Clock-work; shewing to the meanest capacities the Art of calculating Numbers to all sorts of MOVEMENTS; the Way to alter Clockwork; to make CHIMES, and set them to Musical Notes; and to calculate and correct the Motion of PENDULUMS also Numbers for divers Movements with the Antient and Modern History of Clock-Work; And many Instruments, Tables, and other Matters never before published in any other book.*[212]

Derham published his Boyle sermons in a book with the telling title *Physico-Theology*. According to Derham, science had become so good in revealing the great work of God that religious discussions could now finally end. This was done to save religion; but mechanicism was gaining power, and the world of physico-theology became "the Majestic Clockwork," as Bronowski would characterize it.[213] Although the view of Newton's *Principia* was hotly debated in the beginning, around the time of his death, Alexander Pope could write:

> Nature and Nature's laws lay hid in night:
> God said, Let Newton be! and all was light.[214]

This is not to say that there were no dissidents or that the debates did not go on; but now, finally, there was again one dominant world view.

Several generations of French *philosophes* (philosophers) believed that their country was way behind England and should follow its inspiring example. It is this optimistic trust in science that we call the Enlightenment.[215] The French *philosophes* were great popularizers. Who cared that God was now disappearing from the world, because all He had to do was see how the Clock was ticking? So, religious awe for science led to problems for religion.

A new sense of history emerged. The "Middle Ages" were invented to suggest that after the splendor of Athens and Rome, a long and dark time had followed before mankind was able to recover—in the Renaissance—to then reach the modernity of the Enlightenment. Islam and the Arabs disappeared from the tales that were told, as if the moderns had directly inherited civilization from classical antiquity. In popular histories, it was suggested that Harvey and Newton had been mechanical philosophers all the time. Indeed, it was not until 1936 that Newton's alchemical manuscripts became public.

And the soul? Well, who needs an active soul if you are a clock, built to perfection? Wrote De La Mettrie, in a book published in Leyden in 1748:

> The human body is a machine which winds its own springs. It is the living image of perpetual motion. Nourishment keeps up the movements which fever excites. Without food, the soul pines away, goes mad, and dies exhausted.[216]

It is not that De La Mettrie suspended the soul; rather, he made it completely dependent on the food we take, coffee, alcohol, and so on. By doing so, he solved the problems of Descartes and Borelli because there no longer was a separation. But the one world De La Mettrie envisaged was not a world in which we can make things happen. So, Laplace could conclude in 1795:

> We ought . . . to regard the present state of the universe as the effect of its previous state, and as the cause of that which will follow. An intelligence which for a given instant knew all the forces by which nature is animated, and the respective situations of the existences which compose it; if further that intelligence were vast enough to submit these given quantities to analysis; it would embrace in the same formula the greatest bodies in the universe and the lightest atom: nothing would be uncertain to it and the future as the past would be present to its eyes.[217]

These were the years of the French Revolution and Napoleon. But, rest assured, nothing happened—because nobody could make anything happen.

Were these people out of their minds? I don't think so. What they did was to bring the view of mechanism to its extreme: Now everything had become passive and stupid. Logically, that could not make sense. Historically, it opened the way, first, for abolishing the soul from science and, then, for recognizing that matter is not so passive and stupid after all.

The Soul Disappears Altogether

I am back to where I started my venture into the history of movement science about 10 years ago: the history of the spinal frog.[218] I still find that story very instructive because the same experiments were done for well over 300 years, each time creating the same kind of amazement. Now that I have come across Charles' problem, the spinal frog has also acquired a new meaning.

In the medical notebooks of John Locke (1632-1704), there are some isolated remarks, written around 1654:

Take a frog and strip it. You may see the circulation of blood if you hold him up against the sun.

Take out the heart and the frog will leap about a great while after.[219]

Apparently, these notes were written on the occasion of some experiments of Robert Boyle.[220] Contrary to Descartes, Boyle tried to approach the localization of the soul experimentally rather than just through reasoning. He removed the heart from a frog which "being put into the water would swim, whilst I felt his heart beating betwixt my fingers"[221] So, apparently, the seat of the soul was not in the heart. Thus, it should be in the head—as almost everybody already assumed. Boyle removed the heads from frogs, chickens, tortoises, and vipers, and saw that they still could move.

> Now although I will not say, that these experiments prove that . . . the brain may not be confined to the head, but may reach into the rest of the body . . . yet it may be safely affirmed that such experiments as these may be of great concernment in reference to the common doctrine of the necessity of unceasing influence from the brain, being so requisite to sense and motion; especially if . . . we add . . . what we have observed of the butterflies . . . that they may not only . . . survive a pretty time . . . the loss of their heads, but may sometimes be capable of procreation after having lost them. . . .[222]

Boyle was a sceptic, and he did not come with a replacement theory. What he showed, apart from the fact that you don't need your head for procreation, was that the accepted views of mechanicism failed to capture animal motion.

About a century after Boyle and Locke, a dispute over headless animals broke out between Robert Whytt (1714-1766), in Edinburgh, and Albrecht von Haller (1708-1777), in Göttingen. Whytt was of the opinion that even after decapitation, there would still be some drops of soul juice in the body:[223]

> If then the soul in pigeons, frogs, vipers, and tortoises, is not confined to the brain, but can continue for a long time to actuate their bodies independent of that organ . . . why should we deny that, in man and such animals that resemble him most, the parts may continue to be actuated by the soul or sentient principle for some few minutes after their communication with the brain has been cut off?[224]

Von Haller was very angry. He believed that muscles have their own "irritability," quite independent of the "empire" of the soul:

> It is true that Mr Whytt renders the time of death rather shrewdly uncertain, and he believes that the animal still has life even when it has appeared dead for a long time. . . . Since, however . . . the soul, when the head has been cut off, loses its empire over the rest of the body, . . . since, furthermore, irritability remains perfect notwithstanding these circumstances . . . it becomes clear . . . that irritability does not depend on the soul.[225]

An Edinburgh student was to write that neither of the gentlemen was "deficient in irritability."[226] Apart from being amused, I find von Haller's position interesting. He appears to argue that you can get rid of the soul of mechanicism only if you grant activity (goal-directedness) to the body itself.

That was to be the main point of Eduard Friedrich Wilhelm Pflüger (1829-1920), again a century later. Pflüger was one of those great decapitators of frogs who have had so much influence in medical teaching. "When a pair [of copulating frogs] is captured, and one only grips the male, the female will be pulled out of the water as well because the male strongly holds [her] enclosed. . . . When the spinal cord of the male is cut, between the atlas and the second vertebra . . . he does not let go. . . . If . . . she attempts to withdraw, he just holds her stronger."[227] And then, Pflüger does his famous experiment. Drop some acetic acid on the body of the spinal animal (figure 1.15, I), and it will remove the acid with one leg (II). Cut off that leg (III), and drop acid again. The stump of the original scratching leg will move aimlessly for a short while, and the frog scratches the acid off with another leg (IV). What more proof would one want of the active nature of the headless animal!

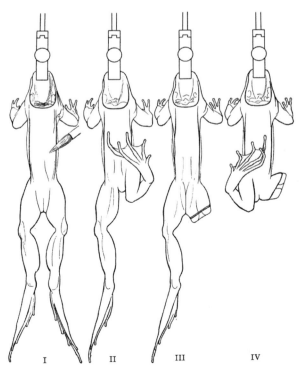

Figure 1.15
Pflüger's frog (Verworn, M., 1907, *Physiologisches Praktikum für Mediziner*, Jena: Gustav Fischer, p. 198).

Thomas Huxley (1825-1895), friend of Charles Darwin, immediately recognized the importance of this experiment and offered a lecture to the Metaphysical Society on the question: "Has a frog a soul; and of what nature is that soul, supposing it to exist?"[228] In his lecture, Huxley discussed Pflüger's experiments and concluded that he was "unable to see in what respect the soul of the frog differs from matter."[229] Some years later, Huxley would state that animals are "intelligent" automata.[230] Archbishop Manning was furious:

> A chest of carpenter's tools is inactive, and has neither invention nor product without the mind and will of the carpenter. What have the brain and the hand more than the lathe and the chisel, without the Agent from whom they derive guidance and activity?[231]

To me, it seems that Manning got the question right but the answer wrong: The whole issue of Pflüger's frogs has to do with the nature of the body itself.[232] Huxley could not do much more than just suspend the soul and hint at the possible "intelligence" of automata. In fact, he did not have a clue how to model an "active" body and still be scientific.

Well, now, "I shall not stick to tell you how this may be done."[233]

"Speelruimte" *(Spielraum)*

Today, when I finish this closing section, it is August 4, 1999, time to prepare for the millennium. During the last millennium, people were eagerly awaiting the coming of Christ. And now, I am told that I should worry about a computer bug. Times they are a-changing. Are they?

Once again, Europe is trying to form one united empire, with Brussels as its capital. Charles V would have liked that, Flemish as he was.[234] Are we still bothered by his problem?

By definition, Charles' problem arises only if one accepts mechanism. In that respect, I see two very important developments for 20th-century movement science.

First, Nikolai Aleksandrovich Bernstein (1896-1966) discovered that coordination should *precede* control.[235] You cannot control your body unless it is already coordinated. Nice thought for Charles V, who tried to do it the other way around: Control the clocks into coordination. That, you cannot do. For Bernstein, animals are "active," controlled by a stochastic model of the "needed future."[236] Bernstein was the major source of inspiration for a group of researchers in Moscow who wrote again on the spinal frog, more than 300 years after the first experiments.[237] On September 12, 1980, their paper appeared in *Science:* "The spinal frog takes into account the scheme of its body during the wiping reflex."[238] We learn that "the spinal frog can make complex leg movements according to the scheme of its body . . . [while] central commands . . . define the final hip angle . . . [and] the motor program provides sufficient stiffness of the hindlimb that the influence of gravity on the movement is minimized."[239] Given their Bernsteinian inspiration, I grant these authors that they probably see the animal as active (and thus reject mechanism as I have defined it). But notions such as "scheme" and "program" are clearly reminiscent of machines, and the Bernstein notion of "activity" is not as clear as one would wish. Old habits die hard.

The second important 20th-century development I see starts with Max Planck (1858-1947), player in that fascinating game of theoretical physics (Einstein, Heisenberg) that gave us a new image of the world altogether. Planck discovered that a physical *macroscopy* can have properties that emerge from the *microscopy,* while they cannot be logically deduced from that microscopy.[240] Thus, for the first time, we can develop a unified image of the world in which psychological phenomena have their proper place.[241] Hermann Haken, currently in Stuttgart, added to Planck's view that macroscopic stability can arise only on the basis of *relationships* within the microscopy.[242] These are ideas that, at least in my mind, are a long way from the passive stupidity of mechanism. Sure, for movement science Haken's "synergetics" is still a metaphor, and we do not know exactly how it relates to the coordination of movement[243] or to the organization of the brain.[244] But it is already clear that the new metaphors of 20th-century science are vastly different from those of the past. Sufficiently so? I honestly don't know.

This is an introductory chapter to a historical source book of 20th-century movement science. Supposedly, the reader is now about to digest important 20th-century papers. Please, do not make the mistake of assuming that detailed knowledge in an author reveals deep understanding—it usually does not. Nor should you expect that 20th-century science makes fewer mistakes or is less hilarious than science of the past. Just try to see the conceptual struggle behind each individual paper. And wonder, once in a while, how far the author you were reading is able to solve Charles' problem. If I have succeeded in installing such a feeling of wonder, I have already done my job.

But then, should we not at least have an inkling of the kind of theory that would allow for the solution to Charles' problem? To me, the biological notion of coordination is very different from Huygens' synchrony. Coordination entails the notion that separate processes acquire some form of commonality. The lesson from history appears to be that we failed to understand the commonality because we used the wrong kind of model for the separate processes. The hallmark of biology is that it comes up with workable solutions to problems such that you can always find a different solution if the circumstances change. Biology is about flexibility. Hence, processes that partake in coordination should have their own "Speelruimte" *(Spielraum).* I used to translate that notion as "working space," but it is more than that. The notion of "Speelruimte" can appear in physics (slack), in biology (space to play), or in the social sciences (freedom to negotiate). Speelruimte is when you refuse to have fixed solutions to your problems.

Not so long ago, Hermann Haken presented his "synergetics" to Beatrix, queen of The Netherlands, in the Royal Palace in Amsterdam. We came to speak about the fact that biology prefers "almost-synchrony" to absolute synchrony. That's the way, for instance, jugglers remain flexible[245] rather than getting trapped in one specific, robot-like pattern. The queen smiled. She described how, when she has to inspect the Guard, some military music is usually played at the moment she is supposed to start walking. She then silently hums a melody to herself and waits until the two melodies interact. It is at this point that she starts walking. "Regally," as the newspapers will say. I think that Queen Beatrix understands the solution to Charles' problem.

Translations and Citations

Whenever I translated sources from languages other than French, German, or Dutch, I have given the original in a note. In using citations from other authors, I have sometimes added a comma or started a cited sentence with a capital letter; other changes are indicated in the notes.

Acknowledgments

For much of the present text, I am indebted to whole generations of students and to many of my colleagues at the Faculty of Human Movement Sciences in Amsterdam. In preparing this chapter, I received great help from Maartje Bosman, Piet Eikelenboom, Lieke Peper, Arne Ridderikhoff, and G. Sander de Wolf. For their critical reading of an earlier version, I gratefully acknowledge Peter J. Beek, Ruud J. Bosscher, Sandra Diemel, Claudine J.C. Lamoth, Lev P. Latash, Mark L. Latash, and Harm Slijper. For my Spanish adventures, I particularly want to thank Geoffrey Parker, the *Archivo General* in Simancas, José Ramón-Nieto, Fray Francisco de Andrés, Ignacio González-Tascón, Beatriz Presmanes-Arizmendi, and of course Yang Tit Man.

Endnotes

[1] García-Diego, 1986, p. 144. Milan authorities commissioned Turriano not later than 1548 to make a clock for Charles V; he was paid for his trip in 1551.

[2] Needham, Wang & Price, 1960; Needham & Wang, 1974, in particular pp. 435-546 on clocks.

[3] Hill, 1974, in particular pp. 17-93 on clocks.

[4] The description of the clock (the "Milanese planetarium") is from García-Diego, 1986. Those who want to see a surviving Renaissance clock may visit Prague and admire the Town Hall. Although Copernicus had written already (in 1543; cf. Moore, 1973), the earth was still regarded as the center of the universe, the movements of the planets understood with Ptolemy's system of cycles and epicycles (2nd century A.D.; Moore, 1973). García-Diego wrote: "In the Ptolemaic system there were no basic grounds for the planets moving at the same time along the circles of their equant and their deferent, for the multiplicity of spheres, for the exceptions to the rules. . . . All this was accepted as the will of God. Thus anyone capable of reproducing it was, if not a superman, at least an exalted and extraordinary person" (1986, p. 23).

[5] García-Diego, 1986, pp. 55-58; italics added by the present author. Vida had been appointed bishop of Alba in 1532. The quote is from a speech to the senators of Milan.

[6] Unless indicated otherwise, my understanding of Charles V derives from Parker, 1999.

[7] Kamen, 1997, p. 47.

[8] We know that he was paid for the trip but not when he arrived or how the meeting went.

[9] García-Diego, 1986, p. xi. I assume that "Juanelo's egg" later changed, in the non-Spanish speaking world, into "the egg of Columbus."

[10] González-Tascón, 1998, particularly pp. 350-356.

[11] García-Diego, 1986, p. 54, citing from the same speech of Bishop Vida (note 5).

[12] Note that Charles forgot "minor" territories such as Mexico (captured by Cortés in 1520) and Peru (taken by the Pizarro brothers in 1533).

[13] García-Diego, 1986, pp. 75-76.

[14] I don't know when and where this was agreed upon. Turriano remained relatively independent, traveling to Milan several times. Only in Charles' last years, in Yuste, were they inseparable.

[15] Kamen, 1997, p. 51.

[16] "Su Majestad no tiene en su corte ni quiere tener hombre ninguno señor ni perlado a quien aya de tener respeto ni quiere oyr negoçios ni firmar los pocos que se dispachan entendiendo y occupandose dia y noche en ajustar y conçertar sus relojes que son hartos y tiene con ellos la prinçipal quenta y con otro reloj nuevo que hay inventado y mandado hazer en una vidrieza de una ventana. Y de noche como el no puedo dormir quando quiere hazia levantar muy a menudo a las ayudas de su camara y a otros y ençienden velas y hachas para desbaratar y tornar a conçertar los dichos relojes" (*Archivo General de Simancas*, F 98/274-275, "Memorial de lo quele dicho Nicolas Nicolai en Flandes", sent to Philip in September, 1553, 274, unnumbered pages 3-4). For the transcription and translation, I heavily relied on Parker, 1999. I assume that the clock "he invented" is the one made by Juanelo Turriano.

[17] García-Diego, 1986, p. 82, paraphrasing the French ambassador.

[18] García-Diego, 1986, p. 82, citing the Venetian ambassador.

[19] Williams, 1996, p. 101. I do not know whether this quote derives from a reliable source (if so, possibly from Gachard, L.P., 1854-1856, *Retraite et Mort de Charles-Quint au Monastère de Yuste*, 3 volumes, Brussels) or is just part of the mythology. "*Desbaratar y tornar a conçertar*" (note 16), however, strongly suggests that at least the gist of the quote is correct.

[20] Ramón-Nieto, 1998.

[21] Note 16.

[22] García-Diego, 1986.

[23] Cf. González-Tascón, 1998.

[24] " . . . it seemed very strange that an Emperor should have what we should now call a hobby" (García-Diego, 1986, p. 82).

[25] " . . . la relativa indiferencia que las diversas ingenierías tenían en los negocios religiosos" (González-Tascón, 1998, p. 19).

[26] Needham & Wang, 1974, p. 435, citing Von Bertele, H., 1954, "Precision time-keeping in the pre-Huygens era," *HORJ*, 95, p. 794. The escapement is what partitions continuous energy into discrete ticks.

[27] His grandparents were Maximilian of Austria, Mary of Burgundy, Ferdinand of Aragon, and Isabel of Castilia. Charles' father, Philip the Fair, died in 1506, leaving a widow who became insane (Juana la Loca).

[28] This is the main theme of Yates, 1975. The tales were retold of the "good Roman Emperors," particularly Marcus Aurelius, and of Charlemagne. Note that this was also the time that Thomas More wrote his *Utopia* (1515-1516). Thomas More was a friend of Erasmus.

[29] Erasmus, 1516/1986.

[30] Yates, 1975, p. 22.

[31] De Guevara, 1529/1986. The book was widely read all over Europe.

[32] The French king, for instance, thought that "clocks have been invented, to live and behave by the rule and order of virtue" (1544, García-Diego, 1986, p. 33).

[33] From the first and last page of "The Argument of the Booke called the Diall of Princes" (De Guevara, 1986, pages not numbered).

[34] Throughout the 16th century, this argument was very popular, particularly on the basis of the works of Hermes Trismegistos (see the intermezzo in the subsection on Harvey). "The God makes Eternity, The Eternity the World, The World The Time; but The Time the Generation . . . the Life and the Death" (Hermes Trismegistos, 1975, p. 68).

[35] In an e-mail, June 19, 1999, Geoffrey Parker wrote to me: "I like far more [than my looking for Arabian sources of Charles's conception of power] your perception that Charles's fascination with taking clocks to pieces and then putting them together again may have reflected his own sense of power—or impotence. . . . On the other hand, this is the period when the idea of 'timing' things gains ground. One of Philip II's courtiers claimed that the king 'timed his day to the moment,' and had two clocks in front of him all the time (they are still on his desk at the Escorial), and in the 1570s at least ministers purchased pocket watches so they could keep time better. So the fascination with clocks may just reflect a fascination with time. It may have been more, but I'd like to see some proof." Of course, I agree with Parker's argument that there was a general fascination with time in 16th-century Spain. I express my gratitude for Parker's stimulating reactions to my e-mails. I find his analyses of 16th-century Dutch-Spanish relationships enlightening, convincing, and fascinating (1995, 1996a & b, 1998).

[36] Notes 4 & 5.

[37] The term "coordination" is my understanding of "conçertar" (note 16). When I ascribe to Charles V the idea that control of the individual elements should lead to overall coordination, I am a 20th-century movement scientist looking back at the origin of the problems my science is facing now.

[38] I borrowed the term "impotence" from Parker (cf. note 35).

[39] But see notes 19 & 35.

[40] For a time, I believed that Charles' obsession could be understood as a conception of power through controlling details (Meijer, De Wolf & Lamoth, 1999 a & b). Reading Parker, 1999, convinced me that that was wrong. Charles was not an absolute monarch who could not delegate, or at least he tried not to be like that. Nevertheless, he advised his son in 1543: "Transact business with many, and do not bind yourself to or become dependent upon any individual, because although it may save time, it does no good" (Parker, 1996b, p. 18); and indeed the (implicit) concept of power of Philip II was to control as many details as possible (cf. Parker, 1996b & 1998).

[41] This is the main point of Parker's "The Political World of Charles V," 1999.

[42] In the battle of Mühlberg, Charles won a major victory over the German Protestants.

[43] Taking them apart and putting them back together to bring them in concert (note 16).

[44] Dijksterhuis, 1980.

[45] Dijksterhuis, 1980, p. 543.

[46] I agree with Gelfand and Latash that "the main problem is not describing the mechanics of movement" (1998, p. 306).

[47] Hackforth, 1972, pp. 63-64.

[48] Ibid., p. 69 & pp. 103-104.

[49] Ibid., pp. 105-106, slightly edited for reasons of clarity.

[50] I use the term "mechanicism" for the idea (explicit or not) that mechanics is "the" theory of everything. Mechanicism is an exaggeration of the importance of mechanics. Of course, mechanics has a validity of its own. Movement science could not have developed without the development of mechanics. Nevertheless, the main challenges of movement science, control and coordination, are not of a mechanical nature. Cf. Gelfand & Latash, 1998.

[51] Lovejoy, 1973.

[52] For Aristotle, there is a natural, internal cause of movement, comparable to a "homing device" in pigeons. Note that I first picked up the stone (control by my soul), to then leave it to itself.

[53] When you lose your "heart" in San Francisco, you are using the Aristotelian notion of the heart as the center of sensations.

[54] Peck & Foster, 1965, pp. 475 & 477.

[55] Ibid., p. 523.

[56] Ibid., p. 391.

[57] Peck & Foster, 1965.

[58] Peck & Foster, 1965, pp. 463 & 465.

[59] This is not a very strong argument, and it is fairly easy to imagine machines in which parts grow heavier and lighter (such as buckets in a water wheel). Nevertheless, biological growth and development would be used as anti-mechanicistic arguments in the late 18th century.

[60] This is a "beginning" both as an anatomical origin and as a first cause, a ruler, the soul.

[61] "What-is-in-the-head." Galen's books were translated by Muslims into Syriac and Greek. Especially in Toledo, in Spain, the books were translated back into Latin. I use the Greek terms because most modern translations derive from Greek versions.

[62] Daremberg, 1856, p. 321.

[63] Tellmadge May, 1968, p. 76. Also for Galen, coordination was not a problem but a given.

[64] Ibid., p. 189; I have changed the translation of demiourgos (δημιουργοσ) from "Creator" into "Architect," which I think a bit closer to the original meaning (somebody who makes something for the people). The translation "Creator" is better if one wants to understand how Galen could have been accepted by Muslims and Christians alike.

[65] The term "organon" (οργανον), which led to the modern word "organ," as in "bodily organs," primarily means "tool" or "instrument."

[66] Tellmadge May, 1968, pp. 69-70. The last part of this quote we will meet again, in the late 19th century, when Archbishop Manning attacks Thomas Huxley's statement that animals are intelligent automata (note 231).

[67] Daremberg, 1856, pp. 321-375.

[68] Ibid., p. 339.

[69] Ibid., p. 343. Note that this argument is weak, revealing Galen's tendency to ascribe the to-be-controlled less intelligence than Plato, for instance, had. Interestingly, Braune and Fischer, 1895-1904, will use this same argument to attack the Weber brothers' dynamic view on the swinging leg during walking (cf. Flesher, 1997).

[70] Ibid., pp. 323-324. It was Galen's conception of the one-way movement of the blood that would finally mark his fall (see the subsection on Harvey).

[71] Tellmadge May, 1968, pp. 431-434; italics added by the present author.

[72] I don't want to take any dogmatic position in the debates on the role of external factors in justifying scientific theories. In my mind, it is just the case that people, being who they are, use the metaphors at hand to make their world understandable (cf. Laudan, 1977).

[73] As Newton would "discover" (note 171).

[74] Particularly in the paintings of Giotto (1267-1337). It is interesting to observe that before the 1868 Meiji Revolution, Utamaro (1753-1806) had a similar fascination with visible reality.

[75] Jan van Eyck (1390-1441) and his brother Hubert depicted reality from two different perspectives in the same painting (one for the world of God and one for the world of Nature), and two sets of shadow (one for the light of God and one for the light of Nature). Experts have it that they did not know how to paint well (cf. Van Puyvelde, 1973), but the effect is systematic.

[76] Quoted from the Chinese movie *Temptress Moon*.

[77] Charles was born in Ghent. Vesalius' great-grandfather had been court physician of Charles' paternal grandmother, Mary of Burgundy (cf. Eriksson, 1959). I use the term "Flanders" for all non-French speaking southern provinces of the Low Countries.

[78] Eriksson, 1959, p. 285.

[79] Note 71.

[80] Eriksson, 1959, p. 289.

[81] "De reticulari uerò Galeni plexus nihil hîc entiendum duxi, quod iam cerebri uasorum seriem mihi perspectam esse haud dubitem, ... quòd nouimus Galenum boum dissectione delusum, non homine cerebri, uti neque ipsius uasa, sed boum recensuisse" (Vesalius, 1543, p. 310). I have some trouble in understanding Vesalius' Latin, but I am confident that the gist of my translation is correct.

[82] Cf. Clarke & Dewhurst, 1972. Willis got canonized because of his "discovery" of the real structure of the relevant vessels in the human brain (the "circulus Willisii"). For our present analysis, it remains unclear how much "progress" was made by Willis' transfer of the seat of the soul from the fluids to the substance.

[83] Eriksson, 1959, p. 107.

[84] "Musculum motus uoluntarij . . . esse instrumentum," Vesalius, 1543, p. 219.

[85] Note 58.

[86] García-Diego, 1986 (cf. the section on the clocks of Charles V).

[87] Wiero J. Beek informed me that the palace of the Doge reveals a fascination with clocks comparable to that of Charles V.

[88] García-Diego, 1986, p. 116. The Council of Trent was where the Catholic Church rejected Protestantism and reformulated its own dogmas.

[89] Particularly, of course, the fact that the Council of Trent (note 88) forbade them.

[90] Williams, 1996, p. 107; I have no clue whether this is a true or an apocryphal story, but I think that it accurately describes the spirit of the time. For another quote from Williams, see note 19.

[91] Williams, 1996, p. 126. Again, I don't know if there is any reliable source for this statement.

[92] "Ad divvm Carolvm Qvintvm, Maximvm, Invinctissimvm, qve Imperatorem," Vesalius, 1543, p. *2.

[93] Eriksson, 1959, p. 23. I have tried to locate the relevant documents but have not yet found them.

[94] Szentágothai, 1968, p. 16. One must assume that it was Vesalius who amputated three of Charles' fingers when the pain had become unbearable (note 16).

[95] Ramón-Nieto, 1998. I still don't understand the role of Spain in general, or that of Salamanca in particular. A clear explanation of Spain's modernity in the 16th century, the era of its great expansion, was that it attracted engineers and scientists from all over Europe (González-Tascón, 1998); but still, I would like to know what intellectual debates were going on.

[96] After the death of Charles, Vesalius became physician to the court of Philip II. Difficulties emerged, and he went on a pilgrimage to Jerusalem. He died on the way.

[97] It was only in Italy and Spain that surgery was taught at the universities (Ramón-Nieto, 1998).

[98] "Porque la gota le maltrata y corre a menudo por todos los miembros y junturas y nervios de su cuerpo hasta dalle en la nunca ques lo ultimo. y el catarro le molesta tanto que le llega a los posteros terminos. y quando lo tiene ny puede hablar ni quando habla es oydo o poco entendido por los çircunstantes de su cámara. y las emorroidas se le hinchan y atormentan con tantos dolores que no se puede rodear syn gran sentimiento y lágrimas" (Report of Francisco Duarte, note 16, 274, unnumbered page 1). For parts of this quote, I again made use of Parker's (1999) transcription and translation.

[99] "Biology" as a separate science arose at the end of the 18th century.

[100] Feigenberg & Meijer, 1999.

[101] Apart from the fun of writing down this sentence, I imply by my characterization that the study of anatomy and histology and cells and molecules is not part of movement science per se. Of course, movement science cannot proceed without them (for a similar argument concerning mechanicism, cf. note 50); but movement science, as I see it, is about principles of biological organization rather than the stuff that is being organized (or organizing itself).

[102] *Discours de la Méthode*, quoted from Descartes, 1953, p. 137.

[103] Ibid., p. 147; the original text is in italics.

[104] On June 22, 1633, Galileo had to renounce his Copernican views (Bronowski, 1964, pp. 189-219).

[105] *Discours de la Méthode* (note 102), p. 152.

[106] *Traité de l'Homme*, quoted from Descartes, 1953, p. 807.

[107] *Discours de la Méthode* (note 102), p. 164; italics in the original.

[108] In which Turing stated that computers will be really intelligent if we can no longer distinguish their performance from that of human beings.

[109] Descartes uses "montre," which may be also translated as "watch."

[110] *Les Passions de l'Âme*, quoted from Descartes, 1953, p. 697.

[111] *Quatrièmes Réponses*, quoted from Descartes, 1953, p. 448.

[112] Van den Berg, 1973, p. 24.

[113] *Discours de la Méthode* (note 102), p. 166.

[114] *Les Passions de l'Âme* (note 110), pp. 710-711.

[115] Leibniz, 1695, quoted from 1969, p. 457.

[116] Jorink, 1999, pp. 51-61.

[117] Borelli, 1989.

[118] Borelli, 1989, p. 1.

[119] Ibid., p. 6.

[120] Ibid., pp. 7-8.

[121] Ibid., pp. 34-35.

[122] In the 18th century, Borelli was seen as the founding father of "Iatromechanics," or Iatrophysics, the opposing school of "Iatrochemistry" (inspired by the alchemy of Paracelsus, ±1493-1526). Note that muscular contraction as such was seen as a chemical process by Borelli.

[123] Borelli, 1989, p. 148.

[124] Ibid., p. 181.

[125] Ibid., p. 183.

[126] Ibid., p. 207.

[127] Although probably a coincidence, it is amusing to know that "In the 1930s, an analogy between keratin, the fibre-substance of hair, and myosin, the structural protein of skeletal muscle was suggested. This analogy was based on X-ray diffraction experiments with isolated films of both proteins, which were very similar. Contraction was thought to be produced by the breakdown or modification of certain cross-linkages" (Ridderikhoff, 1999).

[128] Ibid., pp. 210-211.

[129] Ibid., p. 214.

[130] Ibid., p. 219. Note that it is a common mistake to rule out all but one of the possibilities one can imagine, to then conclude that the remaining alternative must be true. Borelli is aware of the critique that "muscles when contracting do not increase in volume" (p. 237) but rejects this firmly: "The muscles actually swell and increase in volume. This is demonstrated by the hardness and obvious increase of the muscle of the heart" (p. 238).

[131] Ibid., p. 232. Note that Borelli writes "may" occur.

[132] Ibid., p. 233.

[133] Also Briggs, author of "Ophthalmographia" (1676), who corresponded with Newton, thought in terms of sneezing: "Similarly, in sneezing at the sight of the sun, the motion is initiated by the nerve by the very small addition of *more subtle matter;* so far as such sharp particles . . . penetrate the fibres like a sting" (translated from the Leyden manuscript, Ridderikhoff, 1999; italics in the original).

[134] Borelli, 1989, pp. 233-234.

[135] Ibid., p. 234. It is amusing to recognize the similarity between these speculations of Borelli's and Paul Weiss' theory, in 1928, that each alpha-motoneuron has an antenna to detect the pattern of electrical frequencies specifically meant for it (Weiss, 1928; cf. Bongaardt, 1996).

[136] Cf. note 115.

[137] Leibniz, 1969, p. 460. Note that in Leibniz's universe, coordination is God-given, but it is impossible to make things happen. The only place where Leibniz's dream was realized was in baroque music (Bach, Vivaldi). Surprisingly, in the second half of the 20th century, Sir John Eccles and Sir Karl Popper undertook to present a new case for dualism, Eccles to save moral responsibility and Popper to make sure that a Platonic "world of knowledge" really exists (Popper & Eccles, 1977).

[138] Logically, this has nothing to do with one's belief, or unbelief, in a soul (but historically, the soul was important). Logically, it is the conception of the world that matters here.

[139] To date, there are two alternatives. First, one may regard the mind as an "emergent" property of the underlying material organization (see the last section). In my opinion, this renders matter already less "passive and stupid" than in classical mechanicism, without, however, fully solving the problems. Second, one may assume that active and passive views are "complementary" (Bongaardt, 1996). Although logically impeccable, complementarity needs to be supplemented with something that makes it understandable how activity and passivity arose in the first place.

[140] For the style of such a frivolous suggestion, that the Arabs were good in alchemy because they liked sweets, I am indebted to Braudel, 1979.

[141] From the Arab *sharbat* (sweet lemonade). Adding snow may have started in Istanbul (brought in from Bursa). In 16th-century Spain, snow was traded everywhere (Braudel, 1966; González-Tascón, 1998). In a good restaurant, the pot with snow was on the table.

[142] Rios & March, 1993.

[143] Note 131. González-Tascón, 1998, shows that gunpowder, as Europe came to know it, was an Arabic invention.

[144] Harvey, 1976.

[145] Harvey, 1976, p. 3.

[146] Ibid., p. 75.

[147] In contrast to Newton, Harvey himself didn't like to perform alchemical experiments (Schouten, 1972, p. 68).

[148] Lindeboom & Van Lieburg, 1993. In the Dutch Republic, Descartes accepted the gist of Harvey's theory but saw the diastole as the phase of the expulsion of the blood (Jorink, 1999, p. 62).

[149] Harvey, 1976, p. 127.

[150] Harvey, 1959.

[151] Harvey, 1959, p. 51.

[152] Symbols (such as the delta) in this and similar quotes from Harvey are directly from his manuscript.

[153] Harvey, 1959, p. 35, pp. 109 & 127.

[154] Note 54.

[155] Harvey, 1959, pp. 143 & 145; italics added by the present author. It is relevant to note that Harvey wrote a separate book, *The Generation of Animals,* first published, anonymously, in 1653 (Harvey, 1981).

[156] Yates, 1964, p. 12.

[157] Hermes Trismegistos, 1975, p. 2.

[158] Yates, 1964, p. 46.

[159] In quotes from Newton's manuscripts, his own spelling is followed.

[160] Dobbs, 1975, p. 207.

[161] Harvey, 1959, pp. 145, 147, & 149. Note that this is not an alchemical quote per se. I have listed Harvey as an "alchemist" because he regarded matter as active and derived his most important metaphors from alchemy.

[162] Ibid., p. 151.

[163] Dobbs, 1975.

[164] For Newton, mercury (Mercurius, as in Hermes Trismegistos) is of a spiritual nature.

[165] An organ that falls off naturally when it has served its function.

[166] For Nicholas Flammel, see Dobbs, 1975 & Westfall, 1983.

[167] Westfall, 1983, pp. 299 & 308.

[168] Ibid., p. 302.

[169] As Harvey had tried to do; but with Newton the search for a synthesis between the two is much more outspoken. I label Newton as an "alchemist" because he derived his concept of a "mediator" (note 160) from alchemy.

[170] Turnbull, 1959, pp. 367-368; italics in the original.

[171] At the time, there were very good arguments that both "action" and "perception" depended on "spirits." Briggs (note 133) offered a beautiful "proof," which I quote from Ridderikhoff, 1999: "Is it not as if, after spinning the body (whether the eyes are open or closed) all things appear to be flung around us, and they are visible for a little while when the eyelids remain closed, even when this agitation of the body is not continued: this is because the animal spirits annex the motion (like the body-fluids), similar to water in a much rotated vessel, which completes the cycles subsequently, although the vessel is in rest."

[172] Turnbull, 1959, pp. 368-369.

[173] Westfall, 1983, p. 376.

[174] Ibid., pp. 402-468. My understanding of Newton's biography derives from Westfall, 1983.

[175] Ibid., p. 538. Most contemporary Englishmen did Newton the favor of remaining silent about this affair (ibid., p. 539). Locke had the unfortunate experience of suggesting a wrong solution. On September 16, 1893, Newton wrote to Locke: "S^r, Being of opinion that you endeavoured to embroil me wth woemen & by other means I was so much affected with it as that when one told me you were sickly & would not live I answered twere better if you were dead" (ibid., p. 534). Later, Newton would regret this letter very much, but never again would his friendship with Locke regain the intensity it had had before.

[176] Ibid., pp. 551-626.

[177] Newton, 1952.

[178] Newton, 1952, pp. 375-376, 378, & 397. I am indebted to Arne Ridderikhoff for drawing my attention to this Query.

[179] Ibid., pp. 353-354.

[180] Note 134.

[181] Westfall, 1983, p. 169.

[182] Huygens, 1932, pp. 183-187.

[183] Huygens, 1893, pp. 243-244. Huygens' clocks had a precision of about 10 seconds per day, so that the 5 seconds observed was less than normal. In a letter of March 6, Huygens suggested that the phenomenon was caused by small vibrations of the chairs (Huygens, 1932, p. 187).

[184] For example, Peper, 1995, p. 3.

[185] If I ask you twice as loud as before to get me a cup of coffee, you don't get me twice as much coffee: The relationship between the controller and the to-be-controlled is nonlinear.

[186] The definition of "complexity" that appeals most to me is that complex systems contain a simplified description of themselves (Pattee, 1973; Gell-Mann, 1994).

[187] Although the mathematical theory of dynamical systems (cf. Andronov & Chaikin, 1949) is deterministic, Haken's dynamically inspired "synergetics" is a stochastic form of physics (cf. Haken, 1977).

[188] Huygens, 1932, p. 187, gives several sources for later discussions of the "sympathy" between clocks. So far, I have not studied these.

[189] Of course, synchronization can also be understood linearly (as in the "vibrations" of Newton's ether, note 179). Still, linear modeling of synchronization would have forced Huygens to accept "sympathy" as a scientific notion. In the next paragraph, I describe why he couldn't.

[190] Kelso, 1995.

191 Huygens was aware that his pendular clocks would have a fixed frequency only if their amplitudes were small, ideally zero; that is, ideally when they did not move. He did not care (cf. the introduction, p. 2, of H.J.M. Bos to; Huygens, 1986).

192 Andriesse, 1993.

193 Andriesse, 1993, p. 148, citing Huygens.

194 Note 183.

195 Egmond, Jorink & Vermij, 1999.

196 Cf. Parker, 1996a, p. 20.

197 Jorink, 1999, p. 52.

198 Schouten, 1972.

199 Galileo, 1954/1638.

200 Which ended 80 years of war with Spain; cf. Bußmann & Schilling, 1998; Israel, 1998.

201 When in July 1853, the fleet of Admiral Perry steamed into Tokyo Bay, the Japanese sent Dutch interpreters to negotiate because they thought that all barbarians from the West spoke Dutch (for a gripping account, see Gray, 1996); up to that time, mechanical teaching in Japan was from Dutch textbooks. I take this amazing fact as evidence that the Dutch indeed have been engaged in exporting mechanicism.

202 Whenever experiments failed to work out properly, Huygens, in contrast to Newton, had a tendency to give up (Andriesse, 1993). Maybe it is typical of trading nations that one does not go too far in developing one's own theories.

203 I owe this example to Mark Latash.

204 Cf. Haken, 1977.

205 For the Glorious Revolution, see **http://www.lawsch.uga.edu/~glorious/index.html**.

206 Note that these events were far from glorious in the eyes of the Catholics.

207 Andriesse, 1993, p. 342; according to Andriesse, the date in the diary entry is hard to read.

208 Romein & Romein, 1971, p. 420.

209 Boyle and Newton were close friends (Westfall, 1983). Boyle attempted to fit alchemy into mechanical philosophy. In that sense, he was doing "chemistry" rather than alchemy.

210 Andriesse, 1993, pp. 343-344, quoting Huygens.

211 Pearson, 1978, p. 285.

212 Ibid., p. 283.

213 Bronowski, 1964, pp. 221-228. Note that the clockwork was now of a very different nature than in the time of Charles V: This was a clockwork with action at a distance.

214 Dobrée, 1961. I assume that these two lines were meant as an epitaph.

215 Gay, 1966.

216 De La Mettrie, 1912, p. 93.

217 Pearson, 1978, p. 656.

218 Meijer, Wagenaar & Blankendaal, 1988.

219 Bodleian Library, Oxford, Locke's Manuscripts, not dated, p. 111.

220 Cf. notes 210 & 212.

221 Boyle, 1663, quoted from Birch, 1772, volume 2, p. 69.

222 Ibid., p. 71.

223 Whytt may have stolen this idea from Borelli, who wrote that "for a short time after being beheaded and their heart excised, turtles can move and contract their muscles, frogs can jump and vipers crawl since the spirituous juices sent by the brain into the nerves so far and the remnants of blood in the pores of the muscle can carry out posthumous effervescence when the nerves are irritated by stinging, as previously they were shaken when stimulated not only in the brain, but even in their filaments" (1989, p. 239).

224 Whytt, 1768, p. 291.

225 Südhoff, 1922, p. 14.

226 French, 1969, p. 11.

[227] Pflüger, 1853, p. 17.

[228] Huxley, 1870.

[229] Huxley, 1870, p. 7.

[230] In 1874; cf. Huxley, 1893.

[231] Manning, 1871, p. 7; cf. note 66.

[232] Pflüger himself concluded that there must be soul in the spinal cord; but if the soul is everywhere, one may as well conclude that it is nowhere.

[233] Newton, in the letter to Oldenburg, where he discusses animal motion (note 170), quoted from Turnbull, 1959, p. 368.

[234] What he could not foresee is that the realms are now kept together through economics. In the days of Charles V, economic cooperation was poorly understood.

[235] Bernstein, 1935/1967 & 1946-1947/1996.

[236] Feigenberg & Meijer, 1999.

[237] Cf. note 227.

[238] Fukson, Berkinblit & Fel'dman, 1980.

[239] Fukson, Berkinblit & Fel'dman, 1980, p. 1261.

[240] Planck, 1910; cf. Bongaardt, 1996, p. 55.

[241] "To me, it appears as if an analogous difficulty offers itself in most problems of mental life" (Planck, 1910, p. 97, quoted from Bongaardt's translation, 1996, p. 55).

[242] Haken, 1977.

[243] Beek, 1989.

[244] Haken, 1996.

[245] Beek, 1989.

References

Andriesse, C.D. (1993). *Titan kan Niet Slapen: Een biografie van Christiaan Huygens* [Titan Cannot Sleep: A biography of Christian Huygens]. Amsterdam: Contact.

Andronov, A.A. & Chaikin, C.E. (1949). *Theory of Oscillations*. Princeton, NJ: Princeton University Press. (Original work published 1937)

Beek, P.J. (1989). *Juggling Dynamics*. Amsterdam: Free University Press. (PhD thesis)

Bernstein, N.A. (1967). The problem of interrelation of coordination and localization. In: N.A. Bernstein (Ed.), *The Co-ordination and Regulation of Movements* (pp. 15-59). Oxford: Pergamon Press. (Original publication 1935)

Bernstein, N.A. (1996). On dexterity and its development. In: M.L. Latash & M.T. Turvey (Eds.), *Dexterity and its Development* (pp. 3-244). Mahwah, NJ: Erlbaum. (Original manuscript written 1946-1947)

Birch, T. (1772). *The Works of the Honourable Robert Boyle*, 6 volumes. London: W. Johnston.

Bongaardt, R. (1996). *Shifting Focus: The Bernstein tradition in movement science*. Amsterdam: printed by the author. (PhD thesis)

Borelli, G.A. (1989). *On the Movement of Animals*. Berlin: Springer. (Original work published 1680-1681, translated from the Latin by P. Maquet)

Braudel, F. (1966). *La Méditerranée* [The Mediterranean Sea], 3 volumes. Paris: Librairie Armand Collin. (I used the Dutch 1991 edition.)

Braudel, F. (1979). *Civilisation Matérielle, Economie et Capitalisme: XVe-XVIIIe siècle* [Material Civilization, Economy, and Capitalism: 15th-18th century], 3 volumes. Paris: Armand Collin.

Braune, W. & Fischer, O. (1895-1904). Der Gang des Menschen [Human gait]. *Abhandlungen der Könichlich Sächsischen Gesellschaft der Wissenschaften, 21, 25, 26 & 28*, 6 volumes.

Bronowski, J. (1964). *The Ascent of Man*. London: BBC.

Bußmann, K. & Schilling, H. (Eds., 1998). *Krieg und Frieden in Europa* [War and Peace in Europe], 3 volumes. Published to the occasion of the exhibition under the same name in Osnabrück and Münster. Münster: Westfälisches Landesmuseum.

Clarke, E. & Dewhurst, K. (1972). *An Illustrated History of Brain Function*. Berkeley, CA: University of California Press.

Daremberg, C. (1856). *Oeuvres Anatomiques, Physiologiques et Médicales de Galien,* volume 2. Paris: Baillière.

De Guevara, A. (1986). *The Diall of Princes*. Amsterdam: Da Capro Press. (Original work published 1529, facsimile of the 1577 English translation)

De La Mettrie, J.O. (1912). *Man a Machine*. La Salle, IL: Open Court. (Original French publication 1748)

Descartes, R. (1953). *Oeuvres et Letters* [Works and Letters]. Paris: Galimard. (Original works from the first half of the 16th century, edited by A. Bridoux)

Dijksterhuis, E.J. (1980). *De Mechanisering van het Wereldbeeld* [The Mechanization of the World-View]. Amsterdam: Meulenhof.

Dobbs, B.J.T. (1975). *The Foundations of Newton's Alchemy: The hunting of the greene lyon*. Cambridge: Cambridge University Press.

Dobrée, B. (Ed., 1961). *Alexander Pope's Collected Poems*. London: Dent.

Egmond, F., Jorink, E. & Vermij, R. (Eds., 1999). *Kometen, Monsters en Muilezels: Het veranderende natuurbeeld en de natuurwetenschap in de zeventiende eeuw* [Comets, Monsters, and Mules: The changing world-view and science in the seventeenth century]. Haarlem, The Netherlands: Arcadia.

Erasmus, D. (1986). *The Education of a Christian Prince*. In: A.H.T. Levi (Ed.), *Collected Works of Erasmus,* volume 27 (pp. 199-288). Toronto: University of Toronto Press. (Original work published 1516, translated from the Latin by Neil M. Cheshire)

Eriksson, R. (1959). *Andreas Vesalius' First Public Anatomy at Bologna, 1540: An eyewitness report*. Uppsala: Almqvist & Wiksell.

Feigenberg, I.M. & Meijer, O.G. (1999). The active search for information: From reflexes to the model of the future. *Motor Control, 3,* 225-236.

Flesher, M.M. (1997). Repetitive order and the human walking apparatus: Prussian military science versus the Webers' locomotion research. *Annals of Science, 54,* 463-487.

French, R.K. (1969). *Robert Whytt, the Soul, and Medicine*. London: The Wellcome Institute for the History of Medicine.

Fukson, O.I., Berkinblit, M.B. & Fel'dman, A.G. (1980). The spinal frog takes into account the scheme of its body during the wiping reflex. *Science, 209,* 1261-1263.

Galileo, G. (1954). *Dialogues Concerning Two New Sciences*. New York: Dover. (Original work published 1638, translated by H. Crew & A. de Salvio)

García-Diego, J.A. (1986). *Juanelo Turriano Charles V's Clockmaker: The man and his legend*. Madrid: Editorial Castalia.

Gay, P. (1966). *The Enlightenment: An interpretation*. London: Wildwood House.

Gelfand, I.M. & Latash, M.L. (1998). On the problem of adequate language in motor control. *Motor Control, 2,* 306-313.

Gell-Mann, M. (1994). *The Quark and the Jaguar*. New York: Freeman.

González-Tascón, I. (1998). *Filipe II, Los Ingenios y las Machinas: Ingenería y obras publicas en la época de Filipe II* [Philip II, Technical Ingenuity and Machines: Engineering and public works in the era of Philip II]. Madrid: Sociedad Estatal para la Commemoración de los Centenarios de Filipe II y Carlos V.

Gray, A. (1996). *Tokyo Bay: A novel of Japan*. London: Pan Books.

Hackforth, R. (1972). *Plato's Phaedrus*. Cambridge: Cambridge University Press.

Haken, H. (1977). *Synergetics: An introduction*. Berlin: Springer.

Haken, H. (1996). *Principles of Brain Functioning: A synergetic approach to brain activity, behavior and cognition*. Berlin: Springer.

Harvey, W. (1959). *De Motu Locali Animalium* [On Animal Movement]. Cambridge: Cambridge University Press. (Original begun around 1627, translated from the Latin by G. Whitteridge)

Harvey, W. (1976). *An Anatomical Disputation Concerning the Movement of the Heart and Blood in Living Creatures*. Oxford: Blackwell. (Original work 1628, translated from the Latin by G. Whitteridge)

Harvey, W. (1981). *Disputations Touching the Generation of Animals*. Oxford: Blackwell. (Original work 1653, translated from the Latin by G. Whitteridge)

Hermes Trismegistos (1975). *The Divine Pimander and Other Writings*. New York: Samuel Weiser. (Translated from the Greek by J.D. Chambers)

Hill, D.R. (1974). *The Book of Knowledge of Ingenious Mechanical Devices by Ibn al-Razzaz al-Jazari.* Dordrecht: Reidel.

Huxley, T.H. (1870). Has a frog a soul; and of what nature is that soul, supposing it to exist? *Papers of the Metaphysical Society, 1 (for 1869-1874),* November 8, 1-7. (Manchester College Library, Oxford)

Huxley, T.H. (1893). On the hypothesis that animals are automata and its history. In: T.H. Huxley (Ed.), *Collected Essays,* volume 1 (pp. 315-320). London: Macmillan. (Original work published 1874)

Huygens, C. (1893). *Oeuvres Complètes de Christiaan Huygens,* volume 5. Den Haag, The Netherlands: M. Nijhoff.

Huygens, C. (1932). *L'Horologe à Pendule* [The Pendular Clock]. *Extrait des Oeuvres Complètes de Christiaan Huygens, Tome 17.* No city or publisher indicated. (Original work 1656-1666, edited by J.A. Volgraff)

Huygens, C. (1986). *The Pendular Clock or Geometrical Demonstrations Concerning the Motion of Pendula as Applied to Clocks.* Ames, IA: Iowa State University. (Original work published 1673, translated from the Latin by R.J. Blackwell)

Israel, J.I. (1998). *The Dutch Republic: Its rise, greatness and fall 1477-1806.* Oxford: Clarendon Press.

Jorink, E. (1999). *Wetenschap en Wereldbeeld in de Gouden Eeuw* [Science and World-View in the Golden Age]. Hilversum, The Netherlands: Verloren.

Kamen, H. (1997). *Philip of Spain.* New Haven, CT: Yale University Press.

Kelso, J.A.S. (1995). *Dynamic Patterns: The self-organization of brain and behavior.* Cambridge, MA: MIT Press.

Kugler, P.N. & Turvey, M.T. (1987). *Information, Natural Law, and the Self-Assembly of Rhythmic Movement.* Hillsdale, NJ: Erlbaum, p. 117.

Laudan, L. (1977). *Progress and its Problems: Towards a theory of scientific growth.* Berkeley, CA: University of California Press.

Leibniz, G.W. (1969). *Philosophical Papers and Letters.* Dordrecht: Reidel. (Original works 1666-1716, edited by L. Loemker)

Lindeboom, G.A. & Van Lieburg, M.J. (1993). *Inleiding tot de Geschiedenis der Geneeskunde* [Introduction to the History of Medicine]. Rotterdam: Erasmus.

Locke, J. (not dated). Manuscripts. (Bodleian Library, Oxford).

Lovejoy, A.O. (1973). *The Great Chain of Being.* Cambridge, MA: Harvard University Press.

Manning, H.E. (1871). What is the relation of the will to thought? *Papers of the Metaphysical Society, 1 (for 1869-1874),* January 11, pp. 1-13. (Manchester College Library, Oxford)

Meijer, O.G., Wagenaar, R.C. & Blankendaal, A.C.M. (1988). The hierarchy debate: Tema con variazioni. In: O.G. Meijer & K. Roth (Eds.), *Complex Movement Behavior: 'The' motor-action controversy* (pp. 489-561). Amsterdam: North-Holland.

Meijer, O.G., De Wolf, G.S. & Lamoth, C.J.C. (1999a). Bewegingscoördinatie: Relevantie voor oefentherapie-Mensendieck [Movement coordination: Relevance for exercise therapy Mensendieck]. *Nederlands Tijdschrift voor Oefentherapie-Mensendieck, 1999-1,* 32-40.

Meijer, O.G., De Wolf, G.S. & Lamoth, C.J.C. (1999b). Bewegingscoördinatie: Een kwestie van niveau [Movement coordination: A matter of level]. *Bewegen & Hulpverlening, 16,* 83-101.

Moore, P. (1973). *Watchers of the Stars.* New York: Putnam's.

Needham, J., Wang Ling & De Solla Price, D.J. (1960). *Heavenly Clockwork: The great astronomical clocks of medieval China.* Cambridge: Cambridge University Press.

Needham, J. & Wang Ling (1974). *Science and Civilisation in China,* volume 4, *Physics and Physical Technology, Part 2: Mechanical Engineering.* Cambridge: Cambridge University Press.

Newton, I. (1952). *Opticks.* New York: Dover. (Original work published 1704)

Parker, G. (1995). *The Army of Flanders and the Spanish Road, 1567-1659.* Cambridge: Cambridge University Press.

Parker, G. (1996a). *The Military Revolution: Military innovation and the rise of the west, 1500-1800.* Cambridge: Cambridge University Press.

Parker, G. (1996b). *Philip II.* Chicago: Open Court.

Parker, G. (1998). *The Grand Strategy of Philip II.* New Haven, CT: Yale University Press.

Parker, G. (1999). The political world of Charles V. In: H. Soly (Ed.), *De Wereld van Karel V* [The World of Charles V] (pp. 113-225, 513-516). Antwerp: Mercator.

Pattee, H.H. (1973). *Hierarchy Theory: The challenge of complex systems.* New York: George Braziller.

Pearson, E.S. (1978). *The History of Statistics in the 17th and 18th Centuries: Against the changing background of intellectual, scientific and religious thought.* London: Charles Griffin.

Peck, A.L. & Foster, E.S. (Trans., 1965). *Aristotle: Parts of Animals, Movement of Animals, Progression of Animals.* Cambridge, MA: Harvard University Press.

Peper, E. (1995). *Tapping Dynamics.* Amsterdam: CopyPrint 2000. (PhD thesis)

Pflüger, E.F.W. (1853). *Die sensorischen Funktionen des Rückenmarks der Wirbelthiere nebst einer neuen Lehre der die Leitungsgezetze der Reflexionen* [The Sensory Functions of the Spinal Cord of Vertebrates, With a New Theory of the Connection Laws of Reflexes]. Berlin: August Hirschwald.

Planck, M. (1910). *Acht Vorlesungen über theoretische Physik* [Eight Lectures on Theoretical Physics]. Leipzig: Hirzel.

Popper, K.R. & Eccles, J.C. (1977). *The Self and Its Brain: An argument for interactionism.* Berlin: Springer.

Ramón-Nieto, J. (1998). Mateo de Vangorla: Maniquí anatómico para práctica de vendajes [Mateo Vangorla: Anatomical model to learn bandaging]. In: L. Ribot (Ed.), *Filipe II, Un Monarca y su Época: Los tierras y los hombres del rey* (p. 296). Madrid: Sociedad Estatal para la Commemoración de los Centenarios de Filipe II y Carlos V.

Ridderikhoff, A. (1999). Newton's Problem: Perspectives on skeletal muscle. Amsterdam: Faculty of Human Movement Sciences. (Master's thesis)

Rios, A. & March, L. (1993). *De Spaanse Kookkunst* [The Heritage of Spanish Cooking]. Amsterdam: De Lantaarn.

Romein, J. & Romein, A. (1971). *Erflaters van Onze Beschaving: Nederlandse gestalten uit zes eeuwen* [The Ones Who Made Us Inherit Our Civilization: Dutch personalities from six centuries]. Amsterdam: Querido.

Schouten, J. (1972). *Johannes Walaeus.* Assen, The Netherlands: Van Gorcum.

Südhoff, K. (1922). *Albrecht Haller: Von den empfindlichen und reizbaren Teilen des menschlichen Körpers* [On the Sensitive and Irritable Parts of the Human Body]. Leipzig: Barth. (Original publication 1753)

Szentágothai, J. (1968). *Andreas Vesalius Bruxellensis: De humani corporis fabrica.* Budapest: Helikon.

Tellmadge May, M. (1968). *Galen: On the usefulness of the parts of the body,* 2 volumes. Ithaca, NY: Cornell University Press.

Turnbull, H.W. (1959). *The Correspondence of Isaac Newton,* volume 1. Cambridge: Cambridge University Press.

Van den Berg, J.H. (1973). *De Reflex* [The Reflex]. Nijkerk, The Netherlands: Callenbach.

Van Puyvelde, L. (1973). *Les Primitifs Flamands* [The Flemish Primitives]. Brussels: Meddens.

Verworn, M. (1907). *Physiologisches Praktikum für Mediziner.* Jena: Gustav Fischer, p. 198.

Vesalius, A. (1543). *De Humani Corporis Fabrica* [On the Construction of the Human Body]. Basel: Oporinus.

Weiss, P.A. (1928). Eine neue Theorie der Nervenfunktion: Nicht durch gesonderte Bahnen, sondern durch spezifische Formen der Erregung schaltet das Nervensystem mit den Muskeln [A new theory of nerve function: It is not through separate connections but through specific stimulation patterns that the nervous system connects with the muscles]. *Naturwissenschaften, 16,* 626-636.

Westfall, R.S. (1983). *Never at Rest: A biography of Isaac Newton.* Cambridge: Cambridge University Press.

Whytt, R. (1768). *The Works of Robert Whytt.* Edinburgh: Balfour, Auld, and Smellie. (Edited by his son)

Wickersheimer, E. (1926). *Anatomies de Mondino dei Luzzi et de Guido de Vigevano.* Paris: Droz, page not numbered.

Williams, M. (1996). *The History of Spain: The bold and dramatic history of Europe's most fascinating country.* Fuengirola, Spain: Ediciones Santana.

Yates, F.A. (1964). *Giordano Bruno and the Hermetic Tradition.* London: Routledge and Kegan Paul.

Yates, F.A. (1975). *Astraea: The Imperial Theme in the Sixteenth Century.* Harmondsworth, England: Penguin.

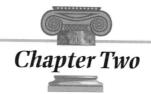
How Bernstein Conquered Movement

R. Bongaardt
Norwegian University of Science and Technology

Revisiting the work of Nikolai Aleksandrovitsch Bernstein

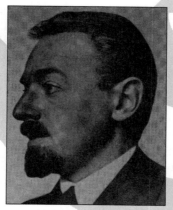

Nikolai A. Bernstein

Bernstein's paper titled "The Problem of Interrelations Between Coordination and Localization" presents a research approach that does justice to the complex characteristics of the human movement system, such as its high degree of integration and nonlinear interactions. Bernstein skillfully maneuvers the reader through the mechanistic views on movement that he aims to overthrow, the reasons behind this effort, and the issues in a new, more dynamic research program for the study of human movement. Bernstein's insights are resourceful and ingenious; his paper, however, is dense and complex.

For the sake of overview, the present introduction sketches the insights that Bernstein included in his 1935 article with reference to the leading Soviet research schools that he was affiliated with and that thus influenced his thinking. Subsequently, the aim is to show how Bernstein molded these insights into an innovative, coherent research program that is still relevant to movement science today.

Context

Nikolai Aleksandrovitsch Bernstein (1896-1966) started his research on human movement in the Soviet Union in the early 1920s, just after the Bolshevik Revolution and the Civil War. At that time the Soviet Union's economy was in turmoil, and many scientists were assigned research tasks aiming for the improvement of the country's industrial output. Bernstein eagerly took up the study of industrial labor movements. He had a laboratory in the Central Labor Institute in Moscow, run by A. Gastev, who aspired to study and train industry laborers as if they were mechanical devices. Contributing to Gastev's mechanistic approach, Bernstein built a film camera, the kymocyclograph, which measured the positions and velocities of moving body segments to a high degree of precision. Profiting from his engineer's eye for detail and his studies in mathematics, Bernstein could determine exactly the kinetic properties of, for example, hammering and filing; and he successfully inferred suggestions for the improvement of the labor process. All the while, however, he also nourished an interest in more fundamental, scientific questions about the organization of human movement.

In the 1920s, while working for Gastev, Bernstein was also affiliated with the Moscow Institute of Psychology. Within the so-called reactology research program of the institute leader, K.N. Kornilov, he studied how movement performance changes in reaction to different (sequences of) tasks. Kornilov's idea was that movement performance could offer a window onto the functioning of the nervous system—the heuristic being that sequences of nervous impulses could be inferred from movement trajectories, via positions and velocities, to accelerations and muscle torques and thus to muscle contractions and ultimately the nervous impulse. Bernstein brought to the Institute of Psychology his detailed knowledge of the kinetics of labor movements. He had learned that movement trajectories or muscle forces do not, in any direct manner, reveal the sequence of nervous impulses. Bernstein realized that the fact that there is an equivocal relation between nervous impulses and movement performance demanded a more sophisticated, nonmechanistic heuristic for the study of the organization of movement.

Many of Bernstein's young colleagues at the Institute of Psychology were emphatically nonmechanistic in their studies of mental behavior. Among them was L.S. Vygotsky, who translated classical books from the Gestalt psychology school, which offered tools for describing overall patterns of mental behavior such as the recognition of problem situations and transfer of problem-solving strategies as a whole. With these tools, Gestalt psychologists had challenged ideas such as that the brain solves problems through step-by-step, associative reasoning. For Bernstein the analogy must have been evident: Movements are not simply sequences of muscle contractions that elicit each other, one after the other, but are constructed as wholes. He argued that these wholes in movement are to be understood in terms of coordination. A useful tool to capture wholes was topology, the kind of geometry that studies the properties of patterns and shapes that are invariant even when lengths, angles, or surfaces change. The idea was that movements with the same topological pattern reveal the same neurophysiological organization of coordination, with respect to both the interplay of nervous impulses and their points of origin, that is, their localization in the brain. Thus Bernstein refined the heuristic for inferring brain organization from observable movements, to what he would come to call the principle of "lines of equal simplicity" (discussed further on).

Creating a new theoretical synthesis, Bernstein did not just jump on any bandwagon that passed by. He was a meticulous researcher, carefully teasing out all the empirical and theoretical ingredients of an answer to a new problem. In his translated works, we see the first signs of Bernstein's awareness of the coordinational patterns of movement in a 1929 article on piano playing, in which he notes that the composition of the arm changes qualitatively with movement frequency (Bernstein & Popova, 1929). But it was not until the mid-1930s that he published the full experimental results—the studies concerned human locomotion, ranging from infant development to military gait, and showed that locomotion instantiates a highly integrated pattern of sensory and motor impulses (Joravsky, 1989; cf. Bernstein, 1936). Thus, in understanding the movement system as Bernstein did, there was no place for the Pavlovian reflex-concept of arbitrary rigid associative links between sensory inputs and motor outputs, engrafted in the brain and functioning as building blocks to which all human behavior was reducible. Given coordination, Bernstein claimed, localization of movements in the brain must be distributed; the organization of movements is not simply decomposable but must be hierarchical; and the inherently changeable outcome of the movement must be liable to corrections through adequate sensory information. Bernstein thus completely disagreed with I.P. Pavlov's research approach and interpretations, and he must have been confident that Pavlov's *conditioned reflexes* would, in the end, make way for his *coordination* as the central concept in movement studies as well as in psychophysiology.

Bernstein often couched his critique of leaders and mainstream thinkers within mitigating formulations. There was good reason for his being politically and diplomatically careful: In 1931, Kornilov was fired as the director of the Institute of Psychology after he had fiercely attacked Pavlov. In 1938, the Central Labor Institute would be closed and its leader Gastev killed. Amid this terror, through which political ideology was being forced onto scientific methodology and which lasted 20 years from 1930 onward, Bernstein came to present his new theoretical and heuristic framework. It is that framework that is condensed in this chapter's classic paper on coordination and localization, published in 1935. In that same year, it was Pavlov's work, though, that received full attention: The 15th International Psychological Congress was held in honor of Pavlov. By that time Bernstein had written a book comparing Pavlov's views with his own. When Pavlov died, in 1936, Bernstein decided not to publish his book (Feigenberg & Latash, 1996). What the exact reason for this was, we can only speculate on—collegial respect, political expedience? Be as it may, from the late 1930s until 1947, Bernstein ran a movement laboratory in the same institute where Pavlov had been the leader for many years. It was not until after World War II that Bernstein infused his views into the mainstream of debates, now openly countering Pavlov's work. Perhaps by then he felt himself sheltered by the practical side of his research; its focus on optimizing labor conditions implied relative political neutrality (cf. Joravsky, 1989).

The Soviet leaders formally acclaimed the practical applicability of his work: Bernstein's 1947 book *On the Construction of Movements* was awarded the highest state prize for academic research. But not long after this triumph, the neo-Pavlovians, having gained hegemony within psychology and physiology, pointed to Bernstein's theoretical revolt against Pavlov, and they smashed his experimental research career (cf. Kozulin, 1984; Feigenberg & Latash, 1996). Despite his initial carefulness, Bernstein was fired; he did not return to the scientific stage until he was partially rehabilitated after Stalin's death in 1953.

Content

In the first section of Bernstein's 1935 paper, a mathematical analysis of the organization of movement serves to show that neither central control nor peripheral interaction alone can generate normal, nonpathological movement performance. Upon this mathematical deduction, Bernstein introduces the physiological concept of integrated circles of information flow within and between the center and the periphery of the movement system—exit the idea of a reflex arc and enter the idea of a reflex circle—more than a decade before Wiener introduced cybernetics (Anokhin, a critical Pavlovian, published a similar alternative in terms of "return afference" just after Pavlov's death; cf. Joravsky, 1989).

The complex organization of movements presents the researcher with the heuristic problem of how to decompose the system so that its organization is revealed, while its integrity is preserved. Bernstein's solution was to discriminate between the temporal and the spatial structure of both coordination and localization. An analysis of each of the four resulting categories of structure is presented in the article, although not all in equal depth: A description of movement performance in terms of summed oscillators serves to capture the temporal structure of coordination (not included in this abridged version of the paper). Analogous to the mathematical analysis in the beginning of the article is Bernstein's reflection on the intricate mix between the comb (top-down) and the chain (peripheral associations) types of implementing the timing of sequences of movements in the nervous system (for the origin of this argument, see Weiss, 1925/1959), that is, the temporal structure of localization. One finds a discussion of the nontopographical, spatially distributed localization of movements, that is, the spatial structure of localization. And, finally, Bernstein discusses the spatial structure of coordination in terms of topology, stressing the difference from Euclidean metrics.

These analyses may reveal how movements are structured and localized in the brain but not what the actual categories of movements are. Approaching this problem, Bernstein concludes the paper with a discussion of the "lines of equal simplicity" heuristic. The relative simplicity with which the structure of coordination is transferred from one movement to another may reveal the localized functional organization of this structure. For example, the text editor on which I write this introduction can just as easily underline words as it checks their spelling; would I now transfer to working on a typewriter, my typing performance would not change much (i.e., would be equally simple), but I would need to use a pen to underline and a dictionary to check spelling (i.e., not equally simple): Observable performance helps us to grasp, at least in part, the system that implements this performance. Therefore, Bernstein concluded that "every new discovery in the field of coordinational [spatial and temporal] structure will at the same time be a new discovery along the lines of localizational structure; and on the day that we understand the one we shall be able to say that we understand the other" (this volume, p. 83).

Relevance

The paper at hand was republished in 1967 in an English translation of papers spanning the last three decades of Bernstein's work. Bernstein himself selected these papers for publication in a book that could provide an overview of his work, both methodologically and theoretically. The book reveals that after his partial rehabilitation in 1953, Bernstein placed his early work on coordination within the larger framework of the "physiology of activity." With the term "activity" at the center of his research, he wanted to attack the problem of how movers choose and accordingly plan movements, thereby implementing the particular coordinational structure that solves the movement problem at hand. The term "physiology" makes clear that Bernstein wanted to formulate a naturalistic theory, grounded in the principles of complex organization that are to be found in nature itself rather than in merely abstract, logical-formal theory or metaphysics (cf. Bongaardt, 1996). Just as in the 1935 paper, this naturalistic approach implied those strands of mathematics and (neuro)physiology that could address the nonmechanistic, dynamic nature of the movement system.

In the West, Bernstein is often quoted for his ground-laying work on movement coordination qua observable performance (e.g., Turvey, 1990). Eastern European and Russian researchers often refer to him as a neuroscientist, stressing the relevance of planning action and taking the initiative (e.g., Feigenberg & Latash, 1996). The title of his classic 1935 paper tells us that for Bernstein, the two approaches were complementary: One cannot study neurophysiology without understanding the relevance of movement behavior, and vice versa (cf. Bongaardt & Meijer, 2000). It is exactly this integrated naturalistic approach that makes Bernstein a pioneer of movement science and a reformer of neuroscience at the same time.

The Problem of Interrelations Between Coordination and Localization

N.A. Bernstein[1]

1. The Basic Differential Equation of Movement

The relationship between movements and the innervational impulses that induce them is extremely complex and is, moreover, by no means unambiguous. The amount of muscle force is a function of both its innervational state E and of its length and velocity at a given time. In an intact organism, the length of a muscle is a function of the joint angle α. On the other hand, one may state that angular acceleration of a limb controlled by a given muscle is directly proportional to the muscle moment F and inversely proportional to the moment of inertia of the limb I.

If there are other forces acting on the segment, the situation becomes somewhat more complicated. Let us consider for simplicity only one external force, namely gravity. In the simplest case of movement of one segment with respect to another motionless segment, the moment due to gravity G is, like the muscle moment, a function of the joint angle. Hence, we get a relation of the following form:

$$I\frac{d^2\alpha}{dt^2} = F\left(E, \alpha, \frac{d\alpha}{dt}\right) + G(\alpha). \tag{1}$$

This is the fundamental equation for the movement of a single segment in the field of gravity under the action of a single muscle activated to the level of innervation E. When a moving system consists of several links and one needs to consider the action of several muscles, equation 1 becomes extremely complex, not only quantitatively but also qualitatively, because mechanical interactions among muscles start to play a role and the moment of inertia becomes a variable. However, despite all the complications, the physiological part of the story does not change much, and the complexities are related to the mechanics and mathematics. So, we will consider only the simplest case of equation 1.

First of all, let us note that equation 1 directly points at a cyclical relation between the muscle moment F and the position of the limb α. The segment changes position under the action of the moment F, while the moment in turn changes because of the changes in joint angle α. Thus, we face a cyclical chain of cause and effect.

This chain would be ideally cyclical if the moment depended solely on α and $d\alpha/dt$, that is, if the movement were completely passive (for example, free fall of the arm). F also depends on the degree of excitation of the muscle E, which explicitly emerges from areas outside the circle we just described. Obviously, there are two possibilities: Either the degree of excitation E depends on α and $d\alpha/dt$ (fully or partially), or it is independent of them and is a function of only time t.

The choice between these two possibilities is clearly of a great physiological significance as will be clearly demonstrated in further sections of this paper. Now, I will only point at some of the consequences of each of the mentioned assumptions. If the degree of excitation E is a function of position and velocity, not of time, then equation 1 turns into a classic differential equation,

$$I\frac{d^2\alpha}{d^2t} = F\left[E\left(\alpha, \frac{d\alpha}{dt}\right), \alpha, \frac{d\alpha}{dt}\right] + G(\alpha), \tag{1a}$$

whose partial integrals depend only on initial conditions. In this case, a movement has to start if appropriate external initial conditions take place, and, once started, it has to proceed with the same precise regularity with which a string oscillates when displaced to a precisely predetermined initial position and then released. Obviously, this assumption does not correspond to physiological reality and effectively ignores the role of the central nervous system.

On the other hand, one may assume that the degree of excitation E is a magnitude which changes with time according to a certain law, depending exclusively on a sequence of impulses from the central nervous system without any relation to the local conditions within the system involving the moving limb. If, according to the first assumption, illustrated with an elastic oscillation of a string, the muscle can be compared to some sort of a string or a rubber band, then, according to the second assumption, it may be viewed as a solenoid which pulls in its core solely in relation to the current supplied by an external source. Changes of the current should be represented in the system of equation 1 as a function of time; in fact, whatever may be the real causes of these changes, the changes themselves are presented to system (1) in a completely finished and independent form. Equation 1 in this case turns into

$$I\frac{d^2\alpha}{d^2t} = F\left[E\,(t),\,\alpha,\,\frac{d\alpha}{dt}\right] + G(\alpha), \tag{1b}$$

which does not allow any definite solution.

It is important here to draw attention to the following. Despite the fact that the measure of excitation E, as assumed earlier, is independent of α and of $d\alpha/dt$, the muscle moment F still depends on them. Meanwhile, as mentioned above, the action of the moment, and consequently the entire course of a movement, will vary with the initial conditions, which in no way enter the expression for excitation E and, consequently, do not affect its time changes. Hence, the outcome of the interactions resulting from equation 1b cannot be foreseen or regulated in advance, because changes in excitation will be involved in the interplay of forces and dependencies which cannot alter the further course of these changes obeying an independent law. Movements constructed according to equation 1b will necessarily be ataxic.

So, we are forced to accept that muscle excitation E is a function of both time and position and velocity, and should be introduced into equation 1 as:

$$I\frac{d^2\alpha}{dt^2} = F\left[E\left(t,\,\alpha,\,\frac{d\alpha}{dt}\right),\,\alpha,\,\frac{d\alpha}{dt}\right] + G(\alpha). \tag{1c}$$

This purely analytical deduction of the functional form of muscle excitation yields a very straightforward physiological interpretation. The dependence of E on time, stemming from the absurdity of the alternative hypothesis (1a), is the cause of changes in excitation directly induced by the activity of the motor areas of the central nervous system. The dependence of the excitation on position of the segment α and its angular velocity dα/dt is the proprioceptive reflex well known to physiologists. Hence, both position and velocity have to influence changes in the measure of muscle excitation directly and independently; both these effects have been firmly established in physiological studies.

Thus, we have formulated, within the basic equation of movement, a superposition of two cyclical connections of different orders, possessing different topics. The first cyclical connection is the mutual interdependence between the position α and the moment F; its nature is purely mechanical as mentioned earlier. The second connection uses the first one as a foundation; it represents a similar interdependence between the position α (and also of the velocity) and the degree of excitation E; this connection is based on reflexes and is related to the activity of the central nervous system.

It is not hard to grasp the basic significance of the aforementioned conclusions. The traditional view, implicitly accepted and retained by many physiologists and clinicians, considers a skeletal link as an obedient element under the control of central impulses. Within this scheme, a central impulse *a* always produces movement *A*, while impulse *b* always produces movement *B*, which naturally leads to viewing the cortical motor area as a distribution panel with push-buttons. However, equation 1b indicates that one and the same impulse E(t) (which ignores the state of the periphery) can produce completely different effects because of an interplay of external forces and variations in the initial conditions. On the other hand, equation 1c shows that a particular motor effect is possible only if a central impulse E is very different under different conditions, being a function of the position and velocity of the limb and leading to different effects within the differential equation depending on initial conditions. Parodying the well known expression about nature, one may say *motus parendo vincitur* (movement is mastered by obedience).

One also needs to point out that external force field is not limited to the force of gravity G(α), and the force of gravity may not even enter the basic equation in such a simple form. Since gravity always affects the position and the velocity of a system which influence changes in E, one has to say that "parendo" of the central impulses is sometimes rather far fetched. The central impulses have to adapt to all the internal and external forces acting on and within the system, while forces that do not directly depend on E may frequently play a central role in the general balance of forces. In such cases (Fig. 1 [*figure 2.1 here*]), if a movement requires force changes in a joint shown by curve B while the resultant force of the external field is represented by curve A, the central nervous system needs to take care only of the residual C which may have no resemblance to the contours of curve

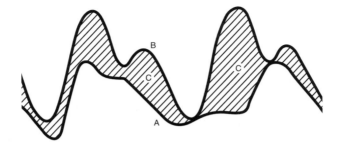

Figure 2.1
A semi-schematic representation of the course of a single central impulse during a rhythmical movement. A, the nonrhythmical curve of changes in external forces; B, the summed rhythmical result; C (hatched area), an impulse bridging the gap between the curve A and the result B.

B, commonly even less resemblance to this curve than changes in the external field A have. And so, it may be said that:

(a) There does not and cannot exist an unambiguous relation between impulses and movements;

(b) This relation is further from being unambiguous for more complex kinematic chains participating in the movement; and

(c) Movements are possible only under the condition of the most precise and continuous correspondence—*unpredictable in advance*—between the central impulses and peripheral events; frequently the peripheral events are quantitatively less dependent on the central impulses than on the external force field.

2. The Integrity and Structural Complexity of Live Movements

The integral unity of movement is the most important feature of what is implied by 'motor co-ordination'. This unity may be detected in very many experimental situations, and significant connections and correlation are observed among various components of the integrated processes. A muscle never participates in a movement as an isolated element. Neither the active increase in tension nor the associated (reciprocal) inhibition in antagonistic[2] subgroups is normally concentrated within a single anatomical muscular entity; rather, there is a gradual, smooth flow from one muscle system to others.

This integration is even more clearly demonstrated in the analysis of automatic rhythmical movements in the phenomenon of the very deep mutual interdependence of system components. Let me only mention the fact that, in rhythmical work with a hammer, the direction of the elbow trajectory (forward or to a side) shows a close correlation to such phenomena, seemingly remote from the elbow, as the relationship of the maximal velocities of the head of the hammer in the swing and striking movements, the angle of hammer inclination with respect to the horizontal during the swing, the relationship between the lengths of the trajectories of the hammer and of the wrist, and so on. A movement never reacts to a detail with a detail; it responds as a whole to changes in each and every minor factor, demonstrating most prominent changes in elements that are sometimes rather far, both spatially and temporally, from the initially changed detail.

While the external expression of coordinating activity leads to patterns of an extreme degree of unity and cooperation, on the other hand, its anatomical structure, according to our present knowledge, also displays a picture of equally highly organized complexity. An impulse in a centrifugal fiber of the last neuron reaching the endplate of a muscle is the resultant of a whole set of independent central impulses which reach the synapses of the anterior horn via different pathways. Centripetal proprioceptive impulses give rise to reactive effector impulses from the cerebellum and from many other structures connected to the spinal cord through the quadrigeminal system. Finally, the decisive role in the production of a movement must be assigned not to centrifugal but to central-processing impulses (an older physiologist would have termed them 'commissural-associative' impulses) travelling along the frontal ponto-cerebellar pathways. One could compile an extensive list of general characteristics of functional specificities of each of these anatomical formations (often the details given by different authors are contradictory); however, this is not my present objective. It is important to emphasize a specific feature, common to all these characteristics: The presence of a qualitatively specific action of each of the central subsystems on one and the same peripheral object.

If we try to reexamine the equation for elementary movements (1c) from this point of view, the following will necessarily follow. As close examination of peripheral processes shows, an innervational impulse E is not unambiguously related to its consequence—a movement—and, therefore, has to be perfectly coordinated with the proprioceptive input reflecting α and $d\alpha/dt$. This impulse is, at the same time, the sum (or another resultant functional form) of a series of impulses that have very different local areas of origin in the brain. Each of the impulse components emerges in a separate nucleus of the brain organized differently from other brain centers. Each nucleus has its particular relationships with other brain centers, its own organization of conducting pathways, a particular degree of proximity and type of connections to the receptors, and, finally, as neurological clinical practice shows, its own manner of action in time and particular means of interaction.

My goal in the first two sections of this paper has been merely to indicate the great difficulties which confront attempts at functional explanation of movement coordination. Already equation 1c is quite different from usual, qualitatively simple ideas of center-periphery interactions. When, however, we are forced to confront their complex interactions resulting from the coordinated activity of an entire system of organs which possess varying degrees of independence, both anatomically and clinically, the resulting overwhelming structural complexity becomes even more striking. This is already fruitful, since a failure to realize the difficulty of a problem frequently defers its solution.

3. The Interrelationship Between Coordination and Localization

The discussion in the preceding sections has already revealed, to a certain degree, the close connection between problems of coordination and localization.

The term coordination itself hints at a common action of separate elements. The subject of the problem of coordination is not in an analysis of the sound and expressive resources of a single instrument in an orchestra but in the technical construction of the score and in the skill of the conductor. Therefore, the main, leading thesis for investigation of coordination must be formulated in the following way. Coordination is an activity which provides a movement with the described earlier homogeneous integration and structural unity. This activity is based not on particular features of processes in individual neurons, but on a certain organization of their common activity. This organization has to be reflected in the anatomy, as a certain localization.

This seems to me an extremely heuristically expedient way of formulating the question. On the one hand, the organization and its forms have to be represented in localized structural forms. Similarly to how one may derive an idea on the function of an electrical circuit from an examination of its diagram, data on localization and anatomy may serve at least as sources of supporting evidence for the analysis of new experimental problems I have put forward—the structural physiology of movement. On the other hand, structural analyses of movements should be equally helpful for critical evaluation of existing and future concepts regarding the type and structure of cerebral localization. It is impossible to imagine a situation when a localizational structure is found to contradict a corresponding organizational structure.

An important point should be made. In no way should one confuse localization with topography. Topography is the geography of the brain, a study of the spatial distribution of its functionally significant points. Localization is a structural plan of anatomical connections among these functional points. If we shuffle in Fig. 2 {17 in 1967} [*figure 2.2 here*] the positions of the centers A, B, C, D, and E, this will change the entire topographical picture, but will not alter the localizational structure. The

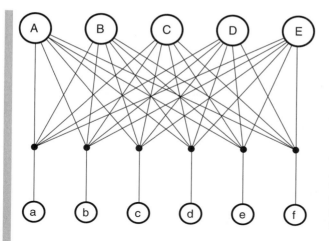

Figure 2.2
The multiplicity of efferent pathways for the control of six muscles a, b, c, d, e, f by five effector centres A, B, C, D, E gives, even in this intentionally simplified case, a complex structural scheme of innervation.

distribution (topography) of the elements in a diagram of a radio receiver is completely different from the topography of these elements in an actual radio set built based on this diagram. And vice versa, for one and the same topography completely different schemes are possible.

Thus, within the problem of localization, we care not about where precisely in the cortex one or another peripheral object or function is reflected, but what exactly and how exactly is represented, and what are the distinguishing characteristics of those objects represented in the cortical hemispheres and in subcortical nuclei. Problems of topography are likely to be largely irrelevant for analysis of the coordinational structure of movements, while the problems of localization are of paramount and principal significance.

This significance may be very well explained using the example of the old concept of localization which has already been mentioned in section 1. Such a concept would have all the rights to exist if every single central impulse unconditionally induced a particular single movement, that is, if there existed a one-to-one correspondence between impulses and movements. In this case, effector impulses would be able to proceed as a pure function of time E(t), always producing one and the same effect independently of what occurs in the periphery. Then, a push-button switchboard model of the cortex, similar in design to an organ keyboard, would be the first to come to mind. However, on the contrary, there is no one-to-one correspondence, and the cerebral motor area executes a planned movement by assuring a precise, flexible balancing among the resultant external forces and inertial events, constantly reacting to proprioceptive signals and simultaneously integrating impulses from separate central subsystems, so that ten repetitions of the same movement require ten different sequences of impulses. I would like to recall here the failure in

1923 of the inventors of "the symphony of whistles". Attempts at converting steam whistles into musical instruments with an organ keyboard failed because any given whistle did not agree to produce the same sound on every occasion, and its pitch depended on the steam pressure, on the number of whistles sounding simultaneously, on the degree of opening of the steam tube, etc., so that it was impossible to obtain a one-to-one correspondence between the pressed key and the tone pitch.

Clearly, a statement of complexity or "impracticality", from our point of view, is not a decisive argument for accepting or rejecting a physiological hypothesis. The decisive argument against the theory of direct representation of muscular systems in the cortex comes from a very different, perhaps unexpected, direction. I will present this argument in its most general formulation later; here, I will only use one of its particular versions that fits best the analyzed problem.

Assume that cortical cells of the central gyrus are actually the effector centers for the muscles. Let us take into account that the activity of these cells must be (this is inevitable within the hypothesis) flexibly different from one case to another during repetitions of a movement, depending on changes in the external force field and proprioceptive signals. If we imagine, for clarity, that each excited cortical effector cell lights up like an electric bulb at the moment when its impulse is sent to the periphery, then each movement would be visible on the cortical surface as a zigzag lightning. The absence of a one-to-one correspondence and all the considerations discussed earlier as consequences of equation 1c would obviously lead to different zigzag light-ups during repetitions of a given movement. Now suppose that this movement is an automated act, a realization of motor skill, in other words, a conditioned motor reflex. The aforementioned arguments lead to an unavoidable conclusion that the conditioned motor reflex each time operates via a new zigzag, using different cells; in other words, we arrive at a conclusion that accepting the hypothesis on cellular localization of muscles necessarily leads to rejecting cellular localization of conditioned reflexes. One of the two chess pieces must be sacrificed, and it is very unclear which of the two the old-fashioned localizationalist would rather forfeit.

I do not plan to overthrow the old localizational concept by a single blow, but one should not be silent about the fact that it has already been very seriously marred. It is worth recalling that, after the rejection of phrenology, the idea of localization also appeared for a long time to be seriously compromised, until it gradually became apparent that it was not necessary to throw the baby away with the dirty bath water. Now, after the emergence and establishment of the theory of conditioned reflexes, to deny the structural, anatomically engraved specificity of the brain would be equivalent to declaring it absolutely beyond human understanding.

Our present experimental goal is to find correct formulation for categories that may actually be represented in brain centers. The key to the search for genuine categories should apparently be in structural analysis of both the receptor side, as it is reflected in experiments with conditioned reflexes, and the effector side, as it is reflected in the coordination of movements.

4. Ecphoria of Movement Engrams

So far, I have considered only phenomena pointing at the instantaneous, extensive structure of motor coordination. It was important to demonstrate that a movement could not be understood as a consequence of a modification of a single impulse, but that it is the result of the simultaneous cooperative functioning of a whole system of impulses; note that the structure of this system—its structural schema—is important for the understanding of the result. There remains only a single step from this position to the central argument of the paper that the innervational and localizational structure is in fact not only non-contradictory to the observable structure of movements of the organism, but has to be an exact reflection of the latter. To move further, we need to address another characteristic of the phenomenon, that is, its changes in time. It is necessary to find out experimentally whether a series of system-related impulses simply coexist in time or there is also a structural interdependence along the time coordinate similar to that described earlier for every separate instant of time.

First, let us consider the aforementioned fact of movement concordance, i.e., its unity and the interrelation among its parts in space and in time. The established representation of a rhythmical movement in the form of a three or four term trigonometric series proves beyond doubt that this concordance exists in time as well; moreover, the origin of the concordance is indeed peripheral or mechanical but originates within the central nervous system. This proves that the central nervous system contains exact formulae of movements (*Bewegungsformeln*) or their engrams, and that, in some brain structure, these formulae or engrams represent the whole movement in its entire course in time. We can therefore claim that, at the moment of movement initiation, there is already, in the central nervous system, a whole set of engrams necessary for the movement to be carried on to its completion. The existence of such engrams is proved by the very fact of the existence of motor skills and of automated movements.

Now, we face a problem regarding structure. Let a given coordinated movement correspond to "N" engrams in the brain. Movement coordination is assured by a successive ecphoria of the engrams, in a certain sequence and with a certain tempo and rhythm. All these N engrams exist in the central nervous system at any given time as long as a motor skill exists; however, they exist in a hidden, latent form. How can one explain that firstly, they do not all undergo ecphoria simultaneously, but in a sequence;

secondly, the order of their ecphoria is not mixed up; and thirdly, their ecphorias are characterized by certain time intervals (tempo) and quantitative relationships among these intervals (rhythm)?

There are two basic possibilities, two "temporal structures": (a) each ecphoria of an engram (or perhaps a proprioceptive signal of its effect at the periphery) serves as an ecphorator for the next engram; or (b) the mechanism for ecphoria, the ecphorator, is beyond engrams and controls their order as in *Überordnung*. The former hypothesis may be termed the "chain" hypothesis, while the latter one—the "comb" hypothesis (Fig. 3 [*figure 2.3 here*]).

Both hypotheses may be supported by strong arguments. The chain hypothesis emphasizes proprioception, and hence, it can satisfactorily explain maintenance of the tempo and rhythm considering them as reflections of peripheral events. Since this hypothesis views the emergence of each successive ecphoria as a consequence of the preceding one, it is possible to explain both the maintenance of an order of a sequence of engrams and the impossibility of gaps within a succession of ecphoria. Finally, it is attractive because of its simplicity and by the lack of necessity to postulate an additional ecphorator.

The arguments in favor of the comb hypothesis are also rather impressive. The presence in the CNS of "a movement plan", and the concordance of its formula and of the movement itself, from the beginning to the end, do not fit well the hypothesis on a fractionated sequence of movement elements, linked among each other only by events at the periphery. The latter view does not present a guiding principle unifying the elements. Further, if we recall the facts discussed earlier, indicating that central impulses only generate additions to the external force field so that a time pattern of central impulses may have very little in common with the movement pattern, the comb hypothesis gets new, important support. The possibility of generating

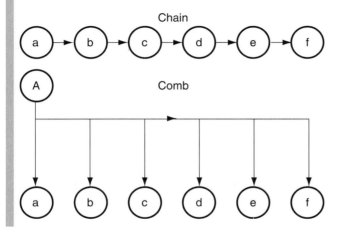

Figure 2.3
Two theoretically possible schemes for successive ecphoria of motor engrams a, b, c, d, e, and f.

a concordant, regular resultant B during movement repetitions requires the existence, within the CNS, of a guiding engram which controls the entire law of the sequence B (see figure 1 [*figure 2.1 here*]). If such a guiding engram exists (we may refer to it as the motor image of a movement), it must be dual: It must contain within itself a united, simultaneously existing entire scheme of the movement time process, like an embryo in an egg or a gramophone record. It must also guarantee the order and the rhythm within a realization of this scheme; in other words, the gramophone record must have some sort of motor to turn it. To pursue this metaphor, what I have called the gramophone record is the directing engram, and what I have compared to a gramophone motor is the ecphorator.[3]

Both these hypotheses are compatible with the structure of the peripheral impulse as reflected by equation 1c, that is, with its dependence of the form $E(t, \alpha, d\alpha/dt)$, but they interpret this dependence differently. Within the chain hypothesis, the critical agents which determine the development of the process are the dependencies of E on α and $d\alpha/dt$, that is, its proprioceptive relationships, while the relation to time, t, is determined only by the tempo and by the activity of each individual element within the chain a, b, c (Fig. 3 [*figure 2.3 here*]). According to the comb hypothesis, the dominant relation is $E(t)$, that is, the independent initiative and the regulating activity of the CNS, while proprioceptive effects provide only corrections to the general whole.

Let us not forget that the hypothesized necessity of an ecphorator mechanism distinct from engrams themselves and, in a sense, dominating over them, is not only related to the comb hypothesis but is equally necessary for both hypotheses. Whatever the regulating engram within the comb hypothesis and elementary engrams a, b, c, . . . , within the chain hypothesis are, they have to contain, in a latent form, the whole movement process during a certain time interval. In other words, they have to assure a dependence of impulse E not only on α and $d\alpha/dt$ but also on t. It makes no difference whether the central mechanism of tempo—the "gramophone motor"—is related in its action to the duration of physico-chemical intracellular reactions or to some other physiological rhythms;[4] it has to exist as a function different from the contents of engrams, because the latter do not contain real time. Further studies will provide support in favor of one of the hypotheses, or maybe in favor of a more complex synthesis incorporating them both. Presently, it is important to emphasize the principal elements, contained in the formulation of the problem itself.

A motor image of a movement (addressed by neurologists as "movement program", *Bewegungsformel, Bewegungsgestalt,* and so forth) must necessarily exist in the CNS in the form of an engram. Such a guiding engram exists not only within the comb hypothesis; indeed, the very fact of successive, established connections among elementary engrams a, b, c, d, e, . . . , within the chain hypothesis is also an engram, drawn as a set of arrows rather than as a circle. This is an engram that determines the law of a succession of ecphoria and, consequently, controls it. This motor image corresponds to the actual movement pattern, that is to curve B in Fig. 1 [*figure 2.1 here*], and in no way to curve C; indeed, its presence makes it possible to adjust the course of impulse C so that a planned performance of a motor skill B is achieved. Therefore, a supreme central organ has to contain an exact representation of what will later occur at the periphery; meanwhile, activity in intermediate operational stages leads to the formation and realization of impulse C, which, as argued earlier, is different from the peripheral effect, and therefore, must also be different from the contents of the guiding engram. Metaphorically speaking, an order issued by a higher center is encoded before transmission to the periphery so that it is completely unrecognizable and, later, is automatically deciphered. In section 3, I have said that the possibility of a motor skill and of a stable conditioned motor reflex requires its unitary localization in central areas, and that such a unity cannot coexist with the theory of muscle representation in higher cortical centers. This thesis is once again confirmed by the previous discussion, now based on considerations of movement time structure; a CNS level which participates in the formation of the centrifugal impulse C and, consequently, where we might expect to find a representation of the muscle system, is not the supreme level of the CNS, and even not the level where elementary engrams a, b, c, . . . , etc. within the comb hypothesis are located. There must be an encoding process, between the comb level and the level of muscle representations, which transforms a motor image into form C. In terms of our equations, this encoding process represents a transformation of the relationship $E(t)$, which dominates in its pure form at the higher level, into a complete dependence of the form $E(t, \alpha, d\alpha/dt)$; that is, a transformation of the impulse based on proprioception.[5]

Thus, the analysis of movement time pattern once again leads us to recognize the structural complexity of a motor act which is represented in terms of localization. The recognition of obligatory existence of a guiding engram and a mechanism of ecphoria demands, by itself, that we postulate a series of hierarchical levels, each having a degree of qualitative independence.

5. Topology and Metrics of Movements: The Motor Field[6]

If we now turn from temporal to spatial movement characteristics, it becomes necessary to consider two factors: the distinction between the metric and topological properties of the psychophysiological space, and specific features of the motor field of the central nervous system.

In any geometrical representation, one should separate topology from metrics. I mean with topology of a geometrical object, the body of its qualitative features irrespective of its size, shape, the curvature of its border, etc. For example, a linear figure may be viewed as possessing such topological features as being open vs. closed, presence of line intersections as in a figure eight or their absence as in a circle, and so on. Besides these properties, which do not possess a quantitative characteristic, we may also consider as topological properties that involve a number, however without including a measure. Among these properties are, for example, having exactly four angles or being a member of the five-pointed star group, and so on. The latter group will be addressed as topological properties of first order, while the former group will be considered properties of zero order. All figures in the upper row in Fig. 4 [*figure 2.4 here*] belong to one and the same topological class of figures of the first order (being, however, very different in their metrics); they are indeed identical with respect to characteristic numbers. All of them have five angles or rays, all of them have five intersections between the lines, and so on. Pattern 6 in this illustration belongs to another first order class containing four angles and one intersection; however, it is in the same class of zero order as are the first five figures, since it is also a closed figure with intersecting lines. To illustrate properties of the first order with a familiar example, let me point out that every printed letter is a separate topological class of the first order, while the letter A class involves A's of all dimensions, fonts, outlines, ornaments, etc. (see 7-14 in Fig. 4 [*figure 2.4 here*]), if one ignores certain purely calligraphic features.

After this general introduction, we may move from geometry to psychophysiology. If we draw the attention of a psychologist or a teacher to our collection of letters A in Fig. 4 [*figure 2.4 here*], he will immediately say that the set displays a common essential characteristic, that is he will admit, without hesitation, that topological characteristics of a figure are of a higher psychologico-pedagogical importance than metric properties. The psychologist or teacher will be absolutely correct, because recognition of letter A does not require the presence of any metric properties and, on the

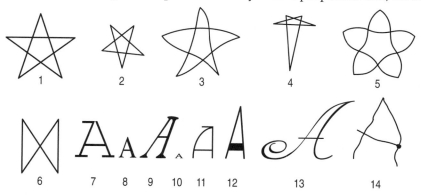

Figure 2.4
1-5, topological class of five-pointed stars; 6, topological class of figure eights with four angles; 7-14, topological class of letters A.

contrary, is entirely dependent on the presence of certain topological cues. This dominating affinity between the process of recognition and topology, which has for a long time been recognized and studied by adherents of Gestalt psychology, is certainly a psychophysiological or even a general biological phenomenon which cannot be deduced from purely geometrical considerations. The biologically specific predominance of topological categories over metric ones may be illustrated with numerous examples. A maple leaf differs from a birch leaf with respect to topological properties of the first order, while, at the same time, all maple leaves belong to one and the same topological class in spite of the thoroughly investigated biometric diversity among separate specimen. The structure of the brain and the location of the main cortical convolutions present another example of an object having the same topology in the presence of all possible metric variations. One may claim confidently that, in the area of biological morphology, cases in which metrics is of importance together with topology (for example, the lens of the eye) are rare exceptions.[7] This domination of topology in living objects may be contrasted with, for example, the morphology of crystals where the essential relationships are all metric.

Until now, insufficient attention has been paid to the fact that movements of living organisms are determined by topological categories to a not lesser degree than their perceptions. This is most clearly illustrated by drawing, perhaps because this type of movement leaves a record that may be conveniently studied. It is easy to draw a five-pointed star, but one can predict with certainty that such a drawing will display only topological but not metric relationships. To prove this, I suggest the reader to draw ten such stars and compare the pictures. I doubt if it is at all possible to draw a metrically perfect copy of such an object without the help of compasses and a ruler; that is, the human motor system seems not to possess any decent degree of metric proficiency, but it is very good in reproduction to topological characteristics of higher orders than first and zero. It is sufficient, for example, to consider handwriting. Earlier, I pointed out letters A belong to a single topological class of the first order no matter how or by whom they are written. However, all letters A written by me are similar to each other and are, at the same time, different from letters A written by other persons. The similarity between my A's is obviously not metrical but topological.

It is of an immense interest for structural analysis of movements that topological specificities of visual perception display both similarities to and significant differences from the topology of motor reproduction. For example, the category of dimension is equally unimportant with respect to visual perception and to movement. I can equally easily recognize a triangle, a star, or a letter independently of its size. It is equally easy for me to draw a star or write a large or a small word on a piece of paper or on a classroom blackboard. It would be interesting to study the quantitative relationship between the variance of these drawings and their size; however, it is safe to say that, for any size, they retain their topological properties not only of the first, but also of higher orders. For example, during writing on a blackboard, all the characteristics of the handwriting of a person on paper are preserved, although the entire muscular-articular structure of the movement is absolutely different in the two cases.

Such analogies and differences may be pursued to great lengths: Their study promises to be extremely fruitful. Within the present article, however, it is time to summarize all that has been said about the topological properties of perception and movements.

First of all, let me note that all the aforementioned facts and characteristics allow us to generalize the body of topological and metric characteristics of movements and their relations with external space under the term "motor field", analogous to the established concept of "visual field". An immediate task of movement physiology is to analyze properties of this motor field. All the discussed material allows us to state that the physiological motor field is as different from objective external space as the visual field is. Characteristic differences of the motor field from the geometrical space, as it is studied in analytical geometry, are, first of all, in the obvious preference of the motor field for topological categories as compared to metric ones; in the presence of apparent tropisms (importance of directions and unimportance of positions); and in the absence of right-left symmetry (inherent to the visual field). The dominance of topology over metrics is also revealed in the fact that straight lines and their differentiation from curved lines are not typical of the motor field (unlike the visual field). Furthermore, the motor field does not demonstrate stable, identical lines; in biomechanics, this is manifested in that successive cyclic movements never exactly repeat themselves (Fig. 5 [*figure 2.5 here*]). The system of coordinates of the motor field should be viewed as different from the Euclidian one in being, first, non-rectilinear, and second, as trembling like a cobweb in the wind. Its "oscillations", however, do not go so far as to destroy topological relationships either of zero order (for example, the "between" category), or of the first and, perhaps, even higher orders.

Some of the grasped properties of the motor field are of a definite importance for the theory of localization. First, there is the deeply rooted indifference of the motor

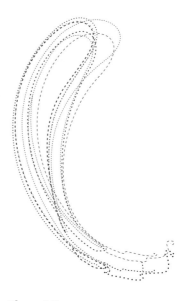

Figure 2.5
Cyclogram of a series of successive poorly automated movements taken on the same plate.

control towards the scale and location of a performed movement. It is obvious that each of the variations of a movement (for example, drawing a large or small circle, directly in front of oneself or to a side, on a horizontal piece of paper or on a vertical blackboard, etc.) demands a very different muscle formula; moreover, it may commonly involve a completely different set of recruited muscles. The almost equal ease and accuracy with which all these variations can be performed provide evidence that all the variations are ultimately determined by one and the same supreme controlling engram with respect to which engrams of dimension and position play secondary roles. Engrams that determine the muscle structure of each of the variations clearly emerge "lower", as described in section 4, in particular in area C of Fig. 1 [*figure 2.1 here*], whereas engrams of dimension and location belong to area B. Hence, we must conclude that the supreme engram, which may be called "the engram of the given topological class", is already structurally extremely remote (and, therefore, probably localizationally remote as well) from any direct relation to joint-muscle schemes; it is entirely geometrical and represents a very abstract motor image of space. This makes us think— for the time being merely as a hypothesis though it forces itself upon us very insistently—that the areas of localization of these supreme motor engrams possess the same topological regularity as the external space or the motor field do (at least, this regularity has nothing to do with the muscular-articular apparatus). In other words, there are good reasons to assume that in the higher motor centers of the brain (very probably in the cortex of their large hemispheres) one can find a localized reflection of a projection of the external space in a form in which the subject perceives the external space with motor means. This projection must be congruent with external space, but only topologically, not metrically. This viewpoint eliminates complexities related to the possibility of compensation for the inversion of retinal projections (section 3) and many other similar problems. It seems that, presently, it is impossible to specify how such a topological representation of space in the CNS may be achieved; however, I think that solving this problem is only a question of time for physiology. It is necessary to emphasize that topological properties of space projections in the CNS may prove to be rather weird and unexpected; one should not expect to find in the brain some sort of a photograph of space, even a very deformed one. Still, the hypothesis that higher CNS levels contain projections of space, not projections of joints and muscles, seems to me more probable than any other view.

6. The Principle of "Equal Simplicity"

It is now time to give a general formulation for a heuristic principle, whose particular case I have already discussed in section 3, and to examine its application to a few examples. I shall call it the *principle of equal simplicity*.

Let me begin with non-physiological examples. I have three devices which can be used to draw a circle: A circular template, compasses, and an ellipsograph. A circle of the same radius as the template may be drawn equally easily with the template and with the compasses; a circle may also be drawn with the ellipsograph, as it is a particular case of an ellipsis, but it will be slightly more complicated than with either the template or the compasses. If we need to draw a circle with another radius, the template immediately becomes useless. The compasses draw circles of all radii with equal ease. A given ellipsograph can only draw a circle with a single radius, and therefore, it is useless just as the template. If we wish to draw an ellipsis, the ellipsograph will require exactly the same effort as during circle drawing, while both the compasses and the template become useless.

In this example, we consider a set of curves of the second order which differ (a) in radius and (b) in eccentricity. One of our instruments, the template, gives us with great simplicity one curve and no others. The second instrument gives us equally easily all variations in radius, but only a single eccentricity, zero, typical of a circle. The third instrument gives us with equal ease (although, quantitatively, it is more complex as compared to the compasses) all eccentricities, but only one radius. A circle of the same radius as the template may be drawn with all three instruments, but the functional relationships between their simplicity and possible variations of the task are quite different for the three tools. The type of this functional relationship is determined by the design of the instrument.

From here, we get to the following formulation of the "principle of equal simplicity": For every structural scheme, which can perform numerous different elementary processes belonging to a certain variety, the lines of equal simplicity correspond to directions within the variety such that motion along these lines changes neither structural nor operational principles of the system. The vague notion of "simplicity" can be substituted with a whole set of similar notions related to particular cases: The notions of speed of performance, degree of accuracy, degree of variance, and so on. For the general formulation, I have selected the notion of simplicity because of its generality and the lack of concrete associations.

The heuristic importance of the principle is clear from the earlier discussion. If we are dealing with a system, whose structure is unknown to us, but whose functioning may be observed under a variety of conditions, then by comparing changes in a variable S (e.g., speed, accuracy, variation, etc.) as a function of each variable describing the conditions, we may draw conclusions related to the system structure which cannot be directly observed.

Imagine, for example, that we watch a movie without having any idea of how cinematography works. We may assume that we are in a puppet show theater (as our great-grandfather might well do). We are astonished by the breadth and variety of the show, which exceeds by far what puppets could do in those days, but we still have the indisputable right to consider what we see on the screen as a greatly improved marionette show. It is true that in a puppet show theater we have never, for example, seen the sea; well (says the great-grandfather), obviously they have invented a very sophisticated mechanical imitation of the sea. In the old puppet show theater, figures could not be made to decrease in size as they moved away, as it happens in the cinema; however, once again, this can also be viewed as a modern achievement of the technology of the marionette theater. All this may be difficult but possible. It is, however, very easy to prove that we are not in a puppet show theater, and to do so exactly with the help of the principle of equal simplicity. It is sufficient, for this purpose, to pick two objects that are very different in their difficulty of representation in the puppet show theater, for example, a rotating wheel and a stormy sea, and then, without asking the movie mechanic (remember that the technical part is inaccessible to us), to turn to the studio's accountant and ask how much it would cost to obtain one-minute representations of these objects on the screen. As soon as we discover that shooting a 20-m piece of film costs about the same for either object (or, to put it more accurately, that the cost of the film is related to some other factors but not to the mechanical properties of objects on the screen), the hypothesis of a puppet show theater collapses.

Everything possible for the cinematography is also possible for the puppet show theater (at least potentially). However, this "everything" is, in principle, unattainable with the same degree of simplicity as seen in the cinema. The described principle promises to be very fruitful in applications to the structural analysis of both receptor and effector functions of the central nervous system. If a circle is drawn with an arm directly in front of the person, then directly out to one side, and then about some intermediate axis, both the muscle and the innervation schemes of the three movements will be very different. However, all three movements are subjectively very much similar in terms of their difficulty and objectively they show approximately the same indices of accuracy and of variability. This allows us to conclude, with a high probability, that the structure of a central complex which controls the production of this series of movements is much more closely related to the spatial pattern than to a muscle scheme, because all three variations of the circular movement lie on lines of equal simplicity with respect to properties of both movements and their patterns, but not with respect to properties of muscle schemes.

In section 3, we discussed a case of incompatibility of the theory of cortical localization of muscles and the idea of a localized conditioned reflex; this example is apparently a particular case of the application of the described general principle of equal simplicity. Further experiments and observations of changes in the accuracy of movements in their different variations and of corresponding changes in the transfer of a motor skill will potentially be able to reveal whole sets of structural regularities of the motor field and of the brain motor functions in their entirety—regularities that cannot be predicted at present. Only one thing can be predicted with certainty: Every new discovery in the field of coordinational structure will, at the same time, be a new discovery in the area of localizational structure; and, on the day when we understand one, we shall be able to say that we have understood the other.

References[8]

Bernstein, N.A. (1923). Studies of the biomechanics of the stroke by means of photo-registration. *Research of the Central Institute of Labour, Moscow 1* (in Russian).

Bernstein, N.A. (1924). A biomechanical norm for the stroke. *Research of the Central Institute of Labour, Moscow 1,2* (in Russian).

Bernstein, N.A., & Popova, T. (1929). Untersuchung über die Biodynamik des Klavieranschlags [Study of the biodynamics of piano playing]. *Arbeitsphysiologie, 1*, 396-432.

Bernstein, N.A. (1929). Clinical Ways of Modern Biomechanics. *Collection of papers of the Institute for Medical Improvement, Kazan* (in Russian).

Bernstein, N.A. et al. (1935). *Studies of the Biodynamics of Locomotions (Normal Gait, Load and Fatigue).* Institute of Experimental Medicine, Moscow (in Russian).

Bethe, A. & Fischer, R. (1927). Die Plastizitat der Nervensysteme [The plasticity of the nervous system]. *Handbuch der normale und pathologische Physiologie, 10.*

Foerster, O. Die Physiologie und Pathologie der Koordination [The physiology and pathology of coordination]. *Zbl. f. die gest Neurol. Psychiatrie 41*, 11-12.

Lewy, F. (1923). *Die Lehre vom Tonus und der Bewegung* [The science of tonus and movement]. Berlin.

Magnus, R. (1924). Die Körperstellung [The body posture]. Berlin.

Monacow, C. (1914). Die Localisation im Grosshirn [The localization in the brain]. Wiesbaden.

Endnotes

Original notes are marked *

[1] Originally published in Russian in Arch. Biol. Sci., 38, 1935. Translated from the original by M.L. Latash; abridged and edited for this volume by R. Bongaardt and M.L. Latash.

[2]* The concept of antagonism may be applied unconditionally only to cases of muscles operating at joints with a single axis of rotation and, further, to those which cross only this one joint. The number of muscles of this type is extremely small; in the skeletal extremities we find as examples of this type only m. brachii and internus, m. pronator quadratus, the short position of m. biceps brachi and m. vastus femoris. All other muscles may be only functionally antagonistic within a given situation and in quite different relationships in other situations.

[3]* It is interesting to note here that the question which I have raised of the ecphoria of movements in a chain system or a comb system is a repetition in new terms in the area of the physiology of movement of the ancient psychological dispute of association (Bleuler, Adler) versus action (Berze) in the manner in which psychological processes are carried on. The chain model corresponds to the concept put forward by the associationists and the comb model is very similar to Berze's hypothesis. I am in no sense a partisan of the latter opinion in view of its deeply idealistic basis (the psychology of voluntarism), but I cannot deny that the attacks made on the opinions of pure associationists were extremely opportune.

[4]* For example, the velocity of the dispersion of waves of excitation through the CNS, time phenomena related to the interference of these waves, rhythmical heart activity, etc.

[5]* The formation and development of new motor habits, that is, the engraphy of conditioned motor reflexes, also appears to be a structurally complex process in the light of the analysis

undertaken in this report. It is in fact the case that new directional engrams with their spatio-temporal details must be built up within the CNS; however, those auxiliary proprioceptive mechanisms which I have just described as "coding" the impulse, and which provide the higher engram with the possibility of an actual detailed existence, must also be built up. The fact that a motor habit is not engraphed in those centers in which the muscles are localizationally represented is at once demonstrated by the fact that an acquired habit may exist while incorporating very different muscles in various combinations. When a child learns to write he can only form large letters, but a literate adult can form either large or small letters with equal ease and write either with straight letters or with skewed ones, etc. Apparently motor directional engrams are developed, generally speaking, later than the auxiliary coding mechanisms and correspond to a higher degree of mastery in the acquisition of a habit.

[6*] The term "topology", as used here, does not coincide exactly with the strict mathematical definition. For the lack of a more adequate expression, I have adopted this term for the whole of the quantitative characteristics of space configurations and of the patterns of movements in contrast to the quantitative, metric ones. A more detailed definition of what is meant here under the term topology will be understood from the text.

[7*] It may never cross the mind of an anatomist or a topographical anatomist that all his life he considers only various topological categories.

[8] This is the original complete references list. The corresponding text references are not present in this abridged version of the paper.

References

Bernstein, N.A. (1936). Die kymocyclographische Methode der Bewegungsuntersuchung [The kymocyclographical method of movement research]. In E. Abderhalden (Ed.), *Handbuch der biologischen Arbeitsmethoden* (vol. 5, pp. 629-680). Berlin: Urban und Schwarzenberg.

Bernstein, N.A., & Popova, T. (1929). Untersuchung über die Biodynamik des Klavieranschlags [Study of the biodynamics of piano playing]. *Arbeitsphysiologie, 1,* 396-432.

Bongaardt, R. (1996). *Shifting focus: The Bernstein tradition in movement science.* Unpublished doctoral dissertation. Vrije Universiteit, Amsterdam.

Bongaardt, R., & Meijer, O.G. (2000). Bernstein's theory of movement behavior: Historical development and contemporary relevance. *Journal of Motor Behavior, 32* (1), 57-71.

Feigenberg, I.M., & Latash, L.P. (1996). N.A. Bernstein: The reformer of neuroscience. In M.L. Latash & M.T. Turvey (Eds.), *Dexterity and its development* (pp. 247-275). Mahwah, NJ: Erlbaum.

Joravsky, D. (1989). *Russian psychology: A critical history.* Oxford: Blackwell.

Kozulin, A. (1984). *Psychology in utopia: Toward a social history of Soviet psychology.* Cambridge, MA: MIT Press.

Turvey, M.T. (1990). Coordination. *American Psychologist, 45,* 938-953.

Weiss, P.A. (1959). Animal behavior as system reaction: Orientation toward light and gravity in the resting postures of butterflies (Vanessa). In L. von Bertalanffy & A. Rappaport (Eds.), *General systems: Yearbook of the society for general systems research* (vol. 4, pp. 1-44). Ann Arbor, MI: Society for General Systems Research. (Original work published 1925)

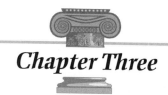

Chapter Three

Human Gait and Joint Mechanics: Is the Pendulum Swinging Back to Passive Dynamics?

Brian L. Davis, Maunak V. Rana, and Ari Levine

Lerner Research Institute, Cleveland Clinic Foundation, Cleveland, United States

Revisiting the work of
W. Braune and O. Fischer

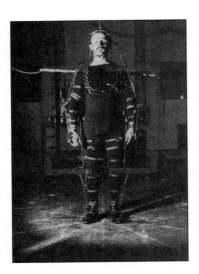

Figure 3.1
Experimental setup used by Braune and Fischer to obtain kinematic information for a single subject during gait.

Human gait is a biomechanical marvel, involving repeatedly losing and then regaining one's balance. Studies on the mechanics of locomotion have covered the spectrum from largely speculative to heavily quantitative. For instance, the work of the Weber brothers in the area of human gait (Weber and Weber, 1894/1992) tended to be more speculative (the only instrument they used was a watch with a second hand), whereas the work of Braune and Fischer (1895-1904/1987) was extremely analytical, involving the design and construction of new equipment (figure 3.1) and years of painstaking calculations (figure 3.2). The methodical manner in which Braune and Fischer conducted their analyses is what sets their work apart from that of other researchers, both then and now.

To determine a coordinate using Braune & Fischer's data, use the following method: *We will calculate a point on the head (vertex) for Experiment II from the right.*

Pick a set of two-dimensional data points $[\zeta_1, \zeta_2]$ from the data set for the proper experiment (in this case Table 2), and find the corresponding three-dimensional data points [x, y] (Table 15).

$\downarrow$

Using the proper equations, calculate z_1 and z_2. In this case, the proper equations for z_1 and z_2 for the left side of the head are (eq. 24):
$$z_1 = (1.46190 - 0.00356 \cdot y) \cdot \zeta_1$$
$$z_2 = (1.57102 - 0.00227 \cdot x - 0.00131 \cdot y) \cdot \zeta_2$$

$\downarrow$

Average the z_1 and z_2 values to obtain z_0

$\downarrow$

Using the proper equations to convert to three-dimensional coordinates, find the Z value. In our case, we use equation (80).
$$z = [z_0] + 87$$

Figure 3.2
Flowchart showing the painstaking mathematical calculations carried out by Braune and Fischer. The equations and tables referenced in this figure refer to those as listed in Braune and Fischer's original text.

The various chapters of Braune and Fischer's work were published on an individual basis in the Proceedings of the Royal Saxon Society for Sciences, and then concatenated into one large work at a later date. In *The Human Gait* (translated 1987), Braune and Fischer rigorously test the Weber brothers' hypothesis concerning the relative contributions of gravity and muscular effort to the motion of the swinging leg. In particular, the Weber brothers postulated that during ambulation the leg that is not contacting the ground mirrors the motion of a pendulum. Gravity, they argued, was the force behind the driving of the leg through an arc of motion.

Who Were the Weber Brothers?

Before we proceed to the work of Braune and Fischer, let us review the work of the Weber brothers. Modern physiology is deeply indebted to these brothers (Ernst, Wilhelm, and Eduard) who led science in new directions (Rothschuh, 1973). Sons of a theologian based in Wittenberg, they contributed greatly to academic knowledge in the second half of the 19th century. Ernst served as professor of anatomy and physiology at Leipzig, beginning his career at 26 years of age. His major areas of research involved utilizing mathematics to explain the inner workings of human physiology, specifically fluid properties and mechanics. He is the author of Weber's law, the result of his studies on touch, temperature, and pressure.

Wilhelm Weber contributed to scientific knowledge as a physicist at Gottingen. His expertise enabled him to study the human body through the use of physical principles. Eduard, the youngest brother, worked with Ernst at Leipzig. There his study centered on the contributions of muscle to the mechanics of the human body. Indeed, it was his monumental work *Mechanik der menschlichen Gehwekzeuge* (loosely translated as *The Mechanics of Human Walking Apparatus*, Weber and Weber, 1894), a collaborative effort with Wilhelm, that paved the way for the interest in analyzing gait and muscle function and for the work of other scientists in this area.

The issue that Braune and Fischer wanted to follow up on is based on the claim of Weber and Weber (1894): "The leg alters its shape when hanging from the trunk and swinging like a pendulum. If it remained extended as it is the instant it is raised from the ground, it would strike the ground and could not swing freely beneath the trunk. Consequently, it is flexed at knee level and thus shortened" (Braune and Fischer, 1987, p. 2). To the Weber brothers the pendulum theory explained why human motion was regular in step length. In essence, they did not consider the effect of muscular activity on the swinging leg during gait. It was this conclusion that prompted Braune and Fischer to expand on prior research by utilizing more sophisticated equipment to study and offer their hypotheses on ambulation qualities.

It is important to note that the Weber brothers proposed many other concepts besides the pendulum theory. In fact, they proposed almost 150 hypotheses (Cavanagh, 1990), including the following:

- The fastest speed of running is about 6.5 m/s (7.1 yd/s).
- The variability during normal walking is less than that during normal running.
- Stride length is greater during running than in walking, but its duration during running is shorter.

Cavanagh (1990, p. 11) makes the point that these postulates are an interesting mixture of "right, wrong and perhaps." The observations on maximum speed were incorrect; the claims regarding variability still need verification; and the statements concerning stride lengths and durations were correct. Cavanagh concludes that the significance of the Weber brothers' work lies not in "what they said, but the fact that they said it."

Braune and Fischer's Approach

Braune and Fischer mathematically quantified the rotatory movement of the leg with the following equation:

$$mx^2 \cdot \alpha = D_m + D_s + D_e$$

where m = mass, x = the radius of inertia with reference to the axis through the center of gravity, and α refers to the angular acceleration. D_m, D_s, and D_e represent the torques exerted by muscles, gravity, and effective forces on the portion of the leg being examined. The effective force is defined as the resultant (geometric sum) of all external forces displaced parallel to the center of gravity. In essence, therefore, Braune and Fischer calculated the net torques acting on the thigh, shank, and foot for the swing phase of gait. By subtracting the components due to gravity, they knew how much torque must have been generated "internally."

The reasoning that Braune and Fischer used to determine which muscles were active and which were not was as follows. They took each limb segment separately and hypothesized which muscles could conceivably have caused the torque acting on it. With regard to the thigh, for instance, at the initiation of swing it was acted upon by a positive torque—the muscles that Braune and Fischer felt could be responsible were the iliopsoas (spanning only the hip), gracilis (crossing both hip and knee), short head of biceps femoris (a knee joint muscle), and gastrocnemius (spanning both knee and ankle). To reduce the number of possible muscles, they then noted what was simultaneously happening to the shank. At the beginning of swing, it also had a positive torque acting on it, so the biceps femoris and gracilis could be eliminated from the initial list because they are only capable of exerting a negative torque on the lower leg. In a similar way, because the foot experiences a positive torque, gastrocnemius was not a likely candidate—leaving iliopsoas as the main contender for explaining the initial motion of the thigh.

Braune and Fischer's Findings

As a result of their studies, Braune and Fischer found values for D_m that were of sufficient magnitude to imply that gravity is not the only force acting on the lower extremity during motion. This led them to make the following statements regarding the work of the Weber brothers (Braune and Fischer, 1987):

- The "pillars on which Weber and Weber built their theory of walking have crumbled" (p. 233).

- Concerning the pendulum theory, "our research demonstrates that this concept cannot be true, even approximately" (p. 431).

- "The much discussed pendulum theory of Weber and Weber is thus erroneous" (p. 437).

Summary of Muscle Activation Patterns

In addition to showing that leg motion is more complicated than originally thought, the researchers were able to determine the activity of muscles during the swing phase of ambulation (figures 3.3 and 3.4). Particularly, they performed an analysis of muscular activity in the various components of the lower extremity. Braune and Fischer carefully looked at the muscle-

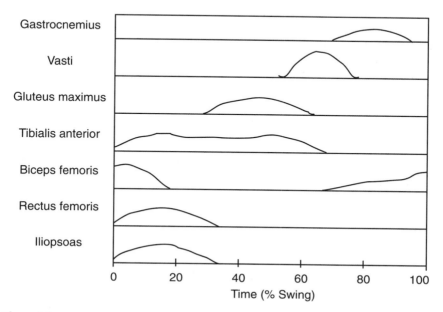

Figure 3.3
Timing of muscle activation sequences inferred from Braune and Fischer's discussion.

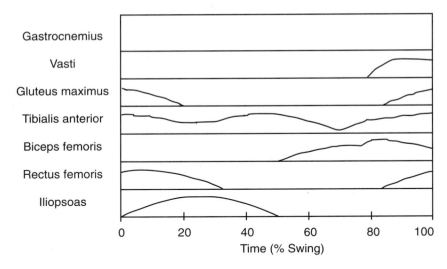

Figure 3.4
Timing of muscle activation sequences obtained from Vaughan et al., 1992. Note the contrast with data shown in figure 3.3.

joint interactions of the leg by examining muscles isolated to the hip, those between the hip and the knee, muscles isolated to the knee, and finally muscles that connected the knee and the ankle. They identified the following muscular activity pattern. Initially in the swing phase, a positive torque is produced by the lower-extremity muscles. With initial motion, Fischer noted that muscles in the flexor compartment of the thigh, the iliopsoas for example, contract to initiate swinging. This was substantiated in a study by the famous scientist Duchenne (1883) as he studied patients with flexor paralysis in the thigh: These patients were not able to swing the lower extremity. The iliopsoas acts with the rectus femoris and tibialis anterior to begin motion. The torque then decreases until the muscles cease their activity. Next, the thigh extensor muscles, for example the gluteus maximus, act with the biceps femoris, the hamstrings, and tibialis anterior to extend the lower extremity. Near the final portion of the swing phase, the gastrocnemius acts to cause a positive torque on the foot. The leg then contacts the ground during the heel strike, at which point the tibialis anterior becomes active again.

In reviewing the work of Braune and Fischer, it is important to note that they reached their conclusions without the aid of technology such as electromyography (EMG). This tool has aided scientists since the 1940s in corroborating the work of the earlier researchers. Inman et al. (1981) raise an interesting point with regard to the use of EMG to analyze muscle activity during gait. They note that the EMG activity has no correlation to the sign of work performed by the muscle, positive or negative. This must be extrapolated from an analysis of angular displacements and moments.

Gluteus Maximus

Winter (1987) has used EMG to look at muscle activation during various phases of human gait and has profiled the actions of various muscles during walking. Gluteus maximus, for example, serves as a hip extensor and stabilizes the pelvis during weight acceptance. Winter notes that it fires during the latter portion of the swing phase, activating to the greatest extent when the foot first contacts the ground. There is also a second, minor, burst early in swing that decelerates the forward-swinging thigh. This pattern is not in agreement with Braune and Fischer's suggestions that gluteus maximus is active after the second third of the swing phase. In fact, the data for gluteus maximus in figures 3.3 and 3.4 are almost mirror images of each other.

Iliacus

Inman et al. (1981) have commented on the iliacus. This muscle connects the iliac crest to the femur. It works with psoas to support and flex the hip. Inman et al. have shown that it has maximal contractile activity at the start of swing, starting the motion of hip flexion. Braune and Fischer noted that it is the action of the iliacus and psoas that in effect initiates the motion of the hip during the swing portion of gait, and they presented concepts that are in agreement with current understanding regarding the actions of iliopsoas.

Hamstrings

The hamstring muscles are located in the dorsal aspect of the lower extremity. The semitendinosus and the semimembranosus are the medial contributions of this group, spanning from the ischial tuberosity to the proximal tibia. These muscles serve as thigh extensors, leg flexors, and medial rotators. Winter (1987) comments that the muscles initiate activity during the latter half of swing, presumably to decrease the motion of the leg as it is traveling forward. The timing proposed by Braune and Fischer, that is, that the muscle becomes active after the second third of the swing, is thus slightly too soon in the cycle (see figure 3.3).

Braune and Fischer were struck by the fact that after about 60% of the swing phase the negative torque on the thigh suddenly decreased, while the torque on the lower leg showed the opposite trend. Rather than ascribing this to action of the hamstrings or any other muscle, they thought that the sudden tensioning of the collateral ligaments of the knee could be responsible. This shows one advantage of using logic over the technique of EMG analysis, since in the case of the latter, one might tend to think that it is only muscles that are responsible for creating joint torques!

Rectus Femoris

Of the components that compose the quadriceps muscle, the rectus femoris is one of the most important used during gait. This muscle spans from the anterior superior iliac spine to the patella and serves as a leg extensor at the knee. It also provides support to the hip and aids the flexing action of the iliopsoas. The rectus femoris has its significant activity just before the heel contacts the ground, and the activity increases to a peak value during weight bearing. Also, this muscle is active after the toes are off the ground, serving to accelerate the leg forward during the swing phase. The early phase of the muscle's activation in swing was correctly identified by Braune and Fischer; however, they did not correctly note that the muscle is active at the end of the swing phase.

Tibialis Anterior

The tibialis anterior connects the lateral portion of the tibia to the medial aspect of the foot at the base of the first metatarsal. This muscle functions to dorsiflex and invert the foot. During the end of the swing portion the tibialis acts to dorsiflex the foot as it completes its motion. The muscle reaches its highest activity after the heel has contacted the ground, counteracting the forces causing the plantar flexion of the foot. It is, however, also important during the swing phase—first serving to keep the foot from "stubbing" the ground and then acting to prepare the foot for landing. Braune and Fischer probably underestimate the function of this muscle during the latter third of swing.

Gastrocnemius

The gastrocnemius is a fleshy muscle of the calf region, composed of a medial and lateral unit. This muscle joins the femur and the calcaneus. The major actions of the gastrocnemius are to plantar flex the foot, raise the heel, and flex the knee. As a result, it has its highest activity after the heel contacts the ground, as the foot pushes off. It is quiescent during swing, though Braune and Fischer thought it was active just prior to heel strike.

As a result of technology such as EMG, much of Braune and Fischer's reasoning has been validated. Certainly one must admire their (in reality Fischer's) attempt to relate their data to functionally important muscle activation sequences. In this regard their work certainly expands beyond Weber and Weber's pendulum theory.

Chapter-by-Chapter Summary of Braune and Fischer's Work

Braune and Fischer begin the first chapter of their monumental work by recapping the prior research of the Weber brothers, Vierordt, Marey, and Muybridge. "Experiments on Man, Loaded and Unloaded" (1895) sets the stage with commentary on the earlier two-dimensional motion studies that were qualitative in nature. Against this background information, Braune and Fischer then present their own three-dimensional quantitative experiments. In particular, they describe the camera apparatus they devised to analyze human motions and the way in which the data obtained translate to landmarks (centers of gravity, centers of joints) on the human body.

Following up on the concept of analyzing centers of motion, in their second chapter (1899) Braune and Fischer study the movement of the total center of gravity and the external forces. They use data presented in the first chapter to analyze the three-dimensional path that the body's total center of gravity follows. Coupled with this tracing is the determination of velocity and acceleration in a three-coordinate system, presented graphically for the reader. This determination of the center-of-gravity motion is critical in that it provides a description of the net external forces, including gravity, ground reaction force, and air friction.

Braune and Fischer turn their attention to the studies of the Weber brothers in the third chapter of their work, titled "Considerations on the Further Goals of Research and Overall View of the Movements of the Lower Extremity" (1900). According to the authors, the conclusions reached by the Webers 70 years earlier are inaccurate—specifically, the notion that during level walking at constant velocity the total center of gravity follows a horizontal path. This idea was rendered obsolete by "the data established by instantaneous photography" (Braune and Fischer, p. 253). The authors then provide body segment and axial angles for the basis of future studies. This chapter is crucial to the further focus of the book as it deals with the mathematics behind the research and goals of this work.

In the fourth chapter of the book, titled "On the Movement of the Foot and the Forces Acting on It" (1901), the authors expand their study from analyzing movement to highlighting the kinetics of ambulation. They present a qualitative description of the forces and moments on the foot, followed by tabulation and a graphical display of the displacement, velocity, and acceleration of the center of gravity of the foot. When these results are multiplied by the mass of the foot, it is possible to determine the effective force on the foot in three dimensions.

In the fifth chapter, "Kinematics of the Swing of the Leg" (1903), Braune and Fischer dissect the theoretical contributions of von Meyer and prove that his conclusions are invalid. Whereas von Meyer stated that the posterior leg must maintain its contact with the floor prior to swing until the center of gravity is above the anterior leg's heel, the authors note that the leg that is traveling through the swinging motion leaves the floor before this moment. Even though Braune and Fischer quantitatively proved their findings, scientists criticized their conclusions, citing unnatural step lengths of their subjects. To refute the charge of a limitation, Braune and Fischer studied the gait patterns of 111 soldiers and students. In this chapter, as a prelude to quantitative conclusions in the final chapter, they present qualitative findings on the forces and moments that act on a swinging leg. Continuing with the data that had been presented in the previous chapter, Braune and Fischer determine the segmental angular velocities and center-of-gravity accelerations of the lower extremity.

In the sixth and final chapter of their analysis of human gait, "On the Influence of Gravity and the Muscles on the Swinging Movement of the Leg" (1904), the scientists utilize their prior data and conclusions to answer the question of muscular involvement in gait. Contrary to the Webers' pendulum theory of gait, Braune and Fischer affirm the role of muscle in ambulation. Utilizing kinematic and kinetic findings and conclusions, the authors state emphatically that a significant muscular contribution is essential to human ambulation.

Could Braune and Fischer Have Improved Their Analyses?

In today's scientific arena, such importance is placed on publishing on a regular basis that researchers find it hard to imagine conducting a single experiment lasting four or five years. Braune and Fischer did just this. In the 1890s their purpose was to investigate whether the leg behaved in a pendular manner during the swing phase of gait. In fact, Fischer died without knowing the final result! The calculations were not even interesting—page after page of repetitive number crunching. Even the equipment these researchers used had to be designed and built by master craftsmen before measurements could be taken. Could they have reduced their labor without sacrificing their results? A branch of statistics dealing with "uncertainty analysis" may throw light on this question.

Briefly, if a quantity (R) is dependent on a number of variables, $x_1, x_2, \ldots, x_n$, each of which is associated with some uncertainty ($\omega_i, 1 \leq i \leq n$), then the uncertainty in R is given by (Kline and McClintock, 1953):

$$\omega_R = \left\{ \left(\omega_1 \frac{\partial R}{\partial x_1} \right)^2 + \left(\omega_2 \frac{\partial R}{\partial x_2} \right)^2 + \ldots + \left(\omega_n \frac{\partial R}{\partial x_n} \right)^2 \right\}^{0.5}$$

Braune and Fischer needed to measure the masses and locations of limb segments and the linear and angular accelerations of these segments. From these measurements they used the "inverse dynamics approach" to calculate ankle, knee, and hip moments. This was no easy task at the turn of the century: Geissler tubes had to be taped to the subject (with precautions to prevent the subject from being electrocuted); these tubes had to be designed to flash rapidly (every 1/26th of a second); and filming had to be done at night, in almost complete darkness. This was just the beginning. After the film had been processed, the joint coordinates were digitized using an instrument custom built for the study by a precision mechanic in Leipzig. The center of gravity for each segment was calculated, and the displacement data were graphically differentiated twice to obtain accelerations.

In their experimental protocol presented in the first chapter of *The Human Gait*, Braune and Fischer used four cameras to determine the x, y, and z coordinates of selected points on the body. Each camera yielded two measurements—coordinates ξ and η—so there were four known quantities for each side of the body. This allowed four variables to be quantified (x, y, and two z values). In terms of checking their methods, the fact that there were two independent calculations for the z coordinates meant that Braune and Fischer could get an estimate of the accuracy of the overall technique. The question to be answered in this example is "Which calculation for 'z' yielded better results?"

In Braune and Fischer (1987), the expressions for z (vertical coordinate of a point P) are

$$z = \frac{(a_1 - y) \cdot \zeta_1}{a_1} \tag{9a}$$

$$z = \frac{(a_2 - x \cos \alpha - y \sin \alpha) \cdot \zeta_2}{a_2} \tag{9b}$$

where a_1 and a_2 are the distances between the origin and the nodal points of the lenses for cameras 1 and 2, respectively. The angle between the direction of gait (i.e., x-axis) and the direction in which camera 2 faces is given by α (which was chosen to be 30°). Finally, ζ_1 and ζ_2 are the measured vertical coordinates on the photographic plates for cameras 1 and 2, respectively.

Clearly, both variations of equation 9 (as referenced in *The Human Gait*) require that x and y be known. In this example it will be assumed that we know these values. (Braune and Fischer deposited the actual x and y data in the archives of the Königlich Sächsische Gesellschaft der Wissenshaften—to make it easy for anyone to take a look at the raw data!) Braune and Fischer calculated a_1 and a_2 to be 410.54 and 599.00 cm, respectively. Let us assume that the uncertainty in these measurements was 0.65 cm since this value had previously been quoted as being small (Braune and Fischer 1895-1904/1987, p. 38). Assume the following at the first time instant:

For the vertex,

$$x = 99.89 \text{ cm}, y = 0.41 \text{ cm (with uncertainties} = 0.25 \text{ cm)}$$

$$\zeta_1 = 74.48, \zeta_2 = 72.73 \text{ (uncertainties} = 0.1)$$

By obtaining partial derivatives for Braune and Fischer's equation 9a, we get

$$\frac{\partial z}{\partial a_1} = \frac{y\zeta_1}{a_1^{2}}$$

$$\frac{\partial z}{\partial y} = -\frac{\zeta_1}{a_1}$$

$$\frac{\partial z}{\partial \zeta_1} = \frac{(a_1 - y)}{a_1}$$

By obtaining partial derivatives for Braune and Fischer's equation 9b, we get

$$\frac{\partial z}{\partial a_2} = \frac{(x \cos \alpha + y \sin \alpha)\zeta_2}{a_2^{2}}$$

$$\frac{\partial z}{\partial x} = -\frac{\zeta_2 \cos \alpha}{a_2}$$

$$\frac{\partial z}{\partial y} = -\frac{\zeta_2 \sin \alpha}{a_2}$$

$$\frac{\partial z}{\partial \alpha} = -\frac{\zeta_2}{a_2}(x \sin \alpha - y \cos \alpha)$$

$$\frac{\partial z}{\partial \zeta_2} = \frac{(a_2 - x \cos \alpha - y \sin \alpha)}{a_2}$$

By substituting values into these equations and using the uncertainty expression described by Kline and McClintock (1953), one can derive predictions for the uncertainty associated with each calculated variable. For the point on the vertex (coordinate Z), table 3.1 gives an example of what the process achieves.

For these data points, the uncertainty for Z_2 is thus always greater than or equal to the uncertainty for Z_1. Publishing "the average values of the two series of coordinates obtained from different sides" (Braune and Fischer, 1987, p. 56) does not account for the fact that some of the calculations yielded

Table 3.1

	Z_1	Z_2	(ωZ_1)	(ωZ_2)
11th data point	74.88	74.32	0.11	0.11
20th data point	77.94	77.52	0.11	0.13
24th data point	75.17	74.81	0.11	0.20

more accurate results than others. For instance, the value of 75.17 for Z_1 is more likely to be correct than the value 74.81 because there is less uncertainty associated with it.

Other Possible "Errors" Made by Braune and Fischer

Braune and Fischer were forced to carry out their data collection and analysis using very archaic methods compared to today's standards. They had no access to even the simplest device to aid in their numerical calculations; everything was completed manually. Taking this into account, it is very probable that the two researchers made errors during their period of data analysis.

Typographical

Braune and Fischer describe three separate experiments—two involving free walking and one with the subject carrying an army-regulation knapsack—that were conducted during the night of July 24/25, 1891. As mentioned before, two cameras each filmed the left and right sides of the subject. For a lay reader it is often confusing to follow the analysis path since data are presented for each experiment for the left leg as viewed by the right camera, the right leg as viewed by the right camera, and so on, in raw (digitized) and scaled (laboratory based) coordinates and finally in true three-dimensional formats. The people who typed up the Braune and Fischer research probably had a difficult time keeping track of this as well! An example of a typographical error is found on page 45 of Braune and Fischer (1987), where Braune and Fischer's equation reference as 21a should be replaced with equation 21b:

$$z_1 = \frac{(410.54 - y) \cdot \zeta_1}{281.55} \tag{21a}$$

$$z_1 = \frac{(410.54 - y) \cdot \zeta'_1}{281.55} \tag{21b}$$

The term ζ refers to scaled coordinates, whereas ζ' refers to coordinates measured on the photographic plates.

Two Dimensions Versus Three Dimensions

The muscle activity patterns described previously, while being reasonable, suffer from the fact that the final processed data are two-dimensional. Because of this, muscles such as gluteus medius, erector spinae, and the adductors are largely ignored. Clearly these are important muscles that control gait movements. Woltring (1989) also makes the point that Braune and Fischer neglect axial rotations of the limbs since only one flashing tube was placed parallel to each limb segment.

Smoothing

Woltring (1989) states that while Braune and Fischer may be regarded as the originators of "analytical close-range photogrammetry," unfortunately no low-pass filtering techniques were available at the turn of the century. As a consequence the researchers were unable to remove noise from their data. The averaging of coordinate values may have reduced some of the noise; but, as stated previously, Braune and Fischer could have weighted their predictions according to the anticipated uncertainty for each data point.

Number of Markers

When reading Braune and Fischer's book, one is struck by the amount of work they performed. It is surprising that the two researchers did not simply put Geissler tubes on the lower extremities—after all, to perform the dynamic analyses to prove the Weber brothers wrong, they needed only data for the lower extremities. Braune and Fischer could therefore have saved themselves a lot of time and effort by omitting the markers on the arms and head (figure 3.1).

Back to Original Pendular Theory of the Weber Brothers

Although the conclusions reached by Braune and Fischer are indeed ingenious given their limited technological assistance, their labeling of the Weber brothers' work as inaccurate may not be correct. While motion is undoubtedly guided by the actions of muscles and the nervous system, researchers in robotics have recently devised robots that can walk without any muscles! Indeed, the motion of these devices is powered by gravity as the lower extremity falls in an arc-like fashion—quite similar to the motion of a double pendulum as described by the Webers.

McGeer (1990), a proponent of this research, has coined the passive-dynamic theory of gait. His theory highlights ambulation as the result of the effects of gravity on springs, not controlled by a feedback mechanism or muscular intervention in the setting of movement. In effect, it is the mechanical structure of the musculoskeletal system rather than the results of the actions of muscles that determines the movements of these passive walkers.

In addition to McGeer, other researchers (Garcia et al., 1998) have been able to develop two-dimensional models and extrapolate to build three-dimensional models of human gait. The beauty of these studies is that power to walk is achieved, as noted above, by gravity. No muscle force is utilized to cause motion. Coleman and Ruina (1997) have even demonstrated how these models can be built with simple Tinkertoy components! (See figure 3.5.)

Conclusions

In viewing the work of Braune and Fischer as a whole, one might decide that their conclusions went beyond what their data covered. They did not collect EMG data, yet they made a number of statements regarding the phasic behavior of gait, only some of which are accurate. Furthermore, their criticism of the Weber brothers seems particularly harsh, especially considering that devices can be built to walk without the need for actuators. The work of Braune and Fischer is held in high esteem by prominent biomechanics researchers. Woltring (1986) regarded Braune and Fischer as having published "classical data." In reviewing the efforts of Braune and

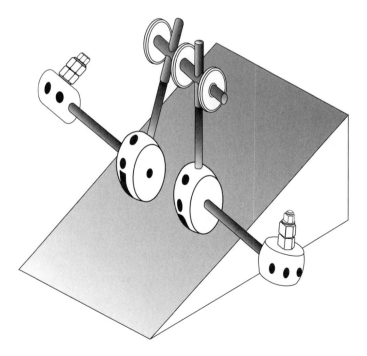

Figure 3.5
Passive-dynamic walkers can ambulate without muscle actuators (Coleman and Ruina, 1997).

Fischer, Cavanagh (1990) states that "the vision of this research was monumental." Brand (1992) maintained that the work of Braune and Fischer "added a new level of sophistication" to the study of gait dynamics. According to Maquet (1992), Braune and Fischer's "mathematical reasoning is unquestionable," and their remarkable work "constitutes a far reaching analysis of human gait." Accolades such as these reflect the fact that Braune and Fischer's work ushered in a new era of quantitative research techniques. The masterpiece is of interest not only to historians: Modern engineers can learn of the complexities of human walking; orthopedic surgeons can appreciate the need for mathematics to describe the behavior of the locomotor system; and researchers can be inspired by Braune and Fischer's determination to succeed despite the obstacles and setbacks they encountered.

Acknowledgment

The authors gratefully acknowledge support from NASA (NAGW 5006) and NSF (EEC 9820538).

References

Brand, R.A. "Assessment of Musculoskeletal Disorders by Locomotion Analysis: A Critical Historical and Epistemological Review." In *Biolocomotion: A Century of Research Using Moving Pictures,* ed. Cappozo, A., Marchetti, M., and Tosi, V., pp. 227-242. Rome: Promograph. 1992.

Braune, W., and Fischer, O. *The Human Gait* (trans. P.G.J. Maquet and R. Springer-Verlag). Berlin: Furlong. 1895-1904/1987.

Cavanagh, P.R. *Biomechanics of Distance Running.* Champaign, IL: Human Kinetics. 1990.

Coleman, M., and Ruina, A. "An Uncontrolled Toy That Can Walk But Cannot Stand Still." *Physical Review Letters,* Nov 18. 1997.

Duchenne, G.B.A. *Selections From the Clinical Works of Dr. Duchenne (de Boulogne)* (trans. and ed. G.V. Poore). London: New Sydenham Society. 1883.

Garcia, M., Chatterjee, A., Ruina, A., and Coleman, M. "The Simplest Walking Model: Stability, Complexity, and Scaling." *ASME Journal of Biomechanical Engineering,* Feb 10, 1998.

Inman, V.T., Ralston, H.J., and Todd, F. *Human Walking.* Baltimore: Williams & Wilkins. 1981.

Kline, S.J., and McClintock, F.A. "Describing Uncertainties in Single-Sample Experiments." *Mechanical Engineering* 1, 3. 1953.

Maquet, P. "'The Human Gait' By Braune and Fischer." In *Biolocomotion: A Century of Research Using Moving Pictures,* ed. Cappozo, A., Marchetti, M., and Tosi, V., pp. 115-126. Rome: Promograph. 1992.

McGeer, T. "Passive Dynamic Walking." *International Journal of Robotics Research* 9, 62-82. 1990.

Moore, K. *Clinically Oriented Anatomy.* Baltimore: Williams & Wilkins. 1992.

Rothschuh, K.E. *History of Physiology* (trans. and ed. G.B. Risse). Huntington, NY: Krieger. 1973.

Vaughan, C.L., Davis, B.L., and O'Connor, J. *Dynamics of Human Gait.* Champaign, IL: Human Kinetics. 1992.

Weber, W., and Weber, E. *Mechanik der menschlichen Gehwerkzeuge.* Berlin: Julius Springer, 1894. Translation by Springer-Verlag, 1992.

Winter, D. *The Biomechanics and Motor Control of Human Gait.* Waterloo, ON, Canada: University of Waterloo Press. 1987.

Woltring, H. "Braune and Fischer Revisited—Estimation of the Instantaneous Helical Axis From Volunteer Knee Motion Data." XVth Symposium of The European Society of Osteoarthrology, Kuopio, Finland, June 25-27. 1986.

Woltring, H. "Book Review: W. Braune and O. Fischer, *The Human Gait.*" *Human Movement Science* 8, 79-83. 1989.

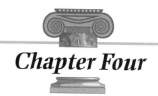

Chapter Four

Involuntary Muscle Contractions Detected by Electromyography (EMG)

Joel A. Vilensky and Sid Gilman

Indiana University School of Medicine, Fort Wayne, United States, and University of Michigan School of Medicine, Ann Arbor, United States

Revisiting the work of
D. Denny-Brown and J.B. Pennybacker

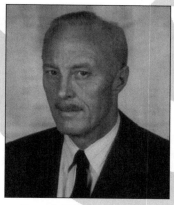

Derek Denny-Brown

Derek Denny-Brown (1901-1981) is well known among contemporary neurologists both for his clinical research, much of it involving movement disorders, and for his influence on neurologic medicine during the second half of the 20th century. This influence, emanating from his position as director of the Harvard University Neurological Unit at Boston City Hospital from 1941 until 1967, was a primary factor in the development of neurology as an independent medical specialty in the United States (Vilensky et al., 1998).

Denny-Brown was born in New Zealand, but in 1924 after earning a medical degree from Otago University in Dunedin, New Zealand, he applied for and received a scholarship to study nervous system physiology in Sherrington's laboratory at Oxford University in England.

While at Oxford, Denny-Brown characterized the distinctive properties of red and white muscles, validated Sherrington's concept of the motor unit, and developed the technique of antidromic stimulation for the analysis of motoneuron responses. His fellowship at Oxford resulted in a DPhil degree, the coauthorship of a classic book, *Reflex Activity of the Nervous System*, and 16 scientific papers. Denny-Brown's work in Sherrington's laboratory also resulted in a lifelong interest in the neurological control of posture and movement.

After completing his fellowship in 1928, Denny-Brown entered classical neurological training at the National Hospital, Queens Square, London, England. Upon completion of this training, he entered clinical practice at the National Hospital and began teaching. He also began to apply his understanding of the physiology of the nervous system and research techniques to clinical neurology. Eventually, Denny-Brown's reputation as an outstanding clinical and experimental neurologist led to his selection as the most-qualified candidate for the position at Harvard, which was originally offered to him in 1939, but which he was unable to accept until 1941 because of his service in the Royal Army Medical Corps during World War II.

The classical paper presented here was written during this period and illustrates the hybrid nature of Denny-Brown's talent. The paper, "Fibrillation and Fasciculation in Voluntary Muscles," is primarily designed to teach clinicians the differences between various types of involuntary muscular contractions but uses the underlying physiology to understand these differences. Originally published in 1938, this paper is still very frequently cited in contemporary reports on the clinical aspects of fibrillation, fasciculation, and cramps in muscles, and the electrical activity that accompanies these movements.

Unfortunately, we know very little about Denny-Brown's coauthor on this paper, J.B. Pennybacker. We believe he was an American and a neurological trainee at the National Hospital while Denny-Brown was a member of the hospital staff.

We have abridged the paper, eliminating sections that were not directly relevant to the main theme. Further, to improve interpretation and understanding of the figures, we have rewritten the legends and corrected grammatical errors wherever we found them. Lastly, we have not altered (except in the figure legends) the article's use of the words "action current" to describe the spikes of activity shown in electromyographic record, despite the fact that contemporary usage would consider the potential voltage differences shown to be termed "action potential."

Definitions

acetylcholine: The neurotransmitter that is released at the synapse between a motor nerve and its muscle (i.e., neuromuscular junction).

amyotrophic lateral sclerosis: A group of disorders that affect both the central and peripheral nerves that innervate muscles. These muscles exhibit progressive atrophy, weakness, and fasciculations.

antidromic: Conducting impulses in a direction opposite to normal.

bromide paper: Light-sensitive paper used to record oscillograph records.

denervate: To cut the nerves that innervate an anatomical structure (e.g., muscle).

galvanometer: An instrument for measuring the strength of an electric current.

hyperhidrosis: Excessive or profuse sweating.

manometer: Instrument for measuring pressure of a liquid or gas.

mylohyoid muscle: A muscle found under the chin.

oscillograph: An instrument for providing a permanent record of changes in electrical voltage over time.

syringomyelia: A disease of the spinal cord that may result in the death of the alpha motoneurons that innervate muscles.

Fibrillation and Fasciculation in Voluntary Muscle*

D. Denny-Brown and J.B. Pennybacker

Involuntary fibrillary twitching of muscle is a phenomenon observed frequently in the course of clinical examination of patients suffering from nervous disorders. It is apparent to the naked eye that what is commonly called "fibrillation" in amyotrophic lateral sclerosis, for example, differs in type from muscle to muscle, and from time to time in the same patient. Of these differing varieties there is little mention in the literature, nor of their relationship to other kinds of involuntary twitching in muscle.

The following study is of myographic and electromyographic records of these various forms of involuntary twitching of muscle fibres.

*Reprinted from Denny-Brown and Pennybacker 1938.

(1) Method of Investigation

The twitching of the muscle has been recorded by concurrent records of the mechanical twitch and the electrical action current of the fibres concerned. The electrical action current has been recorded by inserting a hypodermic needle through the skin into the substance of the muscle being investigated, a superficial portion of the muscle fibre being selected for the purpose. The second electrode in the form of a thin copper wire insulated with cotton winding soaked in celloidin, with silvered perforation at its end, is inserted through the needle just to protrude through its end. Thus the tip of the wire core forms one electrode among the muscle fibres, separated by 1 to 2 mm from the nearest part of the needle, which forms the other electrode. The wire and the hypodermic needle are connected to the input side of a four stage amplifier leading to a Matthews Oscillograph, of which the galvanometer mirror reflects a beam of light on a strip of moving bromide paper. Over the region where the tip of the hypodermic needle lies in the muscle a small cork button or pyramid is stuck to the skin by collodion. Over the button is a balloon lightly inflated with air, and held by adhesive plaster to the body wall or to a metal guard clamped round the limb. Any mechanical movement of the piece of muscle concerned moves the cork, and produces a fluctuation in the air pressure in the balloon which is transmitted by a short length of pressure tubing to a manometer with mirror diaphragm. The movements of the manometer mirror are recorded by a beam of light which is reflected to the same strip of moving paper as records the action currents. The latency of the mechanical system used was 0.004 sec., i.e. the mechanical record lags behind the electrical record by this time interval. In the animal experiments fibrillation was recorded by a very small steel mirror directly applied to the muscular surface.

It cannot be too strongly emphasized that mechanical records made in this manner must be controlled carefully by visual observation of the surface of the muscle.

(2) The Fine Fibrillation of a Muscle Completely Deprived of Its Nerve Supply

Denervated mammalian muscle has long been known to exhibit a fine tremor of its surface (Schiff, 1851, Langley, 1915-16a, Langley and Kato, 1914-15). Usually the tremor is so slight in degree that it is well seen only when the bared surface of the muscle is observed in reflected light. The surface of the muscle is observed to be rippled by a restless agitation without either apparent rhythm or obvious centre of activity. The whole muscle is involved in a confusion of very small twitches. Such fibrillation is related in some way to the wasting following denervation. In the frog, where denervated muscle wastes only very slowly, fibrillation does not occur (Langley, 1915-16a). This phenomenon is most easily observed in man in the tongue when that organ is subject to paralytic atrophy, for here the superficial situation of muscle fibres and thinness of covering facilitate its observation. Where the skin and subcutaneous tissue are thin it can be observed in other skeletal muscles, particularly as a result of damage to peripheral nerves or degeneration of motor anterior horn cells as in poliomyelitis or syringomyelia.

The faint, confused agitation of the surface of the muscle is accompanied by a very fine rapid electrical fluctuation of which a characteristic instance is shown in fig. 1 [*figure 4.1 here*] taken from the mylohyoid muscle of a patient suffering from syringomyelia, with wasting and fibrillation of one half of the tongue and hyoid muscles. These action currents are much smaller than those accompanying motor nervous activity (cf. fig. 11 [*figure 4.9 here*] at the same amplification) and are of such size that they may be each due to the electrical variation of a single muscle fibre.

We have sought to examine this phenomenon further by experimental means by sectioning the sciatic nerve in cats under general anaesthesia, and examining the calf muscles at different periods after the nerve section. For this purpose the animal was decerebrated under deep anaesthesia, after the lapse of an appropriate time interval. The anaesthesia was then allowed to pass off and two hours later the muscle concerned was exposed by skin incision, observed by reflected light, and the electrical record of its action currents made. Langley and Kato (1914-15) have established the onset of fibrillation in denervated muscle of the cat on the fifth day after nerve section and we have confirmed this finding. For the first four days following nerve

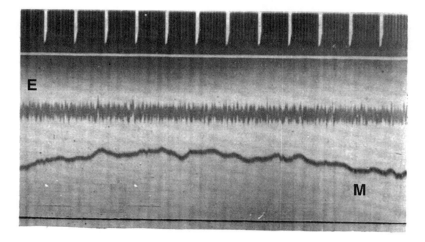

Figure 4.1
Mechanical (M) and electrical (E; electromyogram) record from the mylohyoid muscle of a patient with wasting of this muscle due to syringomyelia. The fibrillation of this muscle, located under the chin, was visible. The vertical white lines at the top of this record and all subsequent records indicate intervals of 0.2 sec. (Reprinted from Denny-Brown and Pennybacker 1938.)

section no fibrillation is observed in the denervated muscle. Its first appearance is in the form of scattered single and very small momentary indentations of the surface of the muscle. Each is accompanied by a single very small diphasic action current (fig. 2 [*figure 4.2 here*]). The electrical change is from 1 to 3 microvolts, but this value is purely relative with needle electrodes. Each twitch can be observed, both by the eye and in the electrical record, to recur at intervals of about two seconds. Fibrillation differs not at all in red and pale muscle fibre in the cat (fig. 3 [*figure 4.3 here*]), as also was noted by Langley and Kato (1914-15). These colour differences, which have been found to be concerned with muscular functions other than the contractile process, (Denny-Brown, 1929) are not affected by the atrophic process until its later stages. When the whole belly of a muscle such as soleus in the cat is observed each indentation is seen to be a momentary tightening in the whole length of a very small part of a muscle fasciculus. It would appear to be the repeated twitching of a single muscle fibre with accompanying very small action current at intervals of two to ten seconds (cf. fig. 2 [*figure 4.2 here*]). Fascicular twitching does not occur.

On the fifth and sixth days few fibres are twitching in this way, and the twitching appears to be confined to those few, the remainder being inactive. Thus only one fibre in a fasciculus may be concerned. On the seventh and later days all fibres are found to have entered upon this phase of recurrent isolated twitchings, and continue to twitch until the muscle is in an advanced state of wasting (fig. 3 [*figure 4.3 here*]). We have not attempted to trace the termination of the process. Langley and Kato (1914-15) observed it up to seventy-one days from time of nerve section.

It is readily ascertained by direct visual observation of the surface of the muscle that the twitches in different fibres have no relationship to each other, the one fibre twitching at a particular rate quite independently of those near or far away. The twitching is inco-ordinate. The final state of confused agitation and the confused action currents of fully developed fibrillation are therefore the result of the combined effect of the irregular mechanical and electrical disturbance in thousands of individual muscle fibres (fig. 3 [*figure 4.3 here*]). In this state it is occasionally possible to observe that one particular twitch or action current is being repeated at intervals of about two-

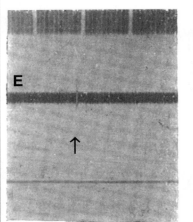

Figure 4.2
Electromyogram from the soleus muscle of a cat six days after denervation. The arrow shows a fibrillation action potential. (Reprinted from Denny-Brown and Pennybacker 1938.)

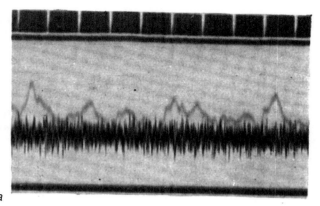

a

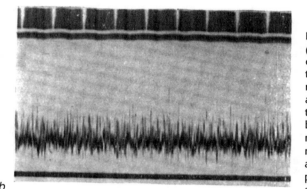

b

Figure 4.3
(a) Mechanical and electrical record of fibrillation in the soleus muscle ("red" muscle) of a cat nine days after denervation. (b) Electrical record of intense fibrillation in the gastrocnemius muscle ("pale" muscle) of a cat nine days after denervation. (Reprinted from Denny-Brown and Pennybacker 1938.)

fifths of a second (fig. 3b [*figure 4.3b here*]). Grouped twitching does not occur until drying or mechanical factors intervene. The electrical action currents become more feeble as the muscle becomes more atrophied.

The appearance of the phenomenon of fibrillation after denervation is associated with the development in degenerating mammalian striped muscle of a particular sensitivity to acetylcholine on the fifth day after denervation, as described by Frank, Nothmann and Hirsch-Kauffmann (1923). The muscle may then enter a spasm of contraction on exposure to an extreme dilution of acetylcholine. Afferent nerve fibres, identical with antidromic vasodilators, distributed in muscle (Hinsey and Gasser, 1930) can by antidromic action liberate a contracting substance, probably acetylcholine, although it is not inhibited by atropine (Frank, Nothmann and Hirsch-Kauffmann, 1923, and Dale and Gaddum, 1930), but fibrillation and atrophy continue in the absence of any sensory or sympathetic innervation. On the other hand, the presence of remaining sensory and sympathetic innervation does not materially alter the process of atrophy in animal experiment (Sherrington, 1892) or in the process of disease in man (poliomyelitis).

It was at first thought that the contracture produced by acetylcholine was not accompanied by action currents (Riesser and Steinhausen, 1923). Schäffer and Licht (1926) and Brown (1937) have found that the contracture is accompanied by fine action currents and have noted that the drug enhances fibrillary contractions. Brown has shown that these small action currents appear with smaller doses, and with a large dose the contracture lasting five to ten seconds occurs, and that this phenomenon is free from action currents. It therefore appeared possible that natural fibrillation may be due to natural acetylcholine.

We observed that a drop of saline containing acetylcholine, diluted 1:500,000, allowed to fall on the surface of a muscle just commencing to fibrillate on the seventh day after nerve section, brought about an immediate local contraction lasting some twelve to twenty seconds (fig. 4b [*figure 4.4b here*]). As the contraction subsided all the muscle fibres in this area remained fibrillating for many minutes, and gradually the disturbance passed by *imperceptible transition* of moderate fibrillation into the original state of a few isolated fibres fibrillating (fig. 4c [*figure 4.4c here*]). Acetylcholine contracture appears therefore to be an intense contraction process of the same essential nature as the phenomenon of fibrillation. It therefore appears likely that true fibrillation is due to the sensitization of the denervated muscle fibre to the small amounts of acetylcholine in the circulating blood. In this connection is of interest that Langley and Kato (1914-15) noted that

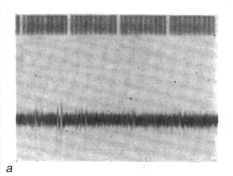

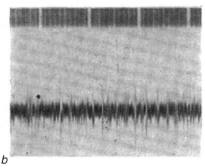

a   b

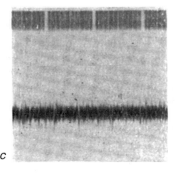

Figure 4.4
(*a*) Electromyogram of the soleus muscle of a cat seven days after denervation. (*b*) Electromyogram immediately after application of 0.1cc of 1:500,000 acetylcholine in saline into the muscle. (*c*) Electromyogram 30 sec later. (Reprinted from Denny-Brown and Pennybacker 1938.)

c

physostigmine (eserine) markedly enhances fibrillation in denervated muscle, but was without effect before the fifth day. In view of the effect of eserine in inhibiting the natural destruction of acetylcholine in the tissues this observation strongly supports our contention that the fibrillation from acetylcholine is not only indistinguishable from spontaneous fibrillation but is identical with it.

We would conclude, therefore, that the fibrillation of muscle undergoing atrophy as a result of denervation is due to periodic rhythmical twitch excitation of each muscle fibre sensitized by neural atrophy. The source of the excitation would appear to be the small amounts of acetylcholine in the normal circulation. We would refer to this phenomenon as "true fibrillation," to distinguish it from other more coarse varieties of muscle twitching to be mentioned below. Such true fibrillation occurs in all voluntary muscles deprived of motor nerve supply. From observations on wasting muscles resulting from diseases affecting motor neurones it would appear that intact sensory nerves to muscle do not influence the phenomenon. In most patients with wasted limb muscles from neuritis or poliomyelitis this fibrillation cannot be observed by clinical examination. When, however, the subcutaneous tissue is unusually thin these muscles can be seen to present the fine characteristic fibrillary tremor. In electromyographic observations (with Dr. S. Nevin) of the wasting muscles of patients suffering from muscular dystrophies including dystrophia myotonica, we have not observed true fibrillation.

(3) The Fasciculation of Muscle in Motor Neurone Disease

Involuntary twitching of muscles has long been recognized as a feature of the course of amyotrophic lateral sclerosis, and its subvarieties, bulbar palsy and progressive muscular atrophy.

The muscles whose nutrition is threatened, or actually damaged, are often jerked by little fibrillary or partial contractions. When this takes place the skin is seen to be raised and depressed as if by the tightening and loosening of delicate cords acting in the direction of the muscles. These contractions are of short duration, but they succeed each other with tolerable rapidity (at intervals of from one to four seconds) and occur in many points of the surface of the muscle. At other times the muscles are agitated with little worm-like movements. In some patients these contractions are almost continuous and occupy a whole limb or a great part of the surface of the body, while in others great attention is necessary to prove their existence, owing to their rarity and weakness, and often they need to be provoked by voluntary or electric stimulation, or by compressing or pinching the muscles. After such stimulation the reflex fibrillary contractions are stronger and more numerous. Partial or fascicular spasmodic contractions sometimes cause little movements of the limbs, especially of the fingers or thumb. Like the foregoing they are short and intermittent, but more rare. (From Duchenne, "L'Electrisation

Localisée," third edition, p. 486, from Selections from the Works of Duchenne, Poore, 1883, London)

In the brief periods of arrest characteristic of the disease, such twitching may disappear for weeks or months at a time. Where it occurs in flat muscles such as pectoralis major it can be readily seen that each twitch involves a bundle of muscle fibres 1 to 3 mm, or more wide, and is a sharp single contraction of that bundle, producing a momentary tightening of its whole length. When the twitching is not too intense it can also be observed that a particular bundle twitches steadily at a particular rate, which varies from one to another with long intervals of five seconds to two minutes. Where the twitching is intense the whole muscle is in continual coarse agitation and the twitching of it in any one place may appear to affect a large muscular bundle in different ways. Each particular shape of twitch is, however, repeated in exact manner after an interval.

In muscles which are extremely wasted, and covered only by a very thin layer of skin and subcutaneous tissue, such as the tongue or the first dorsal interosseous muscle of the hand, this coarse twitching may be seen to be combined with and later replaced by a fine "true" fibrillation such as has been described above for denervated muscle.

Electromyographic records of muscle in this state of coarse twitching (figs. 5 and 6 [*figures 4.5 and 4.6 here*]) show that each fascicular twitch is accompanied by a single large action current. In a long strip of record it can be seen that both the mechanical deformation of the muscle surface, and the accompanying shape of the action current, are individual for each twitch

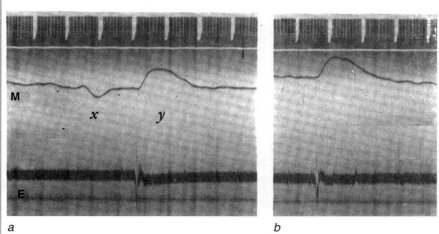

a   b

Figure 4.5
(a) Mechanical and electrical record of the pectoralis major muscle in a patient with amyotrophic lateral sclerosis, with coarse fibrillation. At **x** there occurs a twitch in the underlying intercostal muscle (no action potential in electromyogram) whereas at **y** a twitch occurs in the pectoralis muscle. *(b)* An identical twitch as **y,** but 4.9 sec later. (Reprinted from Denny-Brown and Pennybacker 1938.)

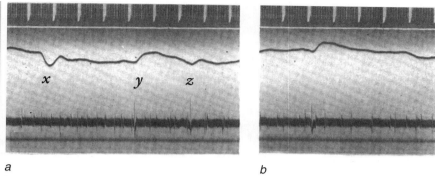

a   *b*

Figure 4.6
(a) Mechanical and electrical record of the pectoralis major in a patient with amyotrophic lateral sclerosis. A slight postural contraction is present, with rhythmical discharge of three small motor units. At **x** there is a twitch in the underlying intercostal muscle (no action potential), whereas those at **y** and **z** are in the pectoralis muscle. *(b)* A continuation of the record showing repetition of the twitch at **y** after an interval of 6.8 sec. (Reprinted from Denny-Brown and Pennybacker 1938.)

and that each particular combination is repeated again and again at long intervals, such as 4.9 and 6.8 seconds for that shown in figs. 5 and 6 [*figures 4.5 and 4.6 here*]. Where the twitching is too complex to identify individual twitches by the naked eye, the electromyographic and mechanical records still show that any one shape of twitch is repeated at relatively long intervals (figs. 7 and 10 [*figures 4.7 and 4.8 here*]).

The regularity in position, size and shape of action current of each involuntary twitch of the "fasciculation" of this disease points to its being *a single impulse contraction in a fixed group of muscle fibres*. The group is smaller than a muscular fasciculus, but much larger than one single muscle fibre. The only functional group of this nature in muscle is the motor unit. If this twitching were the result of the reception of a nerve impulse by the whole

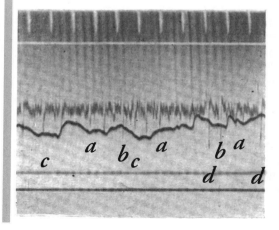

Figure 4.7
Mechanical and electrical record of the triceps muscle of a patient with an advanced stage of amyotrophic lateral sclerosis showing rapid coarse fasciculation and fine fibrillation. The complicated electromyogram shows various shapes of action potentials, marked **a, b, c, d**, being repeated at intervals varying from 0.5 to 10 sec and longer. (Reprinted from Denny-Brown and Pennybacker 1938.)

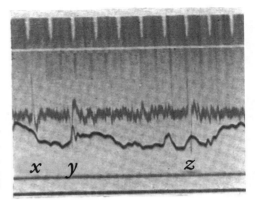

Figure 4.8
Mechanical and electrical record of the triceps from a patient with an advanced stage of amyotrophic lateral sclerosis. Various types of twitches of one large fasciculus are shown. The one marked **x** had occurred 4.4 sec earlier and was repeated 5.4 sec later. The one marked **y** occurred 4.8 sec earlier and recurred 5.4 sec later. The one marked **z** occurred 8.2 sec earlier and recurred 2.3 sec later. (Reprinted from Denny-Brown and Pennybacker 1938.)

group of muscle fibres supplied by a motor nerve fibre, it would follow that the origin of the impulse must be related either to a pathological process in the nerve fibre itself, or in the parent anterior horn cell. From the pathology of this disease we can suspect the latter.

This phenomenon, commonly called "fibrillation," but more properly called "fasciculation," may therefore represent the intermittent involuntary discharge of single nerve impulses by an abnormal motor neurone. These abnormal action currents are in fact comparable in size and shape to the individual discharge of single moderately sized motor units. By instructing the patient to contract the muscle slightly by involuntary effort, the characteristic rhythmical discharge of normal motor units can be made to appear in the electromyogram, accompanying the contraction. A strong or moderately strong willed contraction is accompanied by a confusion of action currents, but by arranging that a very weak contraction is produced, a few simple action current rhythms can be obtained (fig. 11 [*figure 4.9 here*]). Discharge provoked in this way is a rhythmical series of nerve impulses at a rate of five to twenty-five a second. The resulting muscular contraction is a partly fused series of twitches, but the action currents, being much more brief, appear as a regular series of identical shape.

It was of interest to observe if a motor unit which showed "fasciculation" could be excited to normal willed discharge. Normally the *same* motor units always begin the discharge in a very slight muscular contraction—apparently particular units are always the first to contract in the beginning of that particular willed movement. We searched for "fibrillating" units which could thus be possibly called into activity early in slight voluntary movement, and in due course found several examples (fig. 8 [*figure 4.10 here*]). Here there was no doubt that the disordered motor neurone could also discharge a normal series of identical nerve impulses in response to willed effort. It is presumed that the other fasciculating units also did so but came so late into contraction that their discharge was swamped in the

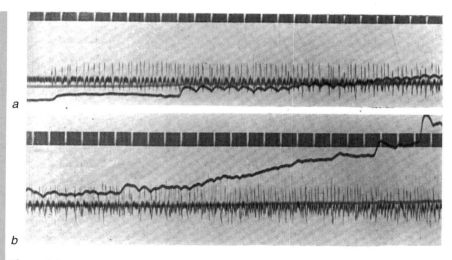

Figure 4.9
Mechanical and electrical record of a normal contraction of biceps brachii. *(a)* The electromyogram shows the rhythmical discharge of motor units becoming more intense by the addition of separate units, each with a slightly larger action potential. *(b)* Continuation of the record after 2.2 sec, showing further increase in activity of motor units. (Reprinted from Denny-Brown and Pennybacker 1938.)

resulting intensity of electrical fluctuation. The units observed in this way were fasciculating at moderately long intervals of five to thirty seconds. Voluntary discharge of the type enhances the "fibrillation" so that in the few seconds following the movement fasciculation is more rapid in that particular unit. This appears to substantiate our conclusion that the site of the abnormality leading to the involuntary twitching is closely related to the excitable portion of the neurone, the cell membrane or the synapse. The disorder is not *directly* related to the process of excitation, for these units are neither more nor less readily excited by voluntary effort than is any random unit sampled by the electromyogram. Their discharge was regular and not subject to abnormal lapses or ease of fatigue. We also observed that percussion and cooling enhanced fasciculation, apparently by also inducing a light voluntary discharge. On account of the naked-eye resemblance of early shivering to this twitching, we do not recommend these procedures for facilitating the observation of the disorder in the clinic, though the electromyographic record is distinctive in shivering (Denny-Brown, Gaylor, and Uprus, 1935), being a grouped sustained discharge.

In the course of a willed movement of moderate degree of any one muscle group at a joint, there occurs complete cessation of tonic and other action currents in the directly antagonistic muscle group. This is not necessarily true for contraction of synergists, but the discharge of the motor neurones is inhibited in the course of direct reciprocal innervation. We have observed

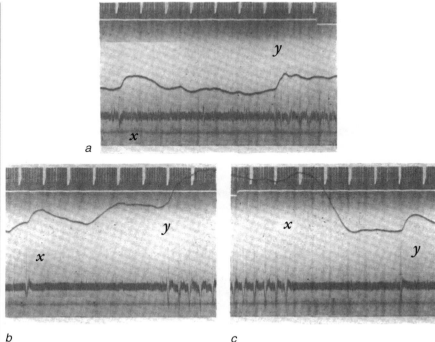

Figure 4.10
Mechanical and electrical record of the pectoralis major in a patient with amyotrophic lateral sclerosis. *(a)* Spontaneous fascicular twitch occurs at **x;** at **y** the patient begins a slight voluntary movement, resulting in repetitive discharge and contraction of the same motor unit. *(b)* Similar spontaneous twitch in another part of the muscle is shown at **x,** and its discharge in response to voluntary movement at **y.** *(c)* The voluntary discharge is seen terminating 1.8 sec after beginning; enhanced fibrillation begins at **y,** and for three irregular beats occurs at intervals of 0.6 sec (not shown). (Reprinted from Denny-Brown and Pennybacker 1938.)

that the motor unit discharge of amyotrophic lateral sclerosis cannot be inhibited in this way by willed contraction of a direct antagonist as prime mover (fig. 9 [*figure 4.11 here*]). We have therefore demonstrated that "central excitatory state" (Sherrington, 1929) can be set up, and the neurone thus caused to discharge naturally, and "central inhibitory state" is unaffected and does not interfere with fasciculation. These processes are related to the synapse. It is to be concluded that the disorder underlying fasciculation is situated in the cell body or its dendrites and not at or outside its surface, and is a precursor of atrophy of the neurone.

In wasting muscles the coarse fasciculation and fine fibrillation are concomitant, which is to be expected from the known true degeneration of the motor neurone which eventually occurs. Here the contrast between the size of the action currents of fibrillation and fasciculation can be seen in the same record (fig. 10 [*figure 4.8 here*]). With needle electrodes only a small

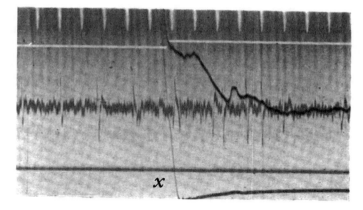

Figure 4.11
Mechanical and electrical record of the triceps muscle from a patient with amyotrophic lateral sclerosis. The patient was strongly contracting the antagonistic elbow flexors before the record began. This contraction ends at **x.** Coarse fasciculation and fibrillation occur irregularly during the effort, which abolishes all other electrical activity in the muscle. (Reprinted from Denny-Brown and Pennybacker 1938.)

electrical field is sampled and the difference in size between muscle fibre action current and motor unit action current is therefore relative and not absolute.

(4) Fascicular Tremor Appearing With Contraction ("Contraction Fasciculation")

Coarse tremors of fasciculi in limb muscles are often observable in subjects of wasting diseases. Such tremor is liable to confusion with the spasmodic fasciculation of amyotrophic lateral sclerosis described above, especially since it may occur in combination with it in that disease, or alone in other affections, or with true fibrillation following poliomyelitis or polyneuritis. It is quite independent of either "true fasciculation" or "true fibrillation" in that it disappears completely with complete relaxation of the muscle.

In characteristic form it is seen as a coarse rhythmical tremor of a fasciculus at a rate of from 5 to 20 a second. The contraction is strong enough sometimes to cause wavering of an extended finger. With stronger contraction other fasciculi show similar tremors, but with moderate to maximal contraction the twitching grows more rapid and may be swamped by the contraction of other fibres in the muscle. In muscles such as pectoralis it can be observed that the contraction involves only part of a fasciculus.

In myographic records the twitching is a regular discharge exactly comparable to that of a motor neurone, though the resulting twitches of the muscle are poorly fused even at higher rates of discharge (figs. 12b, 12c [*figures 4.12, b and c here*]). The individual mechanical twitches are much larger than those of the usual motor units to come early into action in a willed movement, and their discharge is not so rapid. The onset is always at a certain stage in a particular movement in the muscle concerned, sometimes with only slight postural contraction (fig. 12a [*figure 4.12a here*]). The phenomenon is encountered in our experience only where the muscle is notably wasted, but would appear to be the normal discharge of a very large motor unit.

The tremulous motor unit is not necessarily the first to discharge in contraction and when different muscles are observed the tremor is seen to enter the contraction at different stages. As has been stated above, a particular voluntary movement appears to begin always with discharge of the same motor unit. More intense contraction is secured by the addition of more and more units added in a particular sequence (fig. 11 [*figure 4.9 here*]). This "recruitment" of motor units into willed contraction is identical

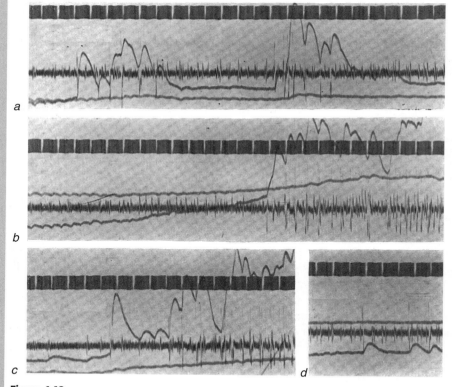

Figure 4.12
Mechanical and electrical record from the atrophied biceps brachii of a patient with progressive muscular atrophy, showing only fasciculations during muscle contraction. (*a*) Occasional periodic twitching during slight elbow flexion. (*b*) Twitching in another unit occurring late in a voluntary movement. (*c*) Twitching occurring early in another voluntary movement. (*d*) Occasional isolated twitches with slight movement such as holding the limb forward. (Reprinted from Denny-Brown and Pennybacker 1938.)

with that occurring in certain reflexes (Liddell and Sherrington, 1923, Sherrington, 1929). The early motor units in normal gradual voluntary contraction are always in our experience small ones (fig. 11 [*figure 4.9 here*]). The larger and more powerful motor units, each controlling many more muscle fibres, enter contraction late. In a muscle wasted by loss of many motor neurones graduation of contraction becomes uneven because large motor units become active without sufficient previous recruitment of small units to smooth their contraction. That they are contracting in the same manner with the rest of the muscle in a normal individual is indicated by the size of the action currents in intense contraction. Their frequency corresponds with that of the muscle sound (15 to 35 a second [Wollaston, 1810]) and appears to us its probable explanation.

We believe that the isolation of large motor units by relatively preponderating atrophy of small ones is an explanation which best serves the facts of "contraction fasciculation."

(5) Coarse Local Tetanic Fasciculation ("False Fibrillation")

Clinicians recognize types of benign "fasciculation" or "fibrillation," which occur in muscles not subject to a wasting disease. Of these a twitching of the orbicularis oculi of the lower lid with fatigue or debility is one type within general experience. Occasional very localized twitching in a calf muscle is also common, and a more generalized form affecting the calf muscles and the small muscles of the feet and hands is described as "myokymia" after Schultze (1895) and Kny (1888). In the latter condition irregular contractions of fasciculi of muscles gives a slow undulation of the surface.

This type of contraction has a longer duration than that of the forms of fibrillation described above. For some one to three seconds the contraction pursues either a rapidly interrupted course as is common in orbicularis oculi, or a deliberate sustained spasm. The contraction appears in the same place at irregular intervals, and is often large enough to make the subject conscious of its occurrence, and he cannot suppress it. It is not related to willed movement.

The *sensation* of twitching appears to result from the size of the structure involved, for other fibrillation is sensible according to its size, and in the type with which we are concerned here the structure involved is of the size of a whole fasciculus.

Records of such twitching confirm the impressions gained from visual observation. Both in the calf (fig. 14 [*figure 4.13 here*]) and in orbicularis oculi (fig. 15 [*figure 4.14 here*]) the twitch is in fact a partly fused muscular contraction with repetitive nervous discharge which is irregular in time interval, and often in shape as well. The irregularity in shape of successive action currents points to a focus of irritation which is not nervous, but affects unevenly a bundle of nerve fibres in the fasciculus.

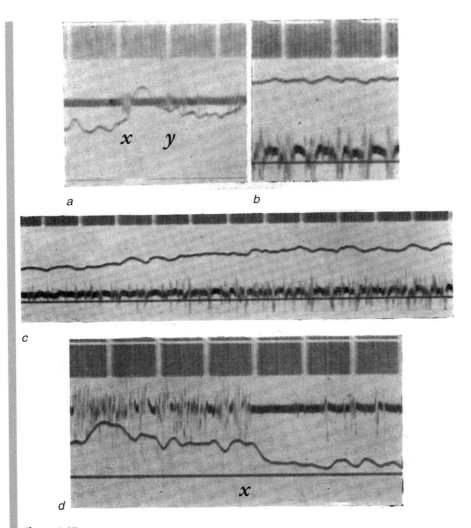

Figure 4.13
Mechanical and electrical record from the gastrocnemius muscle of a patient with myokymia and cramps in both lower limbs. *(a)* A wave of cramps occurs at **x** accompanied by a very rapid electrical discharge lasting 0.4 sec. Some slight normal discharge occurs at **y**. *(b)* Intense cramp with periodic high frequency discharge. *(c)* A voluntary movement develops into a cramp with a modification of a normal action potential into a high frequency discharge. *(d)* A cramp ends suddenly at **x**. (Reprinted from Denny-Brown and Pennybacker 1938.)

In a patient suffering from generalized myokymia, associated with cramps of the legs ("paramyotonia") we obtained records of both phenomena (fig. 14 [*figure 4.13 here*]). In myokymia a fasciculus is suddenly involved in intense high frequency discharge lasting one-twentieth to one-tenth of a second (fig. 14a [*figure 4.13a here*]). The resulting contraction is a

Figure 4.14
Mechanical and electrical record of the lower lid from a patient with involuntary twitching of the orbicularis oculi muscle. A small series of sharp movements is evident in the mechanical record, accompanied by a small repetitive activity in the electrical record. Each wave of activity is indicated by an arrow. At **x**, the patient blinked. (Reprinted from Denny-Brown and Pennybacker 1938.)

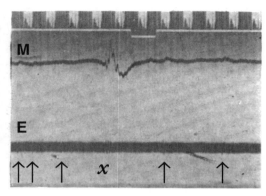

Figure 4.15
Mechanical and electrical record from the biceps brachii of a patient with generalized muscle weakness. A coarse fascicular wave of contraction lasting 1 sec is recorded on a background of slight postural discharge. (Reprinted from Denny-Brown and Pennybacker 1938.)

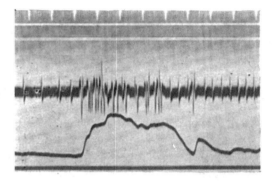

slow wave. This type of contraction occurs in different fasciculi independently and intermittently. A cramp takes the form of rhythmical high frequency discharge of this kind (fig. 14b [*figure 4.13b here*]). We observed the transition of the action currents of willed movement into periodic intense cramp action currents (fig. 14c [*figure 4.13c here*]). Occasionally the intense discharge will last a second or more without intermission, and then cease suddenly (fig. 14d [*figure 4.14d here*]) or become transformed into the intermittent type. The contraction is fascicular, and in our view is but an intense form of the fasciculation of fatigue (fig. 13 [*figure 4.15 here*]).

While further examination of the focus is beyond the means at our disposal, we regard this phenomenon of "false fibrillation" and "myokymia" as one probably related to vascular cramp, or other change in the vessels which supply the fasciculus. Cramps in the same muscles commonly affect the subjects of myokymia. It has not in our experience been relieved by calcium, though improvement in the general health of the subject usually leads to its disappearance.

It is noteworthy in this connection that on the one hand Langley (1915-16b) noted that fascicular contraction occurred in frog muscle at a moderate stage of fatigue, and that on the other Kny and Schultze both noted in generalized myokymia that their patients suffered from greatly enhanced sweating. Excessive perspiration was also a disorder obvious in the two patients suffering from generalized myokymia observed by us. These observations indicate that fatigue may derange the excitability of the motor nerve in or near the muscle, and that disturbance of sodium chloride balance may in particular cause such derangement, in other forms than cramp. It may be stressed therefore that the incomplete relief of the condition by exhibition of sodium chloride indicates that the neurosis or exhaustion state underlying fatigue or hyperhidrosis requires also to be treated in patients subject to this disorder.

Conclusions

(1) Close inspection of spontaneous twitching of muscle fibres reveals characteristics which enable the situation of the disturbance of excitability to be deduced. The single discharges of disordered anterior horn cells are thus distinguishable from the more coarse and longer twitches arising from affections of the intramuscular nerves, and both are distinct from the fine fibrillation of denervated muscle. Combinations of the various types may occur.

(2) Hyperexcitability of motoneurones in diseases such as progressive muscular atrophy or amyotrophic lateral sclerosis results in regularly periodic discharges of single impulses by the motor neurone. The focus of irritation is not at the synapse, but within the neurone. The resulting fasciculation at rest should be distinguished from rapid fasciculation during contraction ("contraction fasciculation").

(3) Denervated muscle fibres contract periodically, and the confused medley of small twitches constitutes true fibrillation. The movement is so slight that it can seldom be seen in the clinic. The twitching appears to be due to heightened excitability of the sarcolemma, or rapidly conducting portion of the muscle fibre, to traces of free acetylcholine in the tissues.

(4) In circumstances of fatigue or excessive loss of sodium chloride involuntary muscular contractions appear. Those due to fatigue are small bursts of contraction in a fasciculus, and are of a type such as would be caused by irregular discharge spreading to and through all the nerve bundles in the fasciculus. Those of myokymia, associated with hyperhidrosis are of similar nature but of more widespread distribution, and more intense discharge. Both are clearly related to muscular cramp. The prolonged discharge, compared with the single twitch of fibrillation and the fasciculation of neurone discharge, give the resulting fascicular movement a slower, undulating appearance.

We wish to acknowledge with gratitude the use of electromyographic apparatus provided by the Medical Research Council, and the permission given by various members of the Medical Staff of the National Hospital, Queen Square, to interest patients under their care in submitting themselves to this investigation.

References

Brown, G.L. (1937), *J. Physiol.,* **89,** 220–237, 438–461.
Dale, H.H., and Gaddum, J.H. (1930), *J. Physiol.,* **70,** 109–144.
Denny-Brown, D. (1929), *Proc. Ray. Soc.,* **104b,** 371–411.
Denny-Brown, D., Gaylor, J.B., and Uprus, V. (1935), *Brain* **58,** 233–237.
Duchenne, G.B.A. (1883). *Selections from the works of Duchenne.* Poore: London.
Frank, E., Nothmann, M., and Hirsh-Kaufmann, H. (1923), *Pflüg. Arch. ges. Physiol.,* **197,** 270–287.
Hinsey, C.H. and Gasser, H.S. (1930), *Amer. J. Physiol.* **92,** 679–689.
Kny, E. (1888), *Arch. Psychiat. Nervenke.,* **19,** 577–590.
Langley, J.N. (1915-16a), *J. Physiol.,* **50,** 404–407.
Langley, J.N. (1915-16b), *Proc. Physiol. Soc.,* **xxvi.**
Langley, J.N., and Kato, T. (1914–15), *J. Physiol.,* **49,** 15–69.
Liddell, E.G.T., and Sherrington, C.S. (1923)., *Proc. Roy. Soc.,* **95b,** 407–412.
Riesser, O., and Steinhausen, W. (1923), *Pflüg. Arch. ges. Physiol.,* **197,** 288–299.
Schäffer and Licht (1926), not provided.
Schiff, M. (1851), *Arch. Physiol. Heilk.,* **10,** 579–593.
Schultze, Fr. (1895). *Deutsch. Z. Nervenheilk.,* **6,** 65–75 and 167–168.
Sherrington, C.S. (1892), *J. Physiol.,* **13,** 621–772.
Sherrington, C.S. (1929), *Proc. Roy. Soc.,* **105b,** 322–362.
Wollaston, W.H. (1810). *Phil. Trans. Roy. Soc. Lond.,* **100,** 1–15.

Summary

Denny-Brown was a pioneer in the use of the electromyograph in clinical medicine. For this paper, he and Pennybacker detail how the electrodes are arranged for use of this device to measure an "action current"; that is, one electrode is the hypodermic needle and the other is a thin copper wire inserted through the canal within the needle. Both are inserted into a muscle, which enables the measurement of the electrical activity that occurs with the firing of the muscle fibers being sampled. Furthermore, Denny-Brown used an ingenious balloon device to measure and record the physical activity of the muscle at the same time.

Denny-Brown and Pennybacker used this methodology to differentiate fasciculation from fibrillation. Fibrillation was shown to be "twitching" of single muscle fibers occurring as a muscle undergoes atrophy, resulting, in turn, from disease of its motor neuron. The authors further suggested that fibrillation occurs as the fibers become sensitized to the small amounts of acetylcholine in the circulating blood. Since publication of this paper it has become common to consider the presence of "sharp wave potentials" characteristic of lower motoneuron disease.

For fasciculations, in contrast, Denny-Brown and Pennybacker used the electromyography records to demonstrate that the data are only consistent with a simultaneous contraction of the group of muscle fibers that constitute a motor unit. Thus, fasciculation represents the intermittent involuntary activity of an abnormal motoneuron. Denny-Brown and Pennybacker also showed in this paper that fasciculations were immune to the cessation of activity that normally occurs in a muscle when its antagonist is activated.

With this report Denny-Brown and Pennybacker were the first to describe the electromyographic features of ordinary muscle cramps. On the basis of these features, they concluded that cramps represent fascicular contractions, probably related to changes in the blood vessels that supply the fascicle.

A principle underlying the orderly recruitment of motor units in a particular muscle is known as "Henneman's size principle," which states that motoneuron size forms the basis of this recruitment. Specifically, smaller motor units are recruited before larger ones. Credit for development of this principle has gone to Henneman, who first published an article on this subject in 1957. However, as is evidenced on page 117 of Denny-Brown and Pennybacker, this idea was actually first developed almost 20 years earlier by these two authors. Thus, the principle should in fact be known as the Denny-Brown and Pennybacker principle (Vilensky and Gilman, 1998).

References

Henneman, E. (1957). *Science,* **126,** 1345–1346.
Vilensky, J.A., and Gilman, S. (1998), *Science,* **280,** 2031.
Vilensky, J.A., Gilman, S., and Dunn, E. (1998), *J. Med. Biol.,* **6,** 73–78.

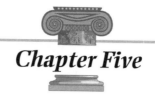
Mechanical Work in Human Movement: Comments on Papers by Fenn and Elftman

Vladimir M. Zatsiorsky

The Pennsylvania State University

Revisiting the work of Wallace O. Fenn, with the assistance of C.A. Morrison, and the work of Herbert Elftman

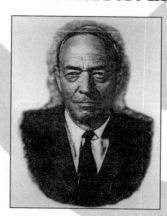

Wallace Osgood Fenn
Reprinted from Fenn 1963.

Wallace Osgood Fenn

Dr. Wallace Osgood Fenn was born on August 27, 1893, in Lanesboro, Massachusetts. He received his bachelor's degree (1914) and his master's degree (1916) from Harvard. During World War I he served in the Sanitary Corps. Upon discharge, Fenn finished his doctoral thesis in 1919 and started an appointment at the Harvard Medical School. From 1922 to 1924 he was a Rockefeller Institute Travelling Fellow along with A.V. Hill and Sir Henry Dale in England. After returning to the United States, he accepted a position as the chair of physiology at the School of Medicine and Dentistry at the University of Rochester, New York. In 1959 he was named a Distinguished Professor of Physiology. He became the director of the Space Science Center of the University in 1962. Dr. Fenn died on September 20, 1971.

Between 1916 and 1972, Dr. Fenn published 267 scientific papers in several scientific fields. He received many academic honors and awards. These included honorary degrees, honorary society memberships, the presidency of many scientific societies, and major scientific prizes. A most unusual award was the dedication of the *Respiration Suite* to him by the Dutch composer Jurriaan Andriessen. The jacket of the recording contained the following statement:

> An understanding of the musical performance of these artists, in a physiological sense, rests to a large extent on the work of Dr. Wallace O. Fenn and his associates on the pressure-volume relationship of the lungs and chest, on the composition of alveolar air during breath holding, and on physiological effects of pressure breathing.

The scientific interests of Dr. Fenn were very broad. He became immediately famous for his study on the heat production of muscle, published in 1924. Before Fenn, it had been believed that muscles behaved in a springlike fashion. If a spring is stretched, it stores a certain amount of potential energy. When the spring is released, part of the potential energy is spent for the production of mechanical work and the rest is dissipated as heat. The total amount of energy liberated by the spring remains constant (work + heat = potential energy). Hence, in springs, the larger the amount of work performed, the smaller the amount of heat dissipated. While studying muscle contraction, Fenn discovered that the amount of heat increased when the muscle shortened; the extra heat production was proportional to the external work done by the muscle. Opposite to the behavior seen in springs, increase in the amount of mechanical work produced in muscles causes concomitant increase in heat production. Consequently, in muscles it was shown that work + heat potential ener gy. Muscle shortening is an active process that requires the supply of energy. In this regard, muscles are not similar to prestretched springs that shorten passively. A.V. Hill was the first to refer to this discovery as the Fenn Effect, and it has been known as such ever since.

Dr. Fenn made several other important discoveries in muscle physiology. He was first to show that potassium is lost from muscle in exchange for sodium during contraction and that in recovery the process is reversed. He also described the force-velocity relationship of muscle (Fenn and Marsh, 1935). In 1942, Dr. Fenn was elected to the National Academy of Sciences. At this time he changed his scientific interests to human respiration. He soon conducted many classic studies in respiratory physiology. He was the first to study pressure-volume diagrams, the work of breathing, pulmonary compliance, airway resistance, the alveolar gas equation, and other topics that can be found in any university-level textbook on respiration. In the 1960s, his scientific interests shifted to the physiology of space flight and underwater physiology. Dr. Fenn's interest in human biomechanics was enduring, and his achievements in this field were substantial (see "Selected Readings").

Dr. Fenn was a man of wisdom and a good sense of humor. The following "fable of the cats" was taken from one of his talks and may serve as an example. The topic of discussion was the relationship between basic and applied science.

> A man called up a veterinarian about his sick cat and described its symptoms. The veterinarian understood "calf" for "cat" and prescribed a pint of castor oil, which was duly administered (more or less). Some days later the veterinarian met his client and inquired about the welfare of the patient. The man threw up his hands in despair and said that the cat had had a hard time and had enlisted the assistance of three other cats. One was digging holes for him, the second was covering them up, and the third was way out in front opening up new territory. We probably need and should have two applied researchers for every one in basic research, but we cannot do without the latter—the fellows who are out in front opening up new fields and developing new interpretations, new products, new ideas, and new methods. (Fenn 1949)

Dr. Wallace O. Fenn was certainly such a man.

Selected Readings

Fenn, W.O. (1924). The relation between the work performed and the energy liberated in muscular contraction. *Journal of Physiology (London), 58,* 373-395.

Fenn, W.O. (1929). Mechanical energy expenditure in sprint running as measured by moving pictures. *American Journal of Physiology, 90,* 343.

Fenn, W.O. (1930). Frictional and kinetic factors in the work of sprint running. *American Journal of Physiology, 92,* 583-611.

Fenn, W.O. (1930). Work against gravity and work due to velocity changes in running. *American Journal of Physiology, 93,* 433-462.

Fenn, W.O. (1932). Zur Mechanik des Radfahrens in Vergleich zu des Laufens. *Pflüger's Archive Für Die Gesamte Physiologie, 229,* 354-366.

Fenn, W.O., & Garvey, P.H. (1934). The measurement of the elasticity and viscosity of skeletal muscle in normal and pathological case: A study of so-called 'muscle tonus.' *Journal of Clinical Investigation, 13,* 383-397.

Fenn, W.O., & Marsh, B.S. (1935). Muscular force at different speeds of shortening. *Journal of Physiology, 85,* 277-297.

Fenn, W.O. (1938). The mechanics of muscular contraction in man. *Journal of Applied Physics,*
19, 165-175.

Fenn, W.O. (1949). Physiology on horseback. *America Journal of Physiology, 159,* 551-555.

Fenn, W.O. (1957). The mechanics of standing on the toes. *American Journal of Physical Medicine, 36,* 153-156.

Herbert Elftman

When we arrived at the idea of publishing a book that would include the
most influential studies in the biomechanics of human motion and motor
control from the last century, we sent an e-mail message to the approximately 3500 users of the BIOMCH-L forum. We asked for opinions on the
studies that should be included in the volume. The work of Dr. H. Elftman
was included in almost all the recommendations. However, when we later
sent a second letter to BIOMCH-L users asking for personal information
on Dr. Elftman, no one was able to help us. We knew that in the 1930s Dr.
Elftman had been with the Department of Zoology at Columbia University, New York. This department no longer exists, so we were unable to ask
anyone from the department for help. We contacted the university library
and university archive, and through the kind help of Kathleen M. Kehoe,
we received the following message:

Dear Colleague:

Herb Elftman was at the Department of Anatomy, College of Physicians and
Surgeons, Columbia University, from sometime in the late 1940s until his
retirement in 1968.

I am not certain precisely when he arrived here, but when I entered as a
graduate student in 1951 he was the Course Director in Gross Anatomy, and
he held that position until retirement. I had the great pleasure of working
under him for a great many years, and he literally, made me a competent
teacher. He passed away some while ago, on the west coast.

Cordially,

Melvin L. Moss, Professor Emeritus, Anatomy and Cell Biology

This is the only information about Herbert Elftman that we were able to
obtain. It is really a pity that the history of our science is so neglected and
that knowledge about its great contributors is not better preserved.

Selected Readings

Elftman, H. (1934). A cinematic study of the distribution of the center of pressure in the human foot. *Anatomical Record, 59,* 481-491.

Elftman, H. (1939). Forces and energy changes in the leg during walking. *American Journal of
Physiology, 125,* 339-356.

Elftman, H. (1939). The function of the arms in walking. *Human Biology, 2,* 529-535.

Elftman, H. (1939). The function of the muscles in locomotion. *American Journal of Physiology,*
125, 357-366.

Elftman, H. (1939). The rotation of the body in walking. *Arbeitsphysiologie, 10,* 477-483.

Elftman, H. (1940). The work done by muscles in running. *American Journal of Physiology, 129,* 672-684.

Elftman, H. (1944). Skeletal and muscular system: Structure and function. *Medical Physics* (pp. 1420-1430). Chicago: Year Book.

Elftman, H. (1966). Biomechanics of muscle with particular application to studies of gait. *Journal of Bone and Joint Surgery, 48-A,* 363-377.

Elftman, H. (1969). Dynamic structure of the human foot. *Artificial Limbs, 13* (1), 49-58.

Frictional and Kinetic Factors in the Work of Sprint Running*

Wallace O. Fenn, with the assistance of C.A. Morrison
From the Department of Physiology, School of Medicine and Dentistry, University of Rochester, Rochester, New York

Received for publication October 30, 1929

[Introduction]

If one divides the energy equivalent of the total excess oxygen consumed as a result of a short sprint at top speed by the number of seconds occupied in the run, one finds[1] (after correcting for the start and the pull up) (cf. Sargent, 1926) that the rate of energy expenditure while running at a maximum speed is about 13 horse power for an average man. From measurements on isolated muscles (Hill, 1926) as well as from calculations made by Furusawa, Hill and Parkinson (1927) on sprinters, it may be concluded that about 40 per cent of this energy was expended during the sprint in the "initial" or anaerobic phase of muscle contraction, the remainder representing the inefficiency of recovery. The present paper is concerned with the disposition of this initial energy which is being expended at a rate of about 5.2 horse power.[2]

The conclusions reached and the problems involved are illustrated in the following diagram:

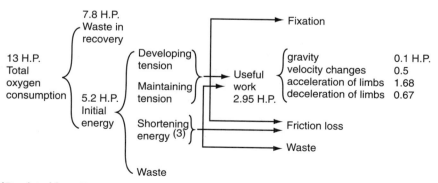

*Reprinted from Fenn 1930.

Some of the arrows in this diagram should be accompanied by question marks. Thus the source of the work is doubtful, whether from shortening energy or previously developed potential (tension) energy. It is also possible that the "shortening energy"[3] is partly wasted or partly used to overcome friction. The point of chief interest in this diagram, however, is the magnitude of the rate of useful work which has actually been measured from moving pictures and was found to be 2.95 horse power. The various items which are included in this figure are shown in the last column and include work against gravity, changes in velocity due to wind resistance and to bringing the foot into contact with the ground, and the kinetic energy changes of the limbs. Marey and Demeney in 1885 made an estimate of the magnitude of these various components of the work. Their estimates for the first two items agree fairly well with ours but their estimate of the kinetic energy of the limbs was 7 or 8 times too small because they measured only the average velocity of the limbs during a swing, neglected movements around the knee and elbow joints and neglected the back swings (ef. Amar, 1923, p. 504). In walking, the work against gravity is a much more important factor than in running and indeed Benedict and Murschhauser (1915) found it to be 23 per cent of the total oxygen consumption in excess of the standing value. Hill (1927), who has discussed in many valuable papers the problems connected with rapid movements of muscles, has regarded frictional loss as a limiting factor in a fast run and as in fact the only item of considerable importance. From the above diagram, however, it is obvious that, after deducting the work, only 5.2 minus 2.95 or 2.25 horse power is left to be divided between the three items of fixation energy, waste heat and frictional loss. The isometric contractions involved in making the body rigid and in fixating the joints, etc., are by no means negligible although there is no method of measuring them exactly; hence the energy left for frictional loss is not so large as has been supposed. In order to show how significant this conclusion is for the theory of muscular contraction, some further discussion of muscle viscosity is necessary.

A New Method of Demonstrating Muscle "Viscosity"

The problem of "muscle viscosity" can be clearly presented as applied to man, by the following experiment in which the muscle tension is measured as it decreases with increasing speed of movement. The subject seats himself on a table with one leg hanging over the edge. Arrangements are made for recording variations in the angle of the knee with time as the leg swings from the knee. This is most easily done by fastening the leg to a light wheel, the horizontal axis of which coincides with the axis of the knee joint. As the wheel revolves with the leg it winds up a thread carrying a short pointer; the thread is held taut by an elastic band. The curve traced by the pointer on a revolving drum as the leg swings indicates angles plotted against time. The slope of this curve represents the angular velocity in radians per second.

If the angular velocity is plotted as a function of time the slope of the resulting graph represents angular acceleration and must be proportional at any moment to the torque applied to the leg at that time. The proportionality factor is the moment of inertia of the leg around the knee axis. This may be estimated with fair accuracy from the measurements of Braune and Fischer (1892) on cadavers and enables us to calculate the net external force exerted by the muscles at any moment in the swing. If the subject endeavors to extend his lower leg when the knee angle is 90° while the torque is measured with a spring balance it is found that he can develop a force of 19 kgm. at a distance of 43 cm. from the knee axis. If the lever arm of the extensor muscle is 4 cm. this indicates a force of $\frac{43}{4} \times 19$ or 204 kgm.

If while the muscles are exerting this torque the experimentor suddenly releases the foot, the torque imparts an acceleration to the lower leg which can be measured from the graphic record. If the moment of inertia of the leg below the knee be taken as 3×10^6 gram and centimeter units, the torque producing the acceleration can be calculated (torque = moment of inertia $\times$ angular acceleration). Analysis of a quick release record obtained in this way shows that before the foot has traveled 2 cm. the force exerted by the extensor muscles (on a 4 cm. arm) has fallen from 204 to 108 kgm. and when the foot has moved to 4 cm. the force has fallen to 55 kgm. When the foot has moved 6 cm. the velocity has become constant; there is no further acceleration and hence no further external force except that necessary to overcome friction in the joint.

In a similar manner a record of a free kick with the lower leg was taken. The angular acceleration was determined from the record and thence the force exerted at different times was calculated. In this case a maximum external force of about 142 kgm. was developed after the foot had moved about 1 cm. but by the time the foot had moved 5.3 cm. of the arc the velocity had become so great that a tension of only 37 kgm. could be maintained.

Critique of Measurements of Muscle "Viscosity"

These results show in a fairly quantitative way how extremely quickly the tension falls off in a muscle after it is suddenly released and how small a tension can be maintained when a muscle is rapidly shortening. This failure to develop tension while shortening may, in this case, be due partly to a reflex cessation of stimulation or a reflex inhibition and there would seem to be every reason for expecting that such a reflex would occur. On the other hand, the loss of tension during shortening may be due to some characteristic of the muscle itself since it has likewise been demonstrated in isolated muscles (Hill, 1926). With this idea in mind it has been called "muscle viscosity." The term implies that some internal rearrangements inside the muscles are necessary before external tension can be displayed and that it is a *mechanical* resistance to these movements which prevents a muscle from re-developing tension, during shortening, rapidly enough to manifest tension externally. But in this case, the delay in the development of tension might equally well be in some chemical reaction involving the mobilization of the necessary energy for the contraction. In such a case the term "viscosity" would be inappropriate. The fact that the process of developing tension during shortening (Fenn, 1923) necessitates an extra liberation of energy (shortening energy) and that within certain limits the faster the shortening the less extra energy developed, suggests this latter interpretation. Hartree and Hill (1928) in their most recent communication on this subject have confirmed in the main the finding that shortening under tension involves extra energy liberation and have taken it more seriously into consideration in their theories than heretofore, suggesting that it has an equal share with viscosity in determining the amount of work a muscle may do at different speeds of shortening. For the reasons here suggested it seems advisable to warn against the simple interpretation of the term "viscosity." There seems to be as yet no certain way of determining how quantitatively important "viscosity" or friction may be in muscular movements in man. By "viscosity," I mean a mechanical as opposed to a chemical delay in the external manifestation of tension.

In 1922 Hill published an important paper on the work of human arm muscles, contracting against different equivalent masses. With a small equivalent mass the contraction was rapid and little work was done and vice versa. It was found empirically that the diminution in work with increasing speeds was proportional to the speed of shortening and the interpretation was suggested that this energy which failed to appear as work was developed as potential energy but degraded into heat in overcoming frictional resistance in the muscles. While there is doubtless some truth in this interpretation, the fact that isolated muscles liberate less heat per second (i.e. for a given duration of stimulus) when shortening rapidly than when shortening slowly, makes it probable that in rapid contractions of the arm muscles less energy per second is actually developed. Hence we are at a loss to know how much of the diminution of tension with high speeds is due to diminished rate of energy expenditure and how much is due actually to frictional loss.

More recently in his experiments at Cornell, Hill (1927) (and Furusawa, Hill and Parkinson, 1927) has made use of a similar idea in studying the equation of motion of a sprint runner (cf. also Gertz, 1929). The runner gradually accelerates until he reaches a constant maximum velocity. It is shown experimentally that his velocity as a function of time can be quantitatively explained by supposing that he is being propelled by a constant force and being resisted by a force which is proportional to his speed. This resisting force is again muscle viscosity (or "something which behaves like viscosity"). There can be no question that the equation derived on these assumptions adequately fits the facts. By means of this equation it is possible to determine the magnitude of the hypothetical propelling force; this force multiplied by the distance traveled gives the work done in the run. Since no appreciable external work is done in the run it is supposed that "the whole of the mechanical energy liberated is used in overcoming the frictional resistance of the body itself, particularly the 'viscosity' of the muscles themselves" (Hill, 1927).

This method resembles the thermodynamic method; it gives us the end results without telling us the mechanism. Assuming that it tells us correctly the total amount of mechanical energy expended it does not tell us in what way it is expended. It certainly is not all expended in overcoming viscosity. In the sentences following the one quoted above, Hill (1927) mentions the kinetic energy of the arms and legs which must alternately be created and destroyed, and uses it to show why the cost of running increases so rapidly with the speed. He does not emphasize, however, that this kinetic energy must be created in *spite* of viscosity and that a high viscosity would assist in destroying it, rather than the reverse. In fact as already mentioned, over one-half of the work as measured by Hill's method is actually used in creation and destruction of kinetic energy in the arms and legs, in changes in velocity of the whole body and in work against gravity.

There is another assumption underlying Hill's equation expressing the motion of a runner; the propelling force is assumed to be constant. The only justification for this is that the runner is making a maximal effort throughout the run. At the start however, the limbs are moving slowly and it seems likely that the force exerted (including the internal force used in overcoming viscosity) might be greater than at the end of the run when the limbs are moving at maximum speed.[4]

In case the possible inconstancy of the propelling force does not invalidate Hill's calculations we are left with the difficulty of explaining how it is possible that the items described as "useful work" should "behave like viscosity" in being proportional to the velocity of the runner. This must be the case or Hill's equation would not fit the fact as it apparently does. One would expect that the kinetic energy of the arms and legs for example would vary as the square of the velocity. An increase of velocity is attained however by increasing the length of the stride, as well as by moving the arms and legs more rapidly. Hence it is possible that there is a considerable range over which this factor may increase so nearly in proportion to the velocity as not to invalidate Hill's equation. Hill's facts therefore lend themselves admirably to the interpretation which he has put upon them but it does not seem certain that they do not lend themselves to some other interpretation equally well.

The remainder of this paper is devoted to the measurement of the work of acceleration and deceleration of the limbs. The measurement of the work against gravity and the velocity changes will be described in a later paper.

The Kinetic Energy of the Limbs

Method of Measurement

The method used was the same as that originally used by Marey and Demeney, i.e., the moving picture. Due to the connection of one of us (C.A.M.) with the Eastman Kodak Company and particularly with the work of making Eastman Teaching Medical Films, this work was much facilitated. In order to be able to make accurate absolute measurements from the film it is necessary to have runners run behind a white wooden lattice work making a coordinate system with squares 1 meter on a side. Figure 1 [*figure 5.1 here*] will show the general arrangement used for this purpose. A telephoto lens was used in taking the photographs so that the camera could be placed 30 meters from the runners. If the runners ran 1/2 a meter behind the lattice work, the error in measuring their horizontal velocity from their positions in relation to the lattice was 1.7 per cent. This correction has been neglected in the calculations. The sharpness of the image on the film depends upon the brevity of the exposure. In the first film taken the exposure was about 0.003 second, but in the second film this was reduced to about 0.001 second with a corresponding improvement in definition.

Timing

Since the camera is turned by hand during the exposure the speed of the film is not known nor is it entirely regular. In order to time the pictures, wooden balls (croquet balls), 4 inches in diameter, were dropped in front of a vertical scale so that they appeared at the side of the film. The scale was graduated in tenths of a second so that the speed of the film could be rapidly determined. One of these balls is seen falling in figure 1 [*figure 5.1 here*].

Subjects

Two films were taken, one in May, 1928 and one in October, 1928. In the first case 19 men made each one run in front of the camera. In the second case 15 men ran each three times. The men ran one behind another as close together as convenient. Except in one or two cases they were all instructed to run at top speed, without any special sprints as they passed in front of the camera. In the first case they ran on a concrete walk and in the second case on the level turf. The general arrangement of the two films is shown in figure 1 [*figure 5.1 here*], the first 3 rows being taken consecutively from the second film and the last row from the first film. In both cases the men were members of some of the regular classes in physical education at the University of Rochester. We are much indebted to Doctor Fauver and his colleagues at the gymnasium for their cooperation in making these runners available for us. With the exception of one first rate sprinter (pictured in figure 1 [*figure 5.1 here*]) in the second group, none of the men was selected in any way. They may be regarded as a fairly representative group of college

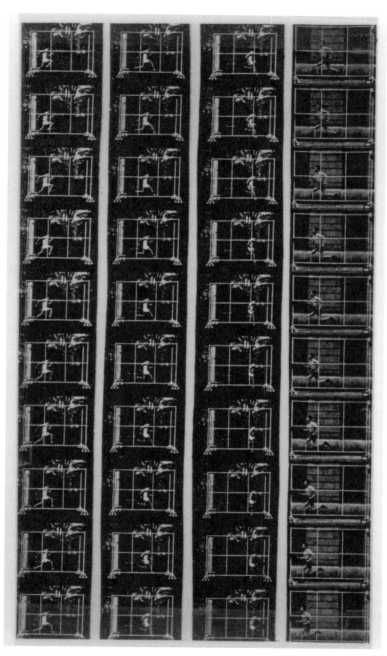

Figure 5.1
Reproductions from strips of the film showing a runner behind the lattice from which measurements were made. (Reprinted from Fenn 1930.)

undergraduates. In order to provide fixed points for measuring the successive positions reached by a runner the men in the second group were provided with markers. The man in figure 1 [*figure 5.1 here*] shows the nature of these. One was a white cloth tied around the neck with a black spot on it. The other was a circular white tag, carrying a black spot which was supported on a stiff wire frame tied firmly around the waist in such a way that no movement in relation to the body was possible.

Measurement of the Films

For purposes of projection and measurement an improvised lantern was used. In the preliminary measurements it turned out that the chief source of error lay in the buckling of the film. To avoid this the film was passed between two glass plates which could be clamped tightly together when the desired frame was brought in front of the lens. The film used was the standard 1-1/4 inch cinematograph film. When projected, one meter on the original lattice behind which the men ran measured 16.6 cm. For the purposes of the data to be described in this paper, measurements were made of the angles of the upper and lower arms and of the upper and lower legs. It proved to be unnecessary to measure every picture in most cases but every other picture was measured. For other purposes the vertical and horizontal positions of the markers were also determined. Where markers were absent the tip of the nose was chosen as the most definite point. It was found that the angles could be estimated within 2 degrees almost without exception. A protractor was merely laid along the longitudinal axis of the image of the limb in question and the angle read off from the intersection of a plumb line hanging from the center of the protractor.

Calculation of Kinetic Energy

For purposes of calculation it is considered that the runner is standing still, as on a tread mill, and is waving his arms and legs as illustrated on the film. This method has advantage that the kinetic energy turns out to be high in that limb where the work is being done. If the kinetic energy is calculated in reaction to the ground, then the limb going backwards has very small kinetic energy although the actual effort on the part of the runner is as great in pushing it backwards as in pushing it forwards. Both methods of course lead to the same result as far as the kinetic energy of the whole runner at any moment is concerned. But the distribution of energy over the body depends upon the point of reference chosen. The use of the runner himself as a reference point has another advantage which will be discussed later; it minimizes the calculated transmission of energy from one moving part to another. It also eliminates the necessity of knowing the momentary forward velocity of the common center of gravity of the body with great accuracy.

The kinetic energy of any part of the body with relation to the body depends upon its translational velocity with relation to the body. To this must be added its energy of rotation. Let the suffix 0 refer to the body as a whole and the suffixes 1, 2, and 3 refer respectively to the trunk, the upper leg (or arm) and the lower leg (or arm). Let m represent the weight and ω the angular velocity, v the linear velocity and s the distance to the center of gravity of the part in question and k its radius of gyration around its center of gravity. s is measured from the hip joint in the case of the upper leg and from the knee in the case of the lower leg, and similarly, *mutatis mutandis* for the arm. Then the kinetic energy of the body as a whole at any moment will be (cf. Fischer and Steinhausen, 1925):

$$\frac{m_0 \, v_0^2}{2} + \frac{m_1 \, v_1^2}{2} + \frac{m_1 \omega_1^2 k_1^2}{2} + \frac{m_2 \, v_2^2}{2} + \frac{m_2 \omega_2^2 k_2^2}{2} + \frac{m_3 \, v_3^2}{2} + \frac{m_3 \omega_3^3 k_3^2}{2} + etc. \quad (1)$$

Here v_0 in the first term represents the velocity of the center of gravity in relation to the ground and is neglected for our present purpose. The variations in v_0 will be discussed in a later paper. v_1, v_2, and v_3 represent velocities in relation to the common center of gravity of the whole body. The values of m are calculated from the weight of the runner according to the factors determined by Braune and Fischer (1894) on cadavers. Thus if the weight of the whole runner is 1.00 the weights of the limbs, m, are as follows:

Table 5.1

	m	s
Upper arm	0.0336	0.47
Lower arm plus hand	0.0312	0.66
Upper leg	0.1158	0.44
Lower leg plus foot	0.0705	0.61

Reprinted from Fenn 1930.

This table also gives values of s in fractions of the length of the limb. The lengths of the limbs were measured from the photographs. The second group of runners was asked to pose for this purpose with the arms and legs conveniently bent and in a plane perpendicular to the camera for greatest accuracy of measurement. The limbs were measured from joint to joint. The lower arm was measured from the elbow to the wrist and the lower leg from the knee to the lower extremity of the tibia. The radius of gyration, k, according to the measurements of Braune and Fischer (1892) on cadavers may be taken with fair accuracy as 0.3 of the length of the limb. For this purpose we have to take into account the length of the hand

and of the foot. Consequently we have added 13 cm. to the length of the lower arm, as measured above, this being the distance from the wrist to the first interphalangeal joint and 6 cm. to the length of the lower leg, this being the "height" of the foot as given by Braune and Fischer (1892). If therefore the length of the lower arm from the elbow to the wrist is 26 cm. the center of gravity of the lower arm plus hand is located 0.66 × 26 or 17 cm. below the elbow and the radius of gyration around the center of gravity is (26 + 13) × 0.3 or 11.7 cm. It was not found possible to measure the lengths of the limbs with great accuracy from the photograph. Our most careful measurements failed to distinguish any constant difference between the lengths of the upper and lower limbs either in the arms or in the legs. Thus the length of the lower arm from the elbow to the wrist is taken as equal to the length of the upper arm from the shoulder to the elbow. Likewise the length of the lower leg from the knee to the ankle is taken equal to the length of the upper leg from the hip to the knee. All of these measurements are approximations but the errors so made cannot appreciably affect the order of magnitude of the results obtained.

In order to calculate the kinetic energy from equation (1) it is, therefore, necessary to measure from the film only the value of the angle α. From this the values of v are calculated in the following manner. Figure 2A [*figure 5.2a here*] represents m_1 and m_2, the latter having an angular velocity of ω_2 and the angular rotation of m_1 being neglected. Its linear velocity in relation to m_1 is therefore $s_2\omega_2 = v_2$, as represented. Its energy of translation with respect to m_1 is therefore $\dfrac{m_2 v_2^2}{2}$ and its rotational energy, around its center of gravity is $\dfrac{m_2 k_2^2 \omega_2^2}{2}$. The sum of these two factors is of course equal to $\dfrac{I_2 \omega_2^2}{2}$ where I_2 is its moment of inertia around the hip joint.

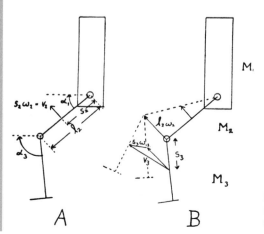

A   B

Figure 5.2
Diagram of body and leg. (Reprinted from Fenn 1930.)

The calculation of the kinetic energy of the lower leg is not quite so simple (fig. 2B [*figure 5.2b here*]). One first determines the linear velocity of the knee joint, which may be called v_l where l is the length of the upper leg. $v_l = l_2\omega_2$. Now if the angular velocity of the lower leg, $\omega_3 = 0$, i.e., if the angle of the lower leg with relation to the horizontal does not change, then all parts of the lower leg, including its center of gravity will move with a velocity v_l as indicated. But if at the moment at which the knee joint moves with a linear velocity v_l, the lower leg is also changing its angle with the horizontal with an angular velocity ω_3, then the true linear velocity of the center of gravity of m_3 will be the resultant of v_l and of $\omega_3 s_3$. This resultant is v_3. The actual determination of v_3 can be done most rapidly by graphical methods rather than by trigonometry. One simply chooses a point of origin on a sheet of coordinate paper and lays off the components in their proper directions and measures the resultant with a millimeter rule. It is convenient for this purpose to let 1 cm. represent a velocity of 100 cm. per second. Knowing v_3, the kinetic energy of the lower leg is calculated by the usual formula,

$$\frac{m_3 \, v_3^2}{2} + \frac{m_3 k_3^2 \omega_3^2}{2}$$

A word should be included about the evaluation of the angular velocities. The data actually obtained are the angular positions of the various members at every other frame (exposure) on the film, or at every 0.016 second approximately. These angles are plotted out against the frame number (time) so obtaining *displacement curves*. These curves are smoothed out graphically with care to preserve all the significant variations. Such displacement curves for the upper and lower arms and the upper and lower legs are shown in figure 4 [*figure 5.4 here*]. The angle which is measured and which is plotted in figure 4 [*figure 5.4 here*] is the angle α illustrated in figure 2 [*figure 5.2 here*], i.e., it is the angle made by the limb with the horizontal line in front of the runner. This convention has the advantage that when α is increasing the leg is going backwards and vice versa. The displacement curves are drawn for one complete cycle. The length of the cycle can be determined either from the contour of the curves or from the interval elapsing between foot-contacts with the ground. The moment when the toe leaves the ground can be determined with somewhat more accuracy than the moment when the foot touches the ground, and this point for the two feet is preferred for determining the cycle length. Care is taken in smoothing out the displacement curves to see that they begin and end at the same angle. Since a runner does not always run with perfectly regular rhythm this sometimes involves a slight violation of the observed data but this change is altogether immaterial and doubtless represents just as fair an average cycle for that runner as the actual movements observed. It is convenient to have the two ends fit in this way in subsequent parts of the analysis. From the smoothed displacement curves the slopes are read off by a straight edge laid tangent to them at every fourth frame, or every 0.03 second approximately. It was found unnecessary to carry through these laborious calculations for every frame measured. With the angular velocities so determined the remainder of the calculation was carried out as indicated.

Now strictly speaking, equation (1) calls for the velocities of the various members of the body in relation to the common center of gravity of the whole body. Then if one can measure the velocity, v_0, of this common center of gravity one can determine the total kinetic energy of the whole moving system. It is not particularly easy to determine precisely the velocity of the common center of gravity because, as will be shown later, the body rocks backwards and forwards to some extent in running and because the position of the common center of gravity inside the body changes with the changing positions of the limbs. The effect of the latter factor can be determined and will be discussed later. It should be noted, however, that the method of calculation given above determines actually the kinetic energy of the legs in relation to the hip joint and the kinetic energy of the arms in relation to the shoulder joint. Besides this, it does not take account of the relative movements of the two shoulder joints. When the arm moves forward the shoulder joint moves forward with it. We have attempted in the case of one runner to take account of this factor by measuring directly from the film the movements forward and backwards of the shoulder joint itself. In this way it is possible to estimate that an allowance for this factor, in the case of the arms, would increase the calculated kinetic energy of the arms about 30 to 50 per cent. The effect due to the movement of the hips would be much less than this. Since the kinetic energy of the arms is rather small in comparison to that of the legs anyway, the total error involved in this factor is not large and tends to make the true figure larger (perhaps 10 per cent) than the calculated, rather than the reverse.

We have also endeavored to make allowance for the movements of the center of gravity within the body due to the varying positions of the limbs and in a number of cases we have corrected our results for the movements of the common center of gravity within the body. Allowance for this factor sometimes makes the observed kinetic energy at any particular moment larger and sometimes smaller but in any case the difference is not large, the velocities with which the center of gravity is shifting inside the body being only about 1/10 of the velocities with which the limbs are moving.

Results

The complete data for the left leg of one of our runners (no. 11) chosen at random, are given in table 1 [*table 5.2 here*] and are plotted in figure 3 [*figure 5.3 here*]. The first column of this table gives the number of the frame on the film. (We have in all nearly 2000 frames each of which has been numbered on the margin in India ink for purposes of identification.) The second

Table 5.2 Kinetic Energy of Left Leg of Runner 11

Frame number	Time	Angles		Angular velocity		Linear velocity				Kinetic energy					
										Upper leg			Lower leg		
		Upper	Lower	Upper	Lower	$v_2 = s_2\omega_2$	$l_2\omega_2$	$s_2\omega_3$	v_3	Translation	Rotation	Total	Translation	Rotation	Total
(1)	(2)	(3)	(4)	(5)	(6)	(7)	(8)	(9)	(10)	(11)	(12)	(13)	(14)	(15)	(16)
	seconds	degrees	degrees	degrees /frame	degrees /frame	cm./ sec.	cm./ sec.	cm./ sec.	cm./ sec.	kgm. m.	kgm. m.	kgm. m.	kgm. m.	kgm. m.	kgm. m.
630	0	30	87	+3.5	-3.2	130	298	166	250	0.59	0.28	0.87	1.32	0.19	1.51
634	0.032	40	78	+2.2	+0.8	82	187	41	225	0.23	0.11	0.34	1.07	0.01	1.71
638	0.064	47	90	+4.2	+3.6	156	357	187	513	0.85	0.40	1.25	5.57	0.24	5.81
642	0.096	67	106	+3.0	+5.5	112	255	286	510	0.44	0.20	0.64	5.51	0.57	6.08
646	0.128	81	127	+5.2	+4.6	194	441	239	630	1.31	0.61	1.92	8.40	0.40	8.80
650	0.160	108	137	+6.5	+0.8	242	553	41	593	2.04	0.96	3.00	7.45	0.01	7.46
652	0.176	119	137	+3.7	+2.0	138	315	104	420	0.66	0.31	0.97	3.74	0.08	3.82
654	0.192	122	148	+0.2	+5.0	7	17	260	275	0	0	0	1.60	0.47	2.07
658	0.224	117	175	-2.7	+6.8	100	230	353	306	0.35	0.16	0.51	1.98	0.86	2.84
662	0.256	107	196	-5.6	+4.6	208	475	239	530	1.51	0.71	2.22	5.95	0.40	6.35
666	0.288	85	210	-6.5	+1.0	242	552	52	580	2.04	0.96	3.00	7.13	0.02	7.15
670	0.320	56	200	-7.7	-4.8	286	654	250	475	2.84	1.33	4.17	4.78	0.43	5.21
672	0.336	37	188	-7.0	-6.0	260	595	312	355	2.35	1.10	3.45	2.68	0.67	3.35
674	0.352	27	172	-4.2	-8.0	156	357	415	240	0.85	0.40	1.25	1.22	1.19	2.41
676	0.368	20	155	-2.0	-8.5	74	170	441	345	0.19	0.09	0.28	2.52	1.35	3.87
678	0.384	18	135	-0.7	-9.5	26	59	493	465	0.02	0.01	0.03	4.58	1.68	6.26
682	0.416	22	98	+3.0	-7.5	112	255	390	520	0.44	0.20	0.64	5.73	1.05	6.78
684	0.432	30	87	+3.5	-3.2	130	298	166	250	0.59	0.29	0.88	1.32	0.19	1.51

Reprinted from Fenn 1930.

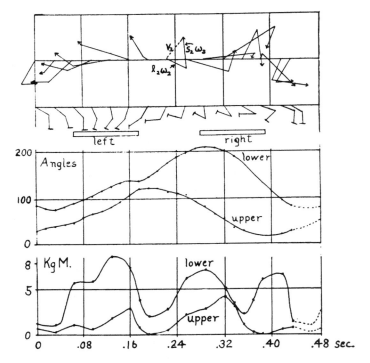

Figure 5.3
Data for the left leg of runner 11. The lower graphs show the kinetic energy of the upper and lower left legs in kg. m. as a function of time. The middle graphs show the angles between the leg (upper or lower) and the horizontal. The dotted portions indicate the beginning of another cycle. The arrows in the uppermost diagram show the magnitude and the direction of the velocities of movement of the upper and lower leg and the resultant v_3. (Reprinted from Fenn 1930.)

column gives the time in seconds as determined from the rate of fall of the croquet balls. Columns 3 and 4 give the angles with the horizontal of the upper and lower legs (femur and tibia) as measured from the film. The slopes of the displacement curve drawn through these points, as graphically determined, are given in columns 5 and 6 in degrees per frame. Columns 7 and 8 are calculated from column 5 by changing to radians per second and multiplying by s_2 and l_2 respectively. Column 10 is the resultant (v_3) of the velocities of columns 8 and 9 which are laid off in directions perpendicular to the angles recorded in columns 3 and 4. Columns 11 and 14 are calculated directly from columns 7 and 10 respectively and represent the translational kinetic energy of the upper and lower legs. Columns 12 and 15 are calculated from columns 7 and 9 and represent the rotational energy of the upper and lower legs respectively. Column 13 is the sum of columns 11 and 12 while column 16 is the sum of columns 14 and 15.

The values of the kinetic energy of the upper and lower legs respectively are given in columns 13 and 16 as they vary with time. These values are plotted in figure 3 [*figure 5.3 here*] in the lower two graphs. The corresponding positions of the leg are shown in the same figure. The graph begins as the left leg starts its backwards movement. The kinetic energy of the *upper leg* is seen to increase slightly until the moment when the foot makes contact with the ground. (At this moment of contact the foot is moving backwards in relation to the body but forwards slightly in relation to the ground.) Contact with the ground causes a slight check to its backwards movement and the kinetic energy falls off slightly. There is a corresponding irregularity at this point in the graph showing the angle between the upper leg and the horizontal. These angles can be measured with an accuracy of 2 degrees so that slight deviations are significant. The kinetic energy then increases again to a still higher level which is reached near the end of the backward stroke, at which point the kinetic energy falls again to zero. During the succeeding forward stroke the kinetic energy passes again through a maximum.

The kinetic energy of the *lower leg* never reaches zero but it starts at a low level as the leg starts backwards. At the point where the foot makes contact with the ground there is a slight hump in the curve, the maximum being reached toward the end of the period of foot contact with the ground. When the thigh starts forward the kinetic energy of the lower leg passes through a minimum but does not become zero because of the flexion of the knee. As this flexion continues, the knee being simultaneously carried forward, the kinetic energy of the lower leg passes through a second maximum which declines as knee flexion gives way to knee extension. As the thigh reaches its extreme forward position the lower leg tends to be thrown rapidly forward and downward thus producing a third maximum in the kinetic energy curve.

As already explained the velocity of movement of the center of gravity of the lower leg depends upon the velocity with which the knee carries it (without change in its angle with the horizontal) and the velocity with which its angle with the horizontal is changing. These two vector quantities are represented in the upper part of figure 3 [*figure 5.3 here*]. Each point is represented by a jointed arrow in two parts. The starting point of each arrow represents the time to which it applies. The first joint represents the direction and velocity of movement of the knee. The second joint, terminating in the arrow head, represents the direction and velocity with which the center of gravity of the lower leg is moving because of its change of angle *with the horizontal*. The resultant of these two vectors is v_3 as indicated in the diagram. It will be noticed that each of these vectors is drawn at right angles to the actual position occupied by the limb in question as illustrated below in figure 3 [*figure 5.3 here*]. Also it will be noticed that where v_3 is large the kinetic energy of the lower leg is also large and vice versa. The rotational energy is sufficiently small to be negligible for purposes of this comparison.

Similar data from runner 1 are plotted in figure 4 [*figure 5.4 here*]. Here the positions of the arms and the kinetic energy of the upper and lower arms are also represented. The displacement curves for both arms and legs showing the angles occupied in successive moments of time are also plotted. On these graphs the points represent the actual measurements taken from

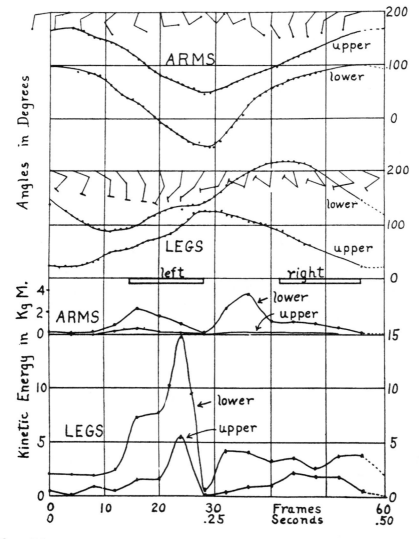

Figure 5.4
Kinetic energy and displacement curves of runner 1. (Reprinted from Fenn 1930.)

the screen and the curves drawn show the extent to which it is necessary to smooth out these curves before calculating slopes. In the case of this runner every frame was measured although as usual, the kinetic energy was calculated only at every fourth frame. It will be seen that the actual measurements in this case do not quite cover the period of a complete cycle so that a slight extrapolation is necessary. In this runner the kinetic energy of the lower leg reached a high peak and then fell off just as the foot left the ground. This great increase in the kinetic energy is coincident with the vigorous push backward given as the foot leaves the ground. The angular velocity of the upper leg becomes high at this moment also as shown by the sudden rise in its displacement curve at frame 25, figure 4 [*figure 5.4 here*]. The low minimum in the kinetic energy reached immediately afterwards is coincident with the cessation of movement of the thigh as it turns forward and the low angular velocity of the lower leg as the ankle extends. The diminution in angular velocity of the lower leg due to extension of the ankle is seen clearly by the flat place on the displacement curve of the lower leg at about frame 25, figure 4 [*figure 5.4 here*].

It is the large distance of the lower leg from the body which makes the work necessary to swing it the most important single item in the total kinetic energy of the limbs. This work can be very appreciably diminished if the knee is flexed as it is when the leg is being brought forward for another step, for in this way the moment of inertia of the leg as a whole is much decreased. Thus, to choose a case at random, it was found that the leg of runner 2 had a moment of inertia of 18.9×10^6 gm. cm.^{2} with the leg extended (knee angle 142 degrees) while the moment of inertia was only 5.5×10^6 gm. cm.^{2} when the knee was flexed (angle 32 degrees). For this purpose the moment of inertia was calculated from the formula of Braune and Fischer (1892).

$$I = m_2 k_2^2 + m_3 k_3^2 + m_2 s_2^2 + m_3 \left(l_2^2 + s_3^2 - 2 l_2 s_3 \cos \beta \right)$$

where β is the angle between the upper and the lower legs at the knee, l is the length of the part and s is measured from above downwards. It should be noted that this formula cannot be used for calculations of the kinetic energy of the whole leg at any particular moment (using the formula $I\omega^2/2$) because it does not enable one to take into account the movement of the lower leg or arm relative to the upper leg or arm; it assumes the whole limb to be a rigid body. Marey and Demeney (1885) took no account of this difficulty nor apparently of the fact that the angular velocity is not uniform throughout the stroke.

On account of the special importance of the lower leg it is necessary to consider how characteristic the lower leg curves of figures 3 and 4 [*figures 5.3 and 5.4 here*] may be. For this purpose similar data from 10 other runners have been plotted in figure 5 [*figure 5.5 here*], at the top of which the approximate positions of the leg are shown diagrammatically.

All of these graphs of figure 5 [*figure 5.5 here*] represent the kinetic energy changes of the lower leg. They are all arranged so that the movement when the foot leaves the ground comes at frame 30. The moment when the foot comes in contact with the ground varies slightly with different runners. In nearly every case there is an irregularity in the curve at this point. Measurements show also that there is always slight bending of the knee to break the shock as the weight of the body comes on the foot. All of these

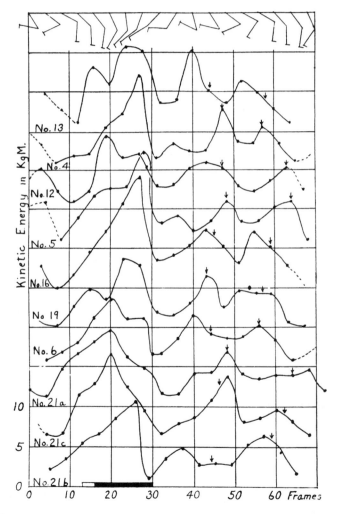

Figure 5.5
The variations of kinetic energy of the lower legs of 10 different runners in 10 different cases. The moment when the foot leaves the ground is made to coincide in each case with frame 30. (Reprinted from Fenn 1930.)

curves are sufficiently characteristic so that it is possible to tell fairly accurately in each case when the foot is on the ground from the shapes in the curve. Each of these curves shows in general three succeeding peaks, which differ somewhat among themselves. (The first of these is the most characteristic and coincided approximately with the period of foot-contact.) The second peak comes as a rule at or a little before the time when the angle made by the lower leg with the horizontal begins to decrease instead of increase (marked by the first arrow on each graph) and also near the point where the forward angular velocity of the thigh is at a maximum. The third of these peaks comes approximately at the point where the thigh reaches its maximum forward position (marked by the second arrow on the graph). The last three of these graphs all come from one runner, no. 21, who was the fastest sprinter in the group, his velocity being 8.3 to 8.5 meters per second.

As a starting point in analyzing these curves and calculating the horse power expended by the runners it may be assumed that each time the kinetic energy of a limb increases there is a corresponding expenditure of energy by the muscles, and each time it decreases, a corresponding amount of energy is dissipated as heat. The total kinetic energy developed during one cycle is therefore the sum of all the *increases* in kinetic energy as taken from the curves. The sum of all these increases for all the limbs divided by the length of the cycle will give the horse power. Data so obtained from all our runners are collected in table 2 [*table 5.3 here*]. The first column gives the runner's number (no. 3 and nos. 22-35 were not analyzed.) Column 2 gives the weight of the runner in kilos. Columns 3 to 6 give the increases in kinetic energy observed in the upper and lower arms during their forward and backward movements, respectively. The sum of columns 3 to 6 is given in column 7. Columns 8 to 12 give the corresponding increases in kinetic energy of the legs, upper and lower. Figures given in parentheses above the line indicate extra increases associated with the making of foot contact with the ground which it was felt ought to be included. Such additional increases are shown in figure 5 [*figure 5.5 here*] for runners 13 and 19 but these have not been included in the calculations. The sum of columns 8 to 12 is given in column 13. Column 14 will be discussed later. Column 15 is the sum of columns 7 and 13 and represents the total kinetic energy developed in one leg and one arm during one complete cycle. Column 16 represents the horse power for both arms and both legs together, calculated by multiplying figures of column 15 by 2, dividing by the length of the cycle and changing units. The *average rate of energy expenditure in the arms and legs alone is seen to be 1.68 horse power*. If the total rate of energy expenditure in the sprint is taken as 13 horse power (from oxygen consumption measurements) then this represents 12.9 per cent.

Discussion

It has been assumed in the interpretation of table 2 [*table 5.3 here*] that when the kinetic energy decreases in a limb it is not stored as potential energy but is degraded to heat. If it were stored temporarily as potential energy it could of course reappear as kinetic energy either in some other part of the body or at some other phase of the cycle in the same member. It is at this point in fact that the interpretation becomes particularly difficult. Consider first the storage of energy in some potential form.

The Effect of Gravity

Energy is of course stored as potential energy whenever a limb is raised. To what extent then does gravity assist in the alternating movements of running and to what extent does it modify the conclusions drawn from table 2 [*table 5.3 here*]?

The original theory of running was that of Weber and Weber (1836) who regarded the movements of the legs as simple pendulum movements. It has been conclusively shown however by Braune and Fischer for a man walking that gravity does not explain the movements and that active muscular contractions must occur to produce the accelerations observed (cf. Amar, p. 504). What is true of walking must be even more true of running where the velocities of the limbs are so much greater. Consider for example the time necessary for the leg to fall by gravity from a horizontal position in front of the body to a vertical position under the body. Let the masses of m_2 and m_3, the upper and lower legs, be respectively 7000 and 4900 grams, $l_2 = 44$, $s_2 = 19$, $k_2 = 13.2$ and $k_3 = 15.0$. To simplify the conditions let the whole mass of the lower leg be considered as located at the knee joint instead of hanging vertically from it as in normal running. The moment of inertia of the whole leg is then 14.3×10^6. The torque due to gravity is $(7000 \times 19 \times 980) + (4900 \times 44 \times 980) = 342 \times 10^6$. The time to fall from the horizontal to the vertical,[5] for a compound pendulum is

$$t = \frac{\pi}{2}\sqrt{\frac{I}{mgl}}\left[1 + \frac{k^2}{4} + \frac{9k^4}{64} + \frac{225k^6}{2304}, etc.\right] \tag{2}$$

where $k = \sin(90 - \alpha)/2$ and α is defined as in figure 2 [*figure 5.2 here*]. For the case where $\alpha = 20°$ this reduces to $1.73\sqrt{\frac{I}{mgl}}$ whence the time for fall is calculated as 0.354 second. The actual time for the corresponding change in position during running is less than half this amount indicating clearly that the muscles must have contributed to the fall.

The effect of gravity needs further consideration. Its relation to the leg movements is of chief importance. In the case of the upper leg, if its mass is 7000 and s is 19 the energy available when it falls from a horizontal to a vertical position is $7000 \times 19 \times 980 = 13 \times 10^7$ ergs = 13 joules. The actual kinetic energy found in the leg after this fall in 7 different runners was 75, 33, 30, 33, 45, 42, and 46 joules or an average of 43 joules, or over 3.3 times as much as could be derived from gravity. This 13 joules (1.33 kgm. m.) must therefore be deducted from the kinetic energy of the upper leg during its back stroke.

It should be emphasized that the weight of the lower leg does not serve to pull the upper leg down. Actually the upper leg would fall more rapidly if the lower leg were absent. Likewise the arm will fall to the side from the horizontal position less rapidly if a heavy weight is carried in the hand than if the hand is empty (provided friction, etc., is negligible). Its natural period as a pendulum is thereby increased. The leg is therefore pushed downwards to some extent to make contact with the ground. On the forward stroke of the upper leg the maximum kinetic energy is reached at an angle of 75° with the horizontal. At this point a negligible fraction (4 per cent) of these 13 joules has been restored to the leg in potential form and the remainder may be assumed to come from the kinetic energy it now possesses. Hence the kinetic energy as listed in table 2 [*table 5.3 here*] requires no correction for gravity at this point.

From table 2 [*table 5.3 here*] it appears that the upper leg develops a kinetic energy of 3.35 kgm. m. on its backward stroke and a similar amount again on its forward stroke. Of the latter, all is produced from muscular activity while of the former, it appears that 1.3 kgm. m. may be assigned to gravity.

Consider now the effect of gravity on the three peaks of the kinetic energy curve of the lower leg as illustrated in figure 5 [*figure 5.5 here*]. When the kinetic energy begins to increase for the first of these three peaks the foot is already practically on the ground and remains so throughout this part of the curve. Hence none of its kinetic energy as recorded in column 10, table 2 [*table 5.3 here*] can have come from the force of gravity. When the toe leaves the ground, the lower leg is raised and at the same time its kinetic energy rises to a maximum. This maximum is reached at about the same time that the lower leg reaches its maximum elevation. Hence the work done against gravity in raising the leg should be added to the kinetic energy produced in this knee flexion (column 11, table 2 [*table 5.3 here*]), which has an average value of 4.33 kgm. m. Measurements show that in the case of runner 1 the center of gravity of the lower leg is elevated 33 cm. during this interval and the work done is therefore 33 cm. × 980 × 4790 gms. or 15.5 × 10^7 ergs or 1.58 kgm. m. The total energy expended by the muscles in moving the lower leg at this period of the cycle is therefore 4.33 + 1.58 or 5.91 kgm. m. The next peak in the kinetic energy of the lower leg comes from when the thigh reaches its maximum forward position. During the interval between this and the preceding peak, the center of gravity of the lower leg remains practically on a level because, as the knee rises, the ankle falls a corresponding amount. Hence none of the potential energy of position which the lower leg possessed at the point of maximum knee flexion can have been transformed into kinetic energy to contribute to this second peak. The figures in column 12, table 2 [*table 5.3 here*], require therefore no correction.

Table 5.3 Increases of Kinetic Energy (in Kilogram Meters) of Arm and Leg During One Running Cycle

Runner	Weight	Arm					Leg							Arm and leg	H.P.
		Upper		Lower		Sum	Upper		Lower			Sum			
		Forward	Back	Forward	Back		Forward	Back	Back	Flex. of knee	Forward	By parts	As a whole		
(1)	(2)	(3)	(4)	(5)	(6)	(7)	(8)	(9)	(10)	(11)	(12)	(13)	(14)	(15)	(16)
	kgm.														
1	68	0.51	0.16	2.33	3.54	6.54	2.26	5.52	12.95	3.85	1.25	25.83	25.65	32.37	1.83
2	65	0.45	0.26	2.06	1.69	4.46	2.13	2.40	4.90	0.82	5.13	15.38	13.59	19.84	1.12
4	67	0.38	0.29	1.41	3.92	6.00	4.31	4.55	11.16	6.10	2.26	28.38	26.65	34.38	1.98
5	63	0.57	0.64	1.45	3.95	6.61	2.93	5.38	11.69	3.99	2.73	26.72	25.15	33.33	1.83
6	66	0.31	0.20	1.01	1.57	3.09	2.24	2.24	9.11	4.60	3.18	21.37	17.64	24.46	1.34
7	64	0.80	0.40	4.02	2.81	8.03	3.59	3.63 (2.43)	8.78	5.16	3.51 (4.03)	24.67	23.86	32.70	1.79
8	64	0.39	0.16	3.04	1.79	5.38	2.11	1.59 (6.86)	10.10	8.91	2.21 (2.45)	31.38	26.38	36.76	2.03
9	61	0.14	0.20	0.49	0.60	1.43	4.14	1.37 (1.68)	6.09	1.30	3.91 (0.88)	20.12	19.43	21.55	1.11
10	67	1.00	0.31	0.86	2.53	4.70	4.54	2.23 (1.25)	8.49	2.95	3.38	24.15	23.64	28.85	1.61

11	52	0.20	0.21	1.45	1.24	3.10	4.17	2.36	7.29	5.08	4.37	24.52	21.89	27.62	1.68
12	58	0.33	0.31	2.57	3.03	6.24	3.70	3.27	9.08	3.06	3.12 (2.79)	22.23	19.34	28.47	1.56
13	70	0.27	0.27	1.59	1.15	3.28	3.57	4.86	9.77	5.30	3.02	29.31	26.29	32.59	2.06
14	70	0.22	0.32	1.39	1.23	3.16	2.46	2.90	5.36	4.15	2.48	17.35	14.41	20.51	1.12
15	64	0.54	0.37	3.80	1.06	5.77	2.31	3.44	10.75	3.83	2.52	22.85	22.58	28.62	1.62
16	73	0.12	0.18	0.97	2.87	4.14	4.11	4.65	14.30	4.36	4.22 (3.35)	31.64	30.10	35.78	1.96
17	70	1.03	0.76	3.60	4.68	10.07	5.73	7.76	17.55	3.00	5.03 (3.59)	42.42	32.90	52.49	2.75
18	70	0.40	0.24	2.77	2.72	6.13	5.26	2.90	13.86	4.30	2.69 (1.35)	32.60	31.55	38.73	1.65
19	59	0.17	0.39	0.80	4.51	5.87	2.79	3.44 (0.78)	8.53	5.29	2.07 (1.08)	23.47	23.02	29.34	1.61
20	61	0.62	0.51	2.68	3.24	7.05	2.88	3.01	9.99	2.81	1.14	21.19	21.08	28.24	1.57
21-a	64	0.35	0.18	2.37	2.83	5.73	3.22	1.65	8.66	5.15	1.09	19.77	17.17	25.50	1.49
21-b	64	0.28	0.21	3.00	1.77	5.26	3.41	2.66	9.20	3.94	3.53	22.74	17.77	28.00	1.53
21-c	64	0.45	0.17	4.08	2.47	7.17	2.44	2.02	10.35	7.34	1.63	23.78	22.13	30.95	1.81
Average		0.43	0.31	2.17	2.51	5.42	3.38	3.35	9.91	4.33	2.93	25.09	22.82	30.50	1.68

Reprinted from Fenn 1930.

On the whole, therefore, corrections for gravity entail a deduction of 1.3 kgm. m. for the upper leg and an addition of 1.58 kgm. m. for the lower leg. Both of these are small amounts and the difference is negligible in comparison to other errors. The effect of gravity on the arms may be neglected as a relatively insignificant item in the total balance sheet for the body.

Storage of Energy in Tendons and Muscles

From the above considerations it is obvious that the storage of energy as potential energy of position and its reappearance as kinetic energy is not an important factor in evaluating the mechanical horse power of sprinting. Is it possible, however, that there could be such storage of energy in stretched tendons and muscles? It seems that the tendons can be dismissed because the actual positions reached by the limbs in swinging are not sufficiently extreme to stretch the tendons without the participation of actively contracted muscles. Likewise the resting muscles could not exert appreciable tensions in the positions occupied by the limbs at the end of their strokes. If the limb were stopped entirely by frictional forces all its energy would be degraded to heat and there would be none to store. Suppose therefore that muscles must contract and exert a tension F against a moving limb for a time t such that Ft equals the decrease in momentum of the limb. In doing so the muscle is stretched and might be supposed to have stored up a certain amount of potential energy. It cannot retain this store of energy, however, without continuous contraction. If it has any potential energy it is continuously losing it at a certain rate and continuously redeveloping it. The balance between those two determines the amount of tension maintained and the energy of maintenance. A muscle may therefore be said to "charge storage" at a rate which would expend the energy value of the stored energy many times over in a few seconds. In the movements of running, a study of the movies shows that the *tension is maintained during the reversal of direction of motion of the limbs* for the acceleration is practically constant during this period. Presumably in this case then the maintenance expenditure is less than the cost of redeveloping the tension and the back stroke must necessarily be somewhat quicker if the tension is already developed.

But however that may be, the energy which the muscles save by thus avoiding the necessity of redeveloping a certain tension for the back stroke is no measure of the amount of potential energy corresponding to that tension; which is the question at issue for the present discussion. Nor can potential energy be measured by the work which the muscle will do when it is allowed to shorten (cf. Fenn, 1923).

The area of the length tension diagram has often been regarded as so much potential energy but one can never recover anything like this amount of energy as work (not over 30 per cent), nor is it certain that the work which is recovered actually came from previously developed potential energy and not from other chemical breakdowns taking place during the performance of work. The excess production of energy observed when work is done favors the latter view. The absence of such excess heat in single twitches has been cited, however, as proof that in this case at least the work must have come from previously developed potential energy (Hartree and Hill, 1928). Although I do not yet feel convinced that this absence of excess heat in single twitches is universally true (since I have observed variations in the initial heat production of muscles with change of load even when stimulated by single twitches under Ringer's solution) nevertheless the result, if true, does not preclude any other hypothesis. One observes simply more energy production during the contraction phase when work is performed, as compared to an isometric contraction, and correspondingly less during relaxation. It may be said that the performance of work accelerates part of the chemical breakdown which otherwise does not appear as heat until relaxation. We have no real means of knowing *where* this same relaxation heat was during the isometric contraction phase— perhaps still in the form of chemical potential energy. Moreover the division of the heat into contraction and relaxation phases is not altogether precise and in any case the relaxation heat is not over half the length-tension area corresponding to the isometric tension developed (Hartree and Hill, 1928). In short many facts fit beautifully into the theory that an isometrically contracting muscle possesses mechanical potential energy like a stretched spring and does work by this means. But it is equally true that the known facts do not altogether preclude another hypothesis according to which the energy needed for muscular work is developed during the actual period of shortening.

In conclusion it appears that during the reversal of a limb, the muscles are continuously innervated so that tension is maintained, redevelopment of tension for the back stroke is avoided and the energy equivalent of a certain amount of oxygen is saved. Such a saving of oxygen does not mean however a saving of mechanical energy. The kinetic energy observed in the return stroke may nevertheless have to be redeveloped *de novo* in spite of the fact that the necessary tension is still there. As a guess it might be said that the storage of energy could not be over 25 per cent of the kinetic energy of the limb before reversal.

Work of Deceleration

The work of deceleration is work necessary to stop a moving limb; it is tension exerted while a muscle is being stretched, or negative work. Measurements have been made in man of the extra oxygen consumption involved in such positive and negative work. Chauveau (1901) found for example that negative work involved 52 per cent as much energy as positive work. Zuntz gave a figure of 40 to 45 per cent. Cathcart and Stevenson

(1922) have reported a considerably higher figure of 71 per cent even after allowing for the energy used in performing movements without a load. Positive work is done in spite of viscosity and negative work with the aid of viscosity. If the external work is A and the viscosity is x, and if the oxygen consumption is assumed proportional to the work, then, using Cathcart's figure, $A + x/A - x = 100/71$ and $x = 1/6$ of A. If Chauveau's figure (52 per cent) is used, then viscosity work is 5/16 of A. Similarly Zuntz's figure (40 per cent) gives 3/7 of A. This estimate is of somewhat doubtful value partly because we never know exactly what the antagonistic muscles are doing in movements in man and partly because we have no proper assurance that the measurements were made either during a steady state or so as to cover completely the period of recovery. Moreover, these figures do not take into account the fact that a muscle loses tension at less than the isometric rate while being stretched and at more than the isometric rate while shortening, so that the necessary rate of tension redevelopment or the heat production is less during stretching than during shortening (Fenn, 1923). Correction for this difference would make the work of viscosity less than 3/7 of A, so that this is probably an upper estimate at the speed employed in the experiments of Zuntz. Also the work against viscosity will vary much with the speed of movement and this factor has not been controlled and is at a maximum in the rapid movements of sprinting. For this last reason it seems safest to choose the lowest of these estimates, (i.e., 40 per cent) in allowing for the work of deceleration of the limbs. *Hence if the rate of work in accelerating the limb is 1.68 horse power, the work of deceleration would be 0.4 × 1.68 or 0.67 horse power*, which would seem to be a conservative estimate.

Transfer of Energy Across Body

When the foot is in contact with the ground in running it is occupied in exerting a force F backwards on the ground for time, t, so that Ft represents the momentum, mv imparted thereby to the body. Much of this goes for example not directly into the body but into the other leg which is being carried forward at a greater velocity than the body. When this leg reaches the end of its forward stroke its momentum must be shared with the body as a whole according to the law of the conservation of momentum. In this way momentum can be transmitted about the body from one part to another, by a series of *inelastic impacts*. It is pertinent to inquire therefore to what extent kinetic energy can disappear from one limb only to reappear in another and so be counted twice in estimating the horse power of sprinting. A partial answer to this question may be suggested in the following manner.

If I_1 is the momentum of inertia of the body around a transverse axis through the two hip joints and I_2 the moment of inertia of the leg around the same axis then, as the leg swings forward with an angular momentum of $I_2\omega_2$, it is checked by the hamstring muscles and an angular momentum $I_1\omega_3$ is imparted to the body, such that

$$I_2\omega_2 = \left(I_1 + I_2\right)\omega_3 \tag{3}$$

both limb and body moving then together with an angular velocity ω_3. The energy gained by the body is then $\dfrac{I_1\omega_3^2}{2}$ and that lost by the leg is $\dfrac{I_2\left(\omega_2^2 - \omega_3^2\right)}{2}$ and the fraction, f, of the energy lost by the leg, which is transferred, is

$$f = \frac{I_1\omega_3^2}{I_2\left(\omega_2^2 - \omega_3^2\right)} \tag{4}$$

From a small cadaver studied by Braune and Fischer (1872, table 2 [*table 5.4 here*]) the following data are obtained.

Table 5.4

	Weight	T	e	I
Body and head	23790	10.57 × 10⁶	30.14 cm.	32.2 × 10⁶
Leg	7840	4.87	32.74	13.2 × 10⁶

Reprinted from Fenn 1930.

I was calculated from the formula $I = T + Me^2$ where M is the weight, T the moment of inertia around the center of gravity and e the distance of the center of gravity from the hip joint. Using these values of I_1 and I_2, ω_3 may be calculated in terms of ω_2 from equations (3). Thus $\omega_3 = \dfrac{13.2}{45.4}\omega_2$ and $\omega_3^2 = 0.085\ \omega_2^2$. This value for ω_3^2 can now be substituted in equation (4) and the fraction of energy transferred becomes equal to $\dfrac{32.2}{13.2} \times \dfrac{0.085}{0.915} = \dfrac{1}{4.4}$. This would seem to be a maximum figure for several reasons. It assumes the knee completely extended and rigid. When the knee is bent I_2 may be 5 × 10^6 whence the fraction transferred is only $\dfrac{1}{8.5}$. Moreover when one leg is going forward the other leg is going back so that the body is being twisted simultaneously in different directions. Thus neither leg will be able to twist the body and hence no energy can be transferred. The body is thus steadied by the opposite limbs in such a way that it behaves as if its moment of inertia or mass were much larger than it is. Hence the energy transfer is far less.

In this connection it is worth pointing out that the body itself has been chosen as a reference. If we had chosen the ground instead of the body as a reference point the problem of this transfer of energy would have involved an inelastic impact between two bodies moving at different speeds, i.e., the body mass m_1 would be moving at velocity v_1 in relation to the ground while the leg of mass m_2 would be moving, during its forward stroke, for example, with a velocity v_2. For the sake of simplicity its angular movement may be neglected. Then $m_2 v_2 + m_1 v_1 = (m_1 + m_2)v_3$ and using values for m_1 and m_2 given above and taking v_1 and v_2 as 7 and 9 meters/sec. respectively

v_3 becomes 7.5 and the fraction of energy transfer is $\dfrac{m_1}{m_2}\left(\dfrac{v_3^2 - v_1^2}{v_2^2 - v_3^2}\right) = 0.87$. As

the leg swings forward it has a relatively high velocity and hence a high kinetic energy in relation to the ground. The above figure shows that at most (7/8) of this energy is not degraded to heat but is transferred to the body which is thus accelerated in stopping the leg. This change in velocity of the body is real and has been measured and its magnitude will be discussed in a later paper. Obviously when the ground is used as a point of reference the danger of counting energy twice is considerable.

The present paper deals, however, only with the kinetic energy of the limbs. To disappear from one limb and reappear in another, energy must be transferred from leg to body and again from body to leg. Utilizing similar

methods in this case, it may be found that $\dfrac{1}{2.4}$ of energy from a body moving

with angular velocity v_3 may be transferred to a stationary leg. Thus the

total energy transferred from leg to leg is only $\dfrac{1}{4.4 \times 2.4}$ or about $\dfrac{1}{10}$.

There remains the important question of transfer of energy from the upper to the lower leg or vice versa. In particular take the case where the thigh is moving forward and is checked while the lower leg continues to move forward. It may be thought of as "snapping" forward like a whip. Whether in this case there is any appreciable energy transfer needs no discussion for it can be answered experimentally from the data at hand. When the kinetic energy disappears from the upper leg a corresponding amount should appear in the lower leg. A study of figure 4 [*figure 5.4 here*] shows that in this runner, at least, the successive increases of kinetic energy in the lower leg cannot be derived in appreciable degree from the upper leg. Instead the kinetic energy contents of both upper and lower legs tend to increase and decrease more or less together. To test this point for all runners the kinetic energy of the whole leg was determined for each point in the running cycle by adding together the figures obtained for upper and lower legs separately. The successive increases in kinetic energy of this combined curve were then determined and added together. The resulting sum is shown in column 14 of table 2 [*table 5.3 here*]. These figures are all slightly less than the corresponding figures of column 13 which were obtained by adding together the separate increases of the upper and lower legs. On the average, however, the difference is small, 22.8 kgm. m. as compared to 25.1 kgm. m. or a 9 per cent difference. Hence *at most 9 per cent of the kinetic energy could have been counted twice.* This does not necessarily mean that 9 per cent *was* in fact transferred from upper to lower leg or vice versa. Possibly therefore the figure 1.68 horse power for the arms and legs is 9 per cent too high and the true figure is 1.53 H.P. This small reduction, however, is completely offset by the previous estimate that the movements of the shoulders if allowed for would increase the observed kinetic energy of the limbs as a whole about 10 per cent.

These considerations make it appear probable that the figure obtained for the kinetic energy changes of the limbs is a fair representation of the actual conditions. Sideways movements of the body have necessarily been neglected as well as the contortions of the face and the contractions of the body muscles, etc. Altogether it seems that the actual output of mechanical energy by the body in sprinting is as large in relation to the oxygen consumption as when the work is measured, for example, on a bicycle ergometer. It would seem as if these mechanical factors had been unduly neglected in preference to viscosity in considering the work of running.

Summary

1. The problem of muscle viscosity is discussed in its relation to the physiology of sprinting in order to show that the available evidence does not preclude the possibility that the actual external work of sprinting (exclusive of work done against viscosity) is a large fraction of the total energy expended.

2. This conclusion is then verified by measurements of moving pictures of sprinters whereby the kinetic energy of the limbs could be calculated and plotted as a function of time.

3. An average sprinter is incurring an oxygen debt at the rate of 13 horse power while he is turning out mechanical work at a rate of 2.95 horse power or with an efficiency of 22.7 per cent. This included work against gravity (0.1 horse power), changes in velocity (0.5 horse power), acceleration of the limbs (1.68 horse power), and deceleration of the limbs (0.67 horse power). It excludes contractions of facial and body muscles, sideways movements of the body and work against viscosity or internal friction.

4. The discussion is concerned chiefly with the possibility of storage of mechanical energy in the muscles and tendons and the transfer of momentum and energy from one part of the body to another. It is concluded that these complications do not seriously interfere with

the accuracy of the figures obtained for the acceleration and deceleration of the limbs.

Bibliography

Amar, J. 1923. Le Moteur Humain, Paris.

Benedict, F. G. and H. Murschhauser. 1915. Pub. of Carnegie Inst. of Washington.

Braune, W. und O. Fischer. 1892. Abh. d. math. Phys. Kl. d. Sachs. Akad. d. Wiss., xviii, 409. 1894. Ibid., xxi, 153.

Cathcart, E. P. and A. G. Stevenson. 1922. Journ. Roy. Army Med. Corps, January.

Chaveau. 1901. C.R. Acad. Sci., lxxxii, 194.

Fenn, W. O. 1923. Journ. Physiol., lviii, 175.

Furusawa, K., A. V. Hill and J. L. Parkinson. 1927. Proc. Roy. Soc. B., cii, 29, 43.

Fischer, E. and W. Steinhausen. 1925. Handbuch. d. norm. u. path. physiol., viii, i, 619.

Gertz, H. 1929. Skand. Arch. f. physiol., lv, 131.

Hartree, W. and A. V. Hill. 1928. Proc. Roy. Soc. B., civ, 1.

Hill, A. V. 1926. Muscular activity. Baltimore.

1927.   Muscular movements in man. New York.

1922.   Journ. Physiol., lvi, 19.

1928.   Proc. Roy. Soc. B., cii, 380.

Marey et Demeney. 1885. C.R. de l'Acad. des Sci., ci, 910.

Marey. 1894. Le Mouvement. Paris.

Sargent, R. M. 1926. Proc. Roy. Soc. B, c, 10.

Weber, E. and W. Weber. 1836. Mechanik der mensch. Gehwerkzeuge. G'ttingen.

Zuntz (quoted by Cathcart, 1922).

A summary of this work was presented before the International Physiological Congress at Boston, August 1929 (Am. J. Physiol., 1929, xc, no. 2).

Footnotes

[1] Unpublished measurements from this laboratory for which I am indebted particularly to Dr. E. Fischer, Mr. H. Brody and Mr. C. I. Wright.

[2] Furusawa, Hill and Parkinson (1927) have found one man in which this figure was 8.5 horse power and Gertz by a somewhat similar method has estimated 6 to 8 horse power for the expenditure of mechanical energy while running at top speed. These men, however, were fast runners. The average speed of our runners was only 8.2 yards per second. Taking an average weight of 150 lbs. and an average propelling force of 0.75 the body weight the horse power would be $8.2 \times 3 \times 150 \times 0.80 \div 550 = 5.4$ horse power.

[3] The shortening energy is the excess heat developed when a muscle is allowed to shorten (Fenn, 1923). Thanks to Professor Hill's sense of humor this is better known in the literature as the "Fenn effect."

[4] Isolated muscles when stimulated with a constant stimulus give off less heat when shortening rapidly under low tension than when shortening under higher tension. (Hartree and Hill, 1928.) This suggests that in rapid running in man less energy is liberated per second and hence less tension exerted. The experiments are not however exactly comparable.

[5] I am indebted to Mr. T. Tomboulian of the Department of Physics, University of Rochester, for this formula.

Forces and Energy Changes in the Leg During Walking*

Herbert Elftman

From the Department of Zoology, Columbia University, New York City
Received for publication October 15, 1938

[Introduction, Methods, and Results]

The study of locomotion yields information not only concerning the mechanics of progression but also concerning the part that muscles play in this intricate activity. Early attempts at a quantitative analysis of human locomotion were made by the Webers, Marey and Otto Fischer, followed in recent years by Bernstein (1927, 1935) and by Fenn (1929, 1930). The present paper is concerned with a detailed analysis of the dynamics of the human leg in walking, providing data concerning muscle function.

In his fundamental investigations of the kinematics of walking, Fischer (1901) was hindered by the fact that he could not determine the point of application of the force exerted by the ground on the foot. The path of this point during the time the foot is on the ground was determined by Elftman and Manter (1934) from cinematic records of pressure distribution in the foot, obtained by a method described by Elftman (1934). For the purposes of the present research, however, a new apparatus has been devised (Elftman, 1938), which gives not only the point of application of this force, but also the magnitude of the force in three components. In addition to solving Fischer's difficulty, this obviates the necessity of dealing with the entire body when one portion, such as the leg, is of immediate interest.

The point of application of this force, as it passes forward during the course of the step, is shown in figure 1 [*figure 5.6 here*]. The force itself is plotted in two components, one in the plane of progression, the other lateral, in the horizontal plane. Only the component in the plane of progression will be considered in the present discussion. It is apparent from the diagram that it has two maxima and that it is at first directed upward and backward against the foot, later upward and forward. This reaction of the platform is plotted in figure 6 [*figure 5.11 here*] in two components, one vertical and the other horizontal, in the plane of progression.

In addition to this knowledge concerning the external force exerted by the platform, it is necessary to know the disposition of the leg in space. This is shown in figure 2 [*figure 5.7 here*] for the left leg during the double step under consideration. The original information was obtained from cinematic records taken at the rate of 92 exposures per second as the subject walked behind a rectangular grid. The timing was obtained by including a vibrating reed of known period in the photographic field. These records were projected on a large sheet of paper and the positions of the axes of the

*Reprinted from Elftman 1939.

hip-, knee- and upper ankle-joints determined. After plotting these positions against time, values were read off at intervals of 0.02 sec. and these were used in all further calculations. The phases are numbered according to the time at which they occurred in hundredths of a second, taking the time of establishment of contact by the foot with the platform as 100. In figure 2 [*figure 5.7 here*] the positions of the axes of the limb are shown at intervals of 0.08 sec. The circles indicate the positions of the centers of gravity of the thigh, shank and foot. They have been determined by applying the proportions given by Fischer (1906) for their positions with respect to the adjacent joints.

Determination of Forces and Torques

The external force and the position of the leg, as portrayed in figures 1 and 2 [*figures 5.6 and 5.7 here*], constitute the fundamental observed data, from which other information, more essential to our purpose, may be derived. The next step is to determine the forces acting on the foot. These are shown in figure 3 [*figure 5.8 here*], which is a free-body diagram of the foot. According to D'Alembert's principle, the reversed effective forces must be in equilibrium with all other forces acting on the body. Consequently if all the forces are known with one exception, that exception can be solved. Upon inspection of the forces, we find that the reaction of the platform is known (figures 1 and 6 [*figures 5.6 and 5.11 here*]). The weight of the foot is known to be 1.14 kgm. by applying Fischer's proportions to the total body weight of 63.4 kgm. The reversed effective force is equal to $-ma$, when m is the mass of the foot in gravitational units and a the acceleration of the center of gravity of the foot. The acceleration is obtained by plotting displacement against time and differentiating graphically, using the prism method, obtaining the velocity. The process is then repeated with the velocity to get the acceleration. The reversed effective force can therefore be calculated; it is plotted in figure 5 [*figure 5.10 here*].

The only force left which is not a member of a couple is the one which acts through the ankle-joint, due to the weight and reversed effective forces of the rest of the body. Since this force must be in equilibrium with the forces already known, it is readily calculated. The ankle-joint force is shown in figure 6 [*figure 5.11 here*], plotted, however, as it acts on the shank, which is opposite to its effect on the foot.

With all the forces determined, it is possible to approach the torques. Since the positions of the forces are known, their lever arms about any desired point can be measured and so their moments, or torques, about that point determined. The reversed effective torque is calculated in a manner analogous to that used for reversed effective forces. The moment of inertia, calculated from Fischer's data, is 0.046 kgm. slug cm.^{2} for the foot. The angular acceleration is obtained by the double differentiation of the angular displacement. The reversed effective torque in walking is quite small; it is plotted in figure 7 [*figure 5.12 here*]. The only torque still unknown

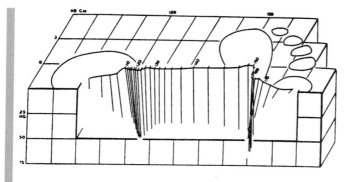

Figure 5.6
Reaction of the platform on the foot and its point of application. The reaction is shown in two components, one in the plane of progression, the other lateral, in the horizontal plane. (Reprinted from Elftman 1939.)

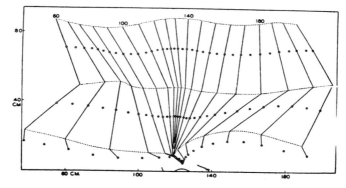

Figure 5.7
Position of the left leg during a double step. The centers of gravity of the thigh, shank and foot are indicated by circles. Time interval between successive positions of the leg, 0.08 sec. The phases are numbered in hundredths of a second, the time of application of the left foot to the platform being taken as 100. (Reprinted from Elftman 1939.)

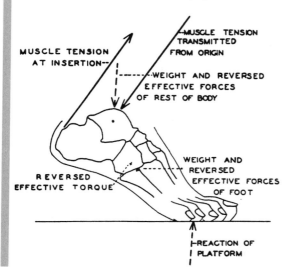

MUSCLE TENSION TRANSMITTED FROM ORIGIN

MUSCLE TENSION AT INSERTION

WEIGHT AND REVERSED EFFECTIVE FORCES OF REST OF BODY

WEIGHT AND REVERSED EFFECTIVE FORCES OF FOOT

REVERSED EFFECTIVE TORQUE

REACTION OF PLATFORM

Figure 5.8
Free-body diagram of foot. (Reprinted from Elftman 1939.)

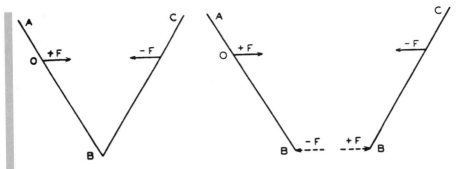

Figure 5.9
Diagram of one-joint muscle. The member *AB* is acted on by the force +*F* of the muscle at its origin. The force –*F* exerted by the muscle at its insertion is transmitted to *AB* through the joint. The two forces constitute a couple. (Reprinted from Elftman 1939.)

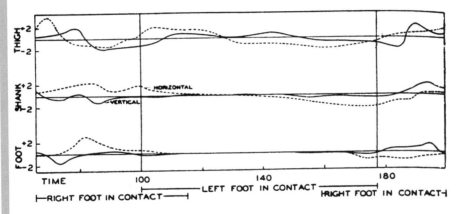

Figure 5.10
Reversed effective forces in kgm. Vertical component, continuous line; horizontal component, dotted. (Reprinted from Elftman 1939.)

is that of the muscles, consequently that can be found by solving the equations for equilibrium.

With the forces and torques acting on the foot completely determined, it is possible to repeat the operations with the shank and the thigh. This is possible because the joint force acting on the member above the joint is equal in magnitude but opposite in direction to the force acting on the member lying below the joint.

The uppermost curve of figure 7 [*figure 5.12 here*] shows the torque exerted by the leg muscles on the trunk. It is possible to calculate this torque because the sum of torques exerted by any muscle must be zero. This is illustrated for a one-joint muscle in figure 4 [*figure 5.9 here*]. The muscle under a tension *F* will exert a force of +*F* at its origin and –*F* at its insertion. When the two members *AB* and *BC* upon which the muscle acts are considered separately,

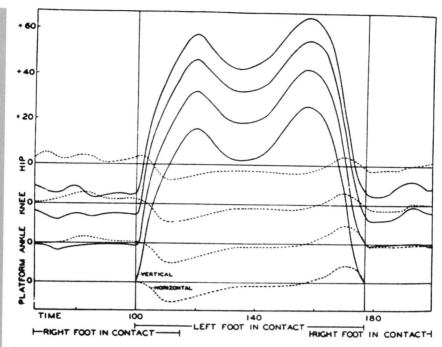

Figure 5.11
Platform reaction and the joint forces which are due to the platform reaction, gravity and effective forces. Forces in kgm. The forces plotted are those which act on the member above the joint. The force on the member below the joint is of the same magnitude but opposite in direction. Vertical forces, continuous line; horizontal forces, dotted. (Reprinted from Elftman 1939.)

it is found the force $-F$ exerted at the insertion is transmitted to AB through the joint B. Since the force on AB at the origin is $+F$ and at the joint $-F$, the two forces acting together constitute a couple, the torque of which is obtained by multiplying the tension by the perpendicular distance between the two forces. It is obvious from the diagram that the torque on BC is equal in magnitude but opposite in direction to that on AB. The sum of the two torques is consequently zero. The same proof may be elaborated for muscles which traverse more than one joint. Consequently the torque exerted by the leg muscles on the trunk must be such that when it is added to the sum of the torques exerted on the foot, shank and thigh the result is zero.

Significance of the Forces and Torques

The reversed effective forces vary with changes in the momentum of the member, since

$$\text{reversed effective force} = -ma$$

$$\text{and } -ma = -\frac{dmv}{dt}$$

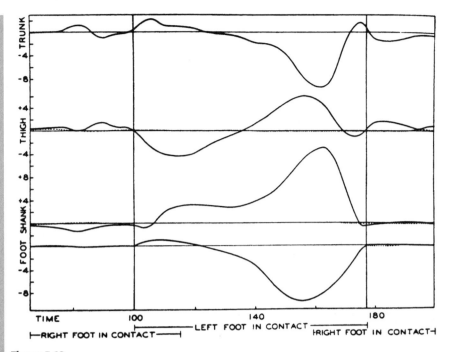

Figure 5.12
Muscle and reversed effective torques in kgm. m. The muscle torques represent the resultant of all muscle torques acting on the member. Positive torques tend to produce counter-clockwise rotation. Muscle torque, continuous line; reversed effective torque, dotted. (Reprinted from Elftman 1939.)

The reversed effective force is consequently the force exerted by the member on the other parts of the system due to a decrease in the momentum of the member. When the momentum of the member is increasing, the reversed effective force is negative. The rate of change of linear momentum of the parts of the leg can consequently be read from figure 5 [*figure 5.10 here*]. While the left foot is in contact with the ground, the horizontal momentum of all parts of the leg first decreases then increases. The vertical momentum varies in a less regular fashion. The time during which the foot is stationary on the ground is indicated by the fact that the reversed effective forces of the foot are zero.

The platform reaction, figure 6 [*figure 5.11 here*], represents the only external force acting on the body while the left foot alone is in contact with the substratum, since air resistance may be neglected at the low velocity of walking. The horizontal component of this reaction is at first negative, pushing backwards against the body, and is later positive. This may also be seen in figure 1 [*figure 5.6 here*]. The vertical component includes the reaction to gravity as well as the reaction to the effective forces transmitted through the left leg. The reaction to gravity is equal to the weight of the body, but is directed upward, for the interval during which the left foot alone is in contact. By subtracting this value from the total vertical reaction, the portion due to acceleration of the body as a whole may be determined and from this, by integration, changes in the momentum of the body as a whole.

The vertical force exerted by the platform describes a characteristic bimodal curve. Both maxima exceed the value for the reaction to gravity, while the intervening minimum is lower than this value.

The forces acting at the joints, due to the platform reaction, gravity and effective forces, are plotted in figure 6 [*figure 5.11 here*] as they act on the member above the joint. There is, of course, an equal but oppositely directed force which acts on the member below the joint. The force plotted here is not the total force acting through the joint, since it does not include the muscle forces. For purposes of dynamics the effect of the muscle forces can best be obtained from a consideration of the couples by means of their torques. If our purpose were the investigation of pressure in the joints, the procedure would be different.

The joint forces for the interval during which the foot is in contact with the platform vary, in general, in the same way as the platform reaction, since this is the largest component entering into their composition. Each vertical component is decreased, as we ascend from the foot to the thigh, by the weight of the parts of the leg which lie below the joint under consideration as well as by the effective forces of these parts. The joint forces are present while the foot is off the ground, at which time the platform reaction is absent.

The reversed effective torques are shown in figure 7 [*figure 5.12 here*] in dotted lines, when they are of sufficient magnitude to be plotted. A positive reversed effective torque represents the rate at which the angular momentum of the member about its own center of gravity is decreasing. In walking, the reversed effective torques are so small that they could be disregarded during the interval of contact of the foot with the ground. In the present research they have been included in all calculations.

The torques of the reversed effective forces and joint forces are not plotted in figure 7 [*figure 5.12 here*]. Since they must be in equilibrium with the muscle torques and reversed effective torques, they must, at each instant, be equal in magnitude to the sum of the muscle and reversed effective torques, but of opposite sign.

The muscle torques, figure 7 [*figure 5.12 here*], represent the resultant torque of all muscles acting on the member. When antagonistic muscles are in action simultaneously, the algebraic sum of their torques will be equal to this resultant torque. The torques are plotted in the usual fashion, a positive torque tending to produce counter-clockwise acceleration of the parts of the leg as they are oriented in figure 2 [*figure 5.7 here*]. If the leg behaved as a conventional compound pendulum, there would be no muscle torques during its swing. This was the basis of Fischer's proof (Fischer, 1904) that the swinging leg does not act as a pendulum. On the basis of figure 7 [*figure 5.12 here*] it is now possible to extend this conclusion to the body as a whole while the foot is in contact with the ground.

The tension in the muscles can be computed from the torque if the lever arms are known. In general, limiting values for tension can be obtained in this way by considering the range in values for the lever arms of various muscles which might be concerned in the production of the resultant torque. The minimum value thus calculated would be exceeded when antagonistic muscles are simultaneously under tension. The maximum torque about the ankle-joint occurred at phase 156, at which time it was 950 kgm. cm. With a lever arm of 4.0 cm. at that moment, the triceps surea was exerting a tension of 237.5 kgm., a value 3.7 times the weight of the individual. This is by no means a maximum value for the muscle, since it occurred while walking at a very moderate rate.

Energy Transfer

The rate at which energy is transferred, or the rate at which work is being done on or by the various components of the system, can be determined since the forces and torques and the velocities of their points of application are known. The results are plotted in figure 8 [*figure 5.13 here*] in kgm. m./ sec., from which the value in horse-power may be derived, if desired, since 1 h.p. = 76.065 kgm. m./sec. The area under each curve represents the total energy involved. A positive area measures the amount of work done by the force on other parts of the system, a negative area the energy receives from the other parts.

The rates of change of potential energy and of kinetic energy due to changes in linear and angular velocity have all been added together and the negative value of this sum plotted. Consequently when the curve labelled K.E. + P.E. is positive, energy is being released from the member, either to be passed on by the joint forces or into the muscles. From the time the left heel leaves the ground (which is indicated by the resumption of muscle power on the foot), through the early part of the swing, energy is being absorbed to increase the combined kinetic and potential energy of the parts of the leg. During the latter part of the swing, shown in the first part of the graph, this energy is given back to the other parts of the system. When considered with respect to the muscle and joint forces, kinetic and potential energy changes in the leg are of more importance when the leg is swinging than when it is in contact with the ground. While the foot is on the ground it is the changes in kinetic and potential energy of the rest of the body which are of importance, as indicated by the curve for the action of the hip-joint forces on the thigh.

The rate of energy transfer due to the joint forces is plotted separately for the forces at the proximal and distal ends of each member. The work done on the member by these forces is the algebraic sum of the areas under these curves, but by plotting them separately it is possible to follow the

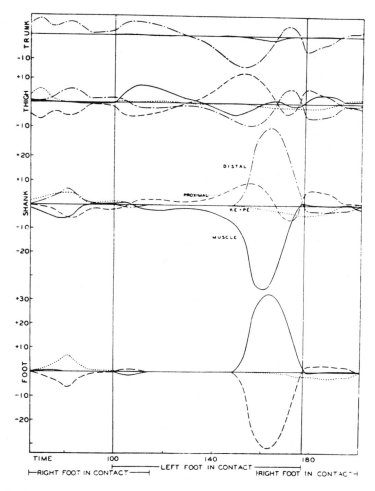

Figure 5.13
Rate of doing work (power) in kgm. m./sec. Positive values indicate that energy is being expended, negative that it is being received. The area under each curve measures the total energy involved. Curves for muscle, proximal and distal joint forces, and contribution of energy from changes in combined kinetic and potential energy of member. (Reprinted from Elftman 1939.)

transfer of energy from one member to those adjacent to it. The platform reaction does no work on the foot. The uppermost curve in figure 8 [*figure 5.13 here*] gives the rate at which work is done on the rest of the body by forces acting through the hip-joint.

The rate at which the muscles do work on, or receive energy from, each part of the leg is shown in figure 8 [*figure 5.13 here*] in continuous lines. This does not represent solely the energy received by the muscle in stretching or released in contraction, but also energy which is transmitted by the muscle from one point of attachment to another. The value for the power of the leg muscles acting on the trunk is obtained by multiplying the torque of these muscles, shown in figure 7 [*figure 5.12 here*], by the angular velocity of the trunk. The determination of this torque is equal in accuracy to the determination of the other muscle torques. Difficulty, however, is experienced in measuring pelvic rotation. The values for the power plotted here agree well with those which the author has obtained from unpublished calculations based on Fischer's (1899) data.

Transfer of Energy Between the Leg and the Rest of the Body

Before considering in detail the transfer of energy within the leg, it is advantageous to consider the leg as a whole. In figure 9 [*figure 5.14 here*] are plotted the combined values for the foot, shank and thigh of rates of energy change due to the action of muscles on the leg and of decrease in kinetic and potential energy of the leg, liberating energy for other purposes. The only joint force now present is the force at the hip-joint, acting on the leg.

In the latter part of the swing of the leg, which occupies the first portion of the graph, the leg is losing combined kinetic and potential energy, and this energy is available for other purposes. Since both the muscle and the hip-joint curves are negative at this time, the energy liberated must be absorbed by the muscles and by the rest of the body, in the relative amounts indicated by the curves. The disposition of the energy received by the rest of the body cannot be traced without considering the right leg, which at this time is in contact with the ground. The energy received by the leg muscles is taken up by the muscle tissue, either for storage or dissipation. The other possibility is for these muscles to expend energy on the trunk, but the power of the leg muscles on the trunk is negligible at this time.

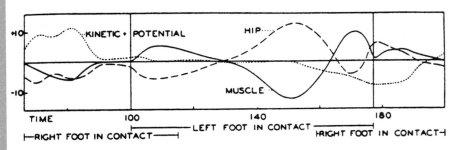

Figure 5.14
Power curves for the left leg as a whole, kgm. m./sec. The muscle curve shows the rate at which muscles contribute to, or subtract from, the energy of the leg; the hip curve the rate of energy change due to joint forces at the hip; and the kinetic and potential curve the rate at which energy is contributed by the decrease in combined kinetic and potential energy of the leg. (Reprinted from Elftman 1939.)

After the foot comes into contact with the ground, the combined kinetic and potential energy of the leg continues to liberate energy. The muscles now do work on the leg. The energy released is passed on to the rest of the body, as is indicated by the fact that the hip-joint forces are receiving energy at this time. From the time at which the right foot leaves the ground, the force acting through the hip-joint and the torque of the left leg muscles on the trunk represent the only external forces, in addition to gravity, which act on the rest of the body. We therefore know that energy absorbed by the rest of the body must be used in increasing the sum of its kinetic and potential energies. That the potential energy of the body is increasing may be inferred from the upward displacement of the hip-joint at this time. From the velocity curves published by Fischer (1899), the velocity of the body as a whole is seen to increase as the foot comes into contact with the ground, decreasing, however, before the center of gravity of the body reaches its maximum height.

It is consequently not surprising that the hip-joint forces begin to do work on the leg, as shown in figure 9 [*figure 5.14 here*], before the hip-joint reaches its maximum elevation. This energy, at first contributed by decrease in kinetic energy of the body, later by decrease in potential energy, is only used in small part for the increase in combined kinetic and potential energy of the leg. By far the greater part of it is received by the muscles of the leg.

During the last 0.1 sec. of contact of the foot with the ground, it is the muscles of the leg which are releasing energy. This is used chiefly in increasing the kinetic and potential energy of the leg. Some of this energy, however, is transferred to the rest of the body, although towards the end of the period of contact the rest of the body is again contributing energy to the leg.

During the early portion of the swing, the leg is increasing its combined kinetic and potential energy. This energy is contributed by the muscles and by the rest of the body, in proportions which vary as the values in figure 9 [*figure 5.14 here*] indicate.

Transfer of Energy Within the Leg

During the latter portion of the swing, shown at the left in figure 8 [*figure 5.13 here*], the foot is decreasing its combined potential and kinetic energy and to this is added a small amount of work done by the muscles acting on the foot. The energy thus made available is transferred to the shank by the joint forces in the ankle, since they receive energy from the foot (dashed line) and contribute it to the shank, where they constitute the distal joint forces (dashed-dot line). In addition to receiving energy from the foot, the shank is also contributing energy from its combined kinetic and potential energy. Part of this energy is passed on to the thigh by the knee-joint force, the rest being received by the muscles. A similar procedure is taking place in the thigh, although there the energy liberated is almost equal to that which is passed on, through the hip-joint to the trunk, leaving little energy exchange to the muscles.

After the foot makes contact with the ground, the chief source of energy is muscle action on the thigh. Part of this energy is passed on to the trunk by the hip-joint force, the remainder to the shank through the knee-joint, although for about 0.05 sec. the knee-joint force transfers energy in the other direction. The energy carried to the shank is absorbed by muscles.

From phase 130 to 150 energy is supplied by the rest of the body through the hip-joint. This energy is partially taken up by the muscles acting on the thigh, partially transferred to the shank to be received by muscles there.

From phase 150 to 165 energy is still being provided by the hip-joint force and is partially taken up by muscles acting on the thigh, except at the close of the interval, at which time the thigh is receiving a small amount of energy from the muscles. The increase in combined kinetic and potential energy of the thigh withdraws a small amount of energy. The remainder of the energy from the hip-joint force is transferred to the shank. The shank also receives a large amount of energy from the foot through the ankle-joint, this energy being released by the muscles acting on the foot. Energy is taken from the shank by the increase of its combined kinetic and potential energy, but by far the larger portion of it is received by muscles.

From phase 165 to 174 energy is being transferred to the rest of the body through the hip-joint from the thigh. Energy is also taken from the thigh by the increase in its combined kinetic and potential energy. The total amount of energy so involved is smaller than it would be if the subject had not been slowing down slightly. The chief source of energy is by transmission from the shank. The only source of energy for the shank at this time is transmission from the foot through the ankle. Enough energy is transmitted in this way for forwarding to the thigh, for increase of the kinetic and potential energy of the shank and for reception by muscle. The source of the energy from the foot is the action of muscles on the foot.

In the first part of the swing of the leg, energy is supplied from the rest of the body through the hip-joint and from the muscles working on the thigh, this energy being transmitted so as to allow the increase in kinetic and potential energy of the shank and foot without appreciable muscular work on those members.

Resume of Energy Changes

Starting with the leg in mid-air, we find that the combined kinetic and potential energies of the foot, shank and thigh are all decreasing, liberating energy for other purposes. Somewhat more than half of this energy is transmitted to the rest of the body, the remainder being received by the muscles, chiefly those acting on the shank.

During the first portion of the period during which the foot is in contact with the ground, the changes in kinetic and potential energy of the leg are small. Muscles acting on the thigh contribute sufficient energy for transmission of a considerable amount to the trunk and a smaller amount to the shank, from which it is taken by muscles.

In the middle portion of the contact period, energy is given to the leg by the rest of the body, to be received by muscles acting on the thigh and shank.

When the heel starts to rise, muscles acting on the foot liberate energy, which is transferred to the shank, to be received by muscles acting on the shank. The rest of the body contributes energy to the thigh, partially transferred to the shank to be received by muscles there. The kinetic and potential energy of the leg is also increasing at this time. Toward the conclusion of the period of contact, the rest of the body is receiving energy from the leg. This energy, together with that which is necessary for the increase in kinetic and potential energy of the leg, is supplied by muscles acting on the foot.

During the first portion of the swing, the kinetic and potential energies of all portions of the leg are increasing. The energy for this increase is supplied by the rest of the body through the hip-joint and by muscles acting on the thigh.

The reception and release of energy by the leg muscles take place in two complete cycles for each double step. The first cycle starts in the middle of the swing, the second while the foot is on the ground.

Discussion

Considered as a locomotor mechanism, the human body represents a compromise between the principles of physical efficiency and the dictates of sound anatomical structure. A wheel rolling upon a level surface need only supply enough energy to overcome friction in order to progress with a uniform velocity. Even on an undulating surface the wheel may roll on without expending extra energy, by converting kinetic energy into potential as it rises, reconverting it into kinetic as it falls. This implies changes in velocity but not of total energy.

The human mechanism overcomes the problem of external friction by not rolling, but introduces difficulties of a more serious nature. Not only does the combined center of gravity move in such a fashion that no exact conversion of kinetic into potential energy is possible, but the limbs must swing forward and backward with consequent flux of energy.

Muscles not only provide forces which guide the limbs into trajectories impossible for compound pendulums, but they also regulate the energy distribution of the body. When the total kinetic and potential energy of the mechanism increases, the energy is supplied by muscles. When the total energy decreases, it is taken up by muscles. The extent to which the energy received may again be issued is a moot question. If the muscles were perfect accumulators and were able to exert force without the expenditure of chemical energy, then the efficiency of human locomotion would approach that of the rolling wheel, the friction of the joints and resistance to deformation of the tissues supplanting the friction of the ground. It is consequently not the innate mechanical structure of the body which limits locomotor efficiency as much as it is the imperfect qualification of muscle tissue for the functions it is called upon to perform.

Summary

1. By recording the reaction of the ground and its point of application, together with motion pictures of the displacement of the body, it is possible to study the kinetics of the leg without the necessity of considering the entire body.

2. The method of determining the instantaneous value of the forces and torques acting on each part of the leg is described. By this means the torques exerted by the muscles on the foot, shank and thigh, and of the leg muscles on the trunk, are found.

3. The transfer of energy within the leg and between the leg and the rest of the body is followed by means of the activity of the forces and torques.

4. The total kinetic and potential energy of the leg increases as the leg is swung forward, decreasing again from the middle of the swing until the foot is in contact. This increase and decrease in energy is only partially balanced by transfer of energy from or to the rest of the body. The maintenance of energy equilibrium is due to the action of muscles, which alternately receive the excess energy and supply the deficit.

5. The reception and release of energy by the leg muscles in walking take place in two cycles for each double step, the first starting when the leg is in the middle of its swing, the second while the foot is on the ground. The regular alternation of reception and release of energy suggests the possibility of partial storage of energy by the muscles.

References

Bernstein, N. Untersuchungen der Biodynamik des Ganges und des Laufes. Moscow, 1927. Untersuchungen ueber die Biodynamik der Lokomotion. Moscow, 1935.

Elftman, H. Anat. Rec. 59: 481, 1934. Science 88: 152, 1938.

Elftman, H. and J. Manter. Science 80: 484, 1934.

Fenn, W. O. This Journal 92: 583, 1929. This Journal 93: 433, 1930.

Fischer, O. Abh. K. Sächs. Ges. Wiss., Math.-Phys. Classe 25: 1, 1899; 26: 471, 1901; 28: 533, 1904.

Theoretische Grundlagen für eine Mechanik der lebenden Kürper. Leipzig, 1906.

Summary of Fundamental Data and Method of Calculation

Constants of the Subject

The total weight of the subject at the time of the experiment was 63.4 kgm. Using the proportions determined by Fischer (1906) the constants of the parts of the body were as follows:

Table 5.5

	Foot	Shank	Thigh
Weight in kgm	1.14	3.34	7.35
Mass in kgm. slugs (gravitational units)	0.00116	0.0034	0.0075
Moment of inertia in kgm. slug cm.^{2}	0.046	0.33	1.19
Length in cm.	6.4	39.5	40.6
Proportion of distance of center of gravity from lower joint to total length		0.58	0.56

Reprinted from Elftman 1939.

The lengths of the shank and thigh are measured between joint axes; the length of the foot given here is the distance from the ankle joint to the center of gravity of the foot.

Explanation of Table 5.6

The fundamental data from which the quantities discussed in this paper are calculated are given in the table for intervals of 0.1 sec. The actual computations were carried out for five times this number of phases. The x– and z– coordinates are given. The angle ϕ is the angle between the long axis of the member and the vertical axis. Parts of the body are indicated by subscripts: ankle-joint, a; knee-joint, k; hip-joint, h; foot, 7; shank, 5; thigh, 3; trunk, 1. The velocities or first derivatives with respect to time, are indicated by one dot, e.g., $\dot{x}$, and the acceleration, or second derivative by two dots, $\ddot{x}$. The accelerations of the centers of gravity are not given directly, to economize space, since they are multiplied by the mass of the member, which is constant, to give the effective force, denoted by E. The force exerted by the platform on the foot is shown in a horizontal component R_x and a vertical component $(R_g + R_z)$ which includes components due to gravity and effective forces. The final entry is x_r, the coordinate of the point of application of the force exerted by the platform.

Method of Calculation

To illustrate the method of calculation, some of the computations for phase 150 will be presented. Since the joint force, as defined in the text, acting as the proximal, or upper, joint of a member must be in equilibrium with the other external forces acting on the member and the reversed effective force, we may write:

proximal joint force = –(distal force + force of gravity on member + reversed
effective force of member)

Table 5.6

Time	70	80	90	100	110	120	130	140	150	160	170	180	190	200
x_a	66.0	96.7	113.0	118.2	119.0	119.0	119.0	119.0	119.0	120.2	124.4	135.5	153.5	177.5
x_k	84.5	92.8	100.4	109.2	116.2	120.1	122.4	125.0	129.2	137.6	149.9	166.3	184.7	200.9
x_h	62.3	69.6	79.8	90.3	100.8	110.5	117.7	125.8	135.1	144.7	155.0	164.9	173.4	181.9
z_a	16.2	11.0	10.3	9.4	8.6	8.5	8.5	8.5	8.5	10.8	15.0	20.5	23.7	18.7
z_k	51.1	50.3	47.7	47.8	47.9	48.0	47.9	47.5	46.7	46.2	45.0	45.2	47.9	50.5
z_h	85.2	83.6	82.7	83.7	85.5	87.5	88.2	88.1	86.9	86.2	85.3	85.8	86.9	86.4
ϕ_7	+23.0	+56.7	+69.0	+58.5	+52.7	+52.6	+52.6	+52.6	+52.6	+41.4	+16.8	-9.8	-7.4	+14.8
ϕ_5	-28.0	+5.7	+18.6	+13.2	+4.0	-1.6	-4.9	-8.7	-15.0	-26.2	-40.2	-51.3	-52.2	-36.3
ϕ_3	+33.1	+33.6	+30.5	+27.7	+22.2	+13.7	+6.7	-1.1	-8.3	-10.0	-7.2	+2.3	+16.1	+27.9
ϕ_1	-6.5	-7.1	-7.2	-6.7	-5.8	-6.1	-7.1	-7.7	-7.8	-7.3	-6.2	-6.2	-6.9	-7.5
$\dot{x}_7$	+333	+267	+90	+21	0	0	0	0	+1	+11	+31	+125	+236	+298
$\dot{x}_5$	+201	+154	+91	+64	+27	+17	+14	+18	+33	+67	+109	+171	+204	+190
$\dot{x}_3$	+109	+81	+96	+102	+78	+58	+50	+63	+78	+99	+121	+142	+130	+110
$\dot{z}_7$	-74.5	+7.5	-12.0	-24.0	-4.0	0	0	0	+2.0	+22.0	+37.5	+61.0	-2.0	-73.0
$\dot{z}_5$	-29.0	-24.0	-10.0	-0.2	+0.2	0	0	-2.0	-1.6	+10.6	+19.8	+29.7	+21.0	-26.0
$\dot{z}_3$	-5.9	-23.0	-6.9	+10.4	+16.0	+5.0	+1.0	-5.0	-13.4	-9.5	-0.3	+13.2	+19.0	+2.0
$\dot{\phi}_7$	+5.20	+4.82	-0.30	-1.96	-0.57	0	0	0	-0.23	-3.40	-5.16	-3.50	+2.35	+4.90
$\dot{\phi}_5$	+5.02	+4.25	0	-1.72	-1.18	-0.68	-0.55	-0.86	-1.36	-2.82	-2.02	-1.20	+1.20	+4.10
$\dot{\phi}_3$	+1.28	-0.40	-0.27	-0.50	-1.86	-1.34	-1.28	-1.50	-0.93	+0.05	+0.80	+1.64	+2.84	+1.18
$\dot{\phi}_1$	-0.15	-0.05	+0.01	+0.17	+0.11	-0.16	-0.14	-0.07	+0.03	+0.15	+0.15	-0.10	-0.14	-0.06
$\ddot{x}_a$	+302	+252	+91	+28	+2	0	0	0	+2	+28	+59	+160	+221	+266
$\ddot{x}_k$	+127	+73	+91	+92	+46	+27	+22	+34	+53	+95	+145	+179	+192	+138
$\ddot{x}_h$	+83	+87	+101	+109	+101	+79	+71	+95	+97	+103	+102	+112	+81	+89
$\ddot{z}_a$	-90.0	-18.3	-10.0	-15.4	-1.1	0	0	0	+3.0	+39.0	+50.0	+54.0	0	-79.0
$\ddot{z}_k$	+11.5	-36.0	-10.0	+4.5	+3.6	-0.7	-1.9	-5.4	-10.0	-9.8	-5.0	+14.6	+37.0	+17.0
$\ddot{z}_h$	-19.6	-19.0	-4.4	+15.0	+29.6	+12.2	+4.3	-6.4	-15.5	-9.2	0	+12.0	+5.0	-6.0
$\ddot{\phi}_7$	+18.0	-30.3	-40.0	+12.0	+10.0	0	0	0	-5.0	-22.0	-6.0	+52.0	+9.5	+31.5
$\ddot{\phi}_5$	+29.0	-38.0	-25.4	-3.5	+6.3	+5.1	-1.0	-4.4	-6.5	-7.5	+3.5	+17.8	+29.4	+23.4
$\ddot{\phi}_3$	-27.6	-8.0	+3.0	-7.0	-2.8	+2.1	-1.4	+0.8	+9.0	+10.6	+10.8	+8.4	+4.0	-13.5
E_{x7}	0	-2.5	-1.2	-0.6	0	0	0	0	0	+0.2	+0.7	+1.1	+1.0	+0.4
E_{x5}	-1.1	-2.1	-0.9	-1.7	-0.5	-0.2	0	+0.3	+1.24	+1.4	+2.15	+1.7	+0.3	-0.4
E_{x3}	-4.1	+1.0	+1.4	-0.8	-1.6	-1.4	+0.5	+1.0	+1.3	+1.8	+1.3	0	-0.8	-1.7
E_{z7}	+0.3	+0.3	-0.4	+0.2	+0.1	0	0	0	0	+0.1	+0.3	-0.3	-0.9	+0.1
E_{z5}	+0.3	-0.4	+0.4	+0.1	0	-0.1	-0.1	0	+0.3	+0.4	+0.4	+0.4	-1.3	-1.1
E_{z3}	-0.7	-1.7	+1.7	+1.2	-0.8	-0.6	-0.2	-0.2	-0.2	+0.6	+0.8	+1.4	-2.3	-0.8
R_x					-8.4	-6.1	-2.5	-1.5	-1.3	+1.6	+7.9			
$R_g + R_z$					+50.0	+68.4	+56.0	+55.6	+70.0	+76.9	+36.0			
x_r					118.5	119.6	121.5	125.4	131.4	131.9	133.3			

Reprinted from Elftman 1939.

For the foot the distal force is the platform reaction. The force is computed in vertical and horizontal, or z and x components, the term for gravity being present only for the vertical component. For the ankle-joint force, acting on the foot, the z component = $-(70.0 - 1.14 - 0) = -68.86$ or -68.9 kgm. The x component = $-(-1.3 - 0) = +1.3$ kgm. The ankle-joint force acting on the shank is of opposite sign to that acting on the foot, but of the same magnitude. With this force known, the formula given above may be applied to the shank. The z component of the knee-joint force acting on the shank = −(68.86 − 3.34 − 0.3) = −65.22 or −65.2 kgm. and the x component = −(−1.3 − 1.24) = +2.5 kgm. Similarly, the z component of the hip-joint force acting on the thigh = −(65.22 − 7.35 + 0.2) = −58.1 kgm. and the x component = −(−2.5 − 1.3) = +3.8 kgm.

The torque of the muscles acting on the foot must be in equilibrium with the torques due to external forces and the reversed effective torque. Taking moments about the ankle-joint, the lever arm of the vertical component of the platform reaction is the horizontal distance of the point of application of the force from the ankle-joint, or 131.4 − 119.0 = 12.4 cm., and the torque is 70 × 12.4 = +868 kgm. cm. The lever arm of the horizontal component is the distance of the floor from the ankle-joint, or −8.5 cm., and the torque is −(−1.3)(−8.5) = −11 kgm. cm. The lever arms of the forces acting at the mass center of the foot are 6.4 cos 52.6° = +5.1 cm. for the vertical components and −6.4 sin 52.6° = −3.9 cm. for the horizontal component. The torque of gravity is therefore −1.1 × 5.1 = −5; of the vertical reversed effective force, 0 × 5.1 = 0; and of the horizontal reversed effective force, −0(−3.9) = 0. The reversed effective torque is obtained from the moment of inertia and angular acceleration and is −0.046 (−5.0) = 0, since the calculation of the other torques is not carried beyond the decimal point. The sum of the torques is consequently +852 kgm. cm.; since the muscle torque must be in equilibrium with this torque, it must have a value of −852 kgm. cm.

Similar computations can then be made for the shank and the thigh, the lever arms of the forces being obtained from the positions of the joints or from the length of the member and its angle of inclination. The proportionate position of the mass center with respect to the joints allows the calculation of the lever arms of forces acting at the mass center. When these computations are carried out, they yield a value of +755 kgm. cm. for the muscle torque on the shank and of +503 kgm. cm. on the thigh. Since the total torque exerted by any system must be zero, and the muscles of the leg end either in the leg or on the trunk, the torque which they exert on the trunk is −(−852 + 755 + 503) = −406 kgm. cm.

The rate at which the forces and torques are doing work, or their activity, is readily calculated since the velocities of the points of application of the forces and the angular velocities of the members upon which the torques act are known. Taking the thigh as an illustration, the activity of the muscle torque is +503 (−0.93) = −467 kgm. cm./sec.; of the distal joint force, with x and z components, (−2.5 × 53) + (+65.2) (−10.0) = −785; and of the proximal joint force, (+3.8 × 97) + (−58.1) (−15.5) = +1268.

In similar fashion the rates at which the potential and kinetic energies of the thigh are decreasing may be obtained from the activity of the force of gravity and the reversed effective forces and torques. For decrease in potential energy the rate is –7.35 (–13.4) = +99 kgm. cm./sec.; for kinetic energy, giving the x and z components of reversed effective force and the reversed effective torque in order, the rate of decrease is –1.3 × 78 + 0.2 (–13.4) + (–1.19) (+9.0) (–0.93) = –94 kgm. cm./sec. The rate of decrease in combined kinetic and potential energy is consequently 99 – 94 = +5 kgm. cm./sec. The computations for the other parts of the leg are made in comparable fashion.

Mechanical Work in Human Movement

The human body conforms to the law of conservation of energy and must spend chemically bound energy to move. Through diverse metabolic processes, metabolic energy is transformed into mechanical work and heat. The mechanical work of human movements is an important field of biomechanical research. Although the measurement of mechanical work provides only one scalar value (a number), in many cases that number is of paramount importance. The direction of research derives benefits from relying on a basic law of nature: the conservation of energy. Research is inviting when an unbreakable benchmark law exists to test findings and hypotheses against, and such an opportunity does not exist in other areas of biomechanics where fundamental laws have not yet been discovered. In addition to its own merit, the investigation of mechanical energy transformations in human movement bridges a gap between biomechanics on the one hand and physiology and motor control on the other. This is a domain in which interdisciplinary projects will likely emerge.

At the same time, the problem of mechanical work in human movement is difficult to solve. If we take into account that the notion of mechanical work has been known for centuries and that the first estimation of mechanical work in human movement was done as early as 1836 (Weber and Weber, English translation in 1992), it would seem natural to think that by this time the solution to the problem would be well established. However, this is not the case. The determination of mechanical power and work in human movement remains a challenging task. After many years of research and dozens of publications, standard procedures of determining mechanical work in human and animal movement do not yet exist. We still do not know how to compute mechanical work in complex human movement, for example in sprint running, in a nonambiguous way. In the scientific community, frequent misunderstanding and the lack of unified terminology complicate the solution of the problem. There is still a huge discrepancy in the methods used and in the results that have been reported (for recent discussions, see van Ingen Schenau et al., 1997; Zatsiorsky, 1998).

In the papers reproduced in this book, Fenn (1930) and Elftman (1939) suggested and implemented two methods that are regularly used for computing mechanical work in human and animal movement.

Fenn's method, also called the "fraction approach" (Aleshinsky, 1986a; Zatsiorsky, 1986), is based on the determination of changes in the total mechanical energy of human body segments. In this method, the total mechanical energy (TME) of a body segment is represented as the sum of three "fractions": potential energy (PE), kinetic translational energy (KTE), and kinetic rotational energy (KRE):

$$TME = PE + KTE + KRE = mgh + mv^2 / 2 + I\omega^2 / 2$$

where m stands for mass; h is the vertical location of a segment's center of mass; I is moment of inertia of a segment; v and ω are the linear and angular velocity, respectively, of a body segment; and g is acceleration due to gravity. The energy values are measured over a particular time period. The gain in energy provides an estimation of the mechanical work done and, if calculated per unit time, the mechanical power.

Elftman's method (1939), also termed the "source approach," is based on the determination of power and work of joint moments. By definition, the source of energy is any force and force moment acting on the system that develop or absorb mechanical energy during its motion. Joint power is computed as the product of joint angular velocity and the joint moment:

$$P_j = M_j \left(\omega_1 - \omega_2 \right) = M_j \omega_j$$

where M_j is the joint moment, ω_1 are ω_2 are angular velocities of the adjacent segments forming the joint, and ω_j is the joint angular velocity, that is, the relative angular velocity of the adjacent segments with respect to one another. To find the values of the moments in several joints, Elftman was the first to suggest an iteration procedure that is customarily used now.

The two methods are based on straightforward mechanics and perform nicely when applied to one body segment (Fenn's method) or one joint (Elftman's method). They also work fine when simple movements are studied, such as a standing vertical jump without a countermovement. However, ambiguous findings have been reported in complex movements. It follows from the experimental investigations using these different techniques (Pierrynowski et al., 1980; Williams and Cavanagh, 1983; Prilutsky and Zatsiorsky, 1992) that the magnitudes of the discrepancies between the various methods may be as high as ninefold. The reason is that Fenn's and Elftman's methods by themselves ensure only the first step in the mechanical work analysis. During the second step, when the task is to determine the total power or total work performed by a subject, researchers need to use additional information and/or to add additional assumptions. The problems and controversies appear during this stage. One such controversy concerns calculating the total mechanical power/work generated in several joints. From a mechanics standpoint, the task is to compute the work that is produced by several forces/moments that act on several bodies. This is an ill-posed problem. Such a problem cannot be solved in an unambiguous way unless additional information about the forces (are the energy sources independent?) and the system under consideration is provided.

Two approaches are advocated in the literature to compute the total power/work. Some authors (for instance, van Ingen Shenau & Cavanagh, 1990) recommend:

$$P_{tot} = \sum_j P_j,$$

where $P_j = M_j \omega_j$ is the power generated by joint moment M_j at the angular velocity ω_j in joint j, P_{tot} is the total power produced in all the joints under consideration, and $\sum_j$ is the summation across the joints.

In contrast, other authors (for instance, Aleshinsky, 1986a, b; Blickhan & Full, 1992) favor the summation of absolute rather than real values of joint power:

$$P_{tot} = \sum_j |P_j|$$

It is easy to provide arguments for and against both of these methods. For instance, the second method has been criticized because the summation of the absolute values of power is not defined in classical mechanics. Imagine that these two approaches are applied to the following movement. A human with the left arm raised and the right arm lowered is lifting the right arm and simultaneously lowering the left one. The joint power values of all the joints of the right arm are positive, and the joint power values of all the joints of the left arm are negative. In addition, the joint power values for the right and left arm are equal in magnitude, $|P_{left}| = |-P_{right}|$. For such a movement, the value of the total power equals zero if the first approach is used and is equal to 2P when the second approach is applied. Intuitively, since movement takes place, the first approach does not look appealing.

Another example is a slow horizontal arm extension with a load in the hand (figure 5.15). In this example, the mass of the body parts as well as the work to change the kinetic energy of the load is neglected. All of the three values of work—that is, the work performed at the shoulder joint W_{sh}, the elbow joint W_{el}, and the work of the force applied to the load W_{lo}—can be easily computed. During the movement, the muscles of the shoulder joint perform positive (concentric) work: They generate an abduction moment and elevate the arm. The flexors of the elbow produce negative (eccentric) work. The elbow joint extends while producing a flexion moment. The work of the force exerted by the hand on the load is zero. The direction of the gravity force is at a right angle to the direction of the load displacement, and as a result the potential energy of the load does not change. Hence, $W_{sh} + W_{el} = W_{lo} = 0$. The question is what is the amount of *total work* produced? Is it zero? Does the negative work at the elbow joint cancel out the positive work at the shoulder joint? Yes and no. The answer depends on the object of interest and the definition of total work. The total amount of work *done on the system* is definitely zero. However, the total amount of work *performed at the joints* remains unknown unless additional information is provided.

Two extreme cases can be distinguished: those with *noncompensated* and those with *compensated* sources of energy (Aleshinsky, 1986a; Zatsiorsky, 1986). If the sources of energy at the joints (the muscles, engines, torque actuators) are independent, or *noncompensated*, negative work at the elbow joint is dissipated as heat and does not compensate for the positive work at the shoulder. This is the case when only one-joint muscles are acting. The total amount of mechanical energy spent for the movement will not be equal to zero in this case. Contrarily, if two joints are served by one common source of energy, or in other words by sources that are *compensated*, the total energy expenditure in an ideal no-friction condition is zero. An example is two electric motors connected in such a way that the work done by an external force at one joint (negative work of the joint moment) is converted into electric power, transmitted to another joint, and used there. A second example is two-joint muscles.

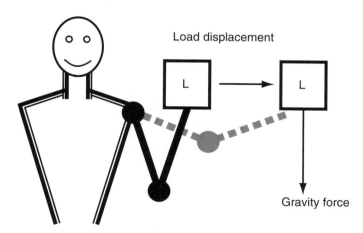

Figure 5.15
A slow horizontal arm extension with a load in the hand. The work done on the load is zero but the work of joint torques is not. (Reprinted from Zatsiorsky & Gregor 2000.)

The preceding examples with compensated or noncompensated sources of energy corroborate the idea that the computation of mechanical work in human movement cannot be performed correctly without a clear-cut understanding of the physical mechanisms of the process. The papers by Fenn and Elftman are excellent in this regard. The authors understood the complexity of the problem and addressed it nicely. Particularly note the discussions of the following issues.

Do the legs move as pendulums during walking and running? The answer is no. Pendulums are conservative systems. In such systems, the total mechanical energy is constant, and the maximal kinetic energy in a cycle equals the maximal potential energy. However, in both sprinting (Fenn, 1930) and walking (Braune & Fischer, 1905, English edition in 1987; Zatsiorsky & Iakunin, 1980), the maximal value of kinetic energy of a leg is several times larger than the leg's potential energy. Therefore, "the storage of energy as potential energy of position and its reappearance as kinetic energy is not an important factor in evaluating the mechanical horse power of sprinting" (Fenn, p. 605). In other words, the legs do not move as pendulums.

What is the role played by muscle viscosity? By assumption, muscle viscosity provides *mechanical* resistance to movement. A suggestion provided by Fenn 70 years ago is still valid: ". . . it seems advisable to warn against the simple interpretation of the term 'viscosity'" (p. 586). Eight years after Fenn's paper, A.V. Hill (1938) arrived at the conclusion that "the 'viscosity' hypothesis must be dismissed" (p. 193) and wrote the following: "The fact that an active muscle shortens more slowly under a greater force is due not to 'viscosity' but, as Fenn has claimed, to the manner in which the energy liberation is regulated" (p. 192). In the 1930 paper, Fenn presented a classical discussion of muscle viscosity (for a recent review, see Zatsiorsky, 1997).

Do muscles exhibit "springlike" behavior? The answer depends on the understanding of the word "springlike." If energy turnover is the point of interest, the answer may be negative. Stretched springs shorten due to the previously accumulated potential energy of deformation. When a spring is released, the supply of additional energy is not necessary for its shortening. Muscles are different. Fenn (1930, p. 606) wrote: "The known facts do not altogether preclude another hypothesis according to which the energy needed for muscular work is developed during the actual period of shortening." In 1938, A.V. Hill confirmed this hypothesis.

Note also a very nice discussion on the transfer of mechanical energy between body parts, the work of deceleration, and energy storage in tendons and muscles. All of these issues are still topics of intensive debate in the contemporary literature (for instance, see the discussion stimulated by a target article of van Ingen Schenau et al., 1997).

This chapter would not be complete without a commendation of the authors for the efforts that were necessary to perform these classical studies. To do such research without digitizers, computers, and other contemporary technical gadgets was by itself a great accomplishment. I do not know whether the next generation of young scientists who will work in the new millennium will gain knowledge from the experiments of Wallace Fenn and Herbert Elftman. I hope, however, that their quest for knowledge will endure.

References

Aleshinsky SY (1986a) An energy 'source' and 'fraction' approach to the mechanical energy expenditure problem—1. Basic concepts, description of the model, analysis of a one-link system movement. *Journal of Biomechanics, 19*, 287-293.

Aleshinsky SY (1986b) An energy 'source' and 'fraction' approach to the mechanical energy expenditure problem—IV. Criticism of the concept of 'energy transfers within and between links.' *Journal of Biomechanics, 19*, 307-309.

Blickhan R & Full RJ (1992) Mechanical work in terrestrial locomotion. In: Biewener AA (Ed.), *Biomechanics: Structures and Systems* (pp. 75-96). New York: Oxford University Press.

Braune W & Fischer O (1987) *The Human Gait*. Berlin, Heidelberg, New York: Springer-Verlag.

Elftman H (1939) Forces and energy changes in the leg during walking. *American Journal of Physiology, 125*, 339-356.

Fenn WO (1930) Frictional and kinetic factors in the work of sprint running. *American Journal of Physiology, 92*, 583-611.

Hill AV (1938) The heat of shortening and the dynamic constants of muscle. *Proceedings of the Royal Society of London, 126-B*, 136-195.

Ingen Schenau GJ van, Bobbert MF & Haan A de (1997) Does elastic energy enhance work and efficiency in the stretch-shortening cycle? *Journal of Applied Biomechanics, 13*(4), 389-415.

Ingen Schenau GJ van & Cavanagh, PR (1990) Power equations in endurance sports. *Journal of Biomechanics, 23*, 865-881.

Pierrynowski M, Winter D & Norman R (1980) Transfer of mechanical energy within the total body and mechanical efficiency during treadmill walking. *Ergonomics, 23*, 147-156.

Prilutsky BI & Zatsiorsky VM (1992) Mechanical energy expenditure and efficiency of walking and running. *Human Physiology, 18*(3), 118-127.

Weber W & Weber E (1992) *Mechanics of the Human Walking Apparatus*. Berlin, Heidelberg, New York: Springer-Verlag.

Williams KR & Cavanagh PR (1983) A model for the calculation of mechanical power during distance running. *Journal of Biomechanics, 16*, 115-128.

Zatsiorsky VM (1986) Mechanical work and energy expenditure in human motion. In: Knets IV (Ed.), *Contemporary Problems of Biomechanics. 3, Optimization of Biomechanical Movement* (pp. 14-32). Riga, Latvia: Zinatne.

Zatsiorsky VM (1997) On muscle and joint viscosity. *Motor Control, 1*, 299-309.

Zatsiorsky VM (1998) Can total work be computed as a sum of the 'external' and 'internal' work? *Journal of Biomechanics, 31*(2), 191-192.

Zatsiorsky VM & Iakunin NA (1980). Mechanical work and energy during locomotion. *Human Physiology, 6*(4), 579-596.

Zatsiorsky VM & Gregor RJ (2000). Mechanical power and work in human movement. In WA Sparrow (Ed.), *Energetics at Human Activity* (pp. 195-227). Champaign, IL: Human Kinetics.

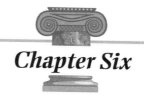

Chapter Six

Contributions of Ragnar Granit to the Understanding of Spinal Mechanisms of Motor Coordination

T. Richard Nichols

Emory University

Revisiting the work of Ragnar Granit

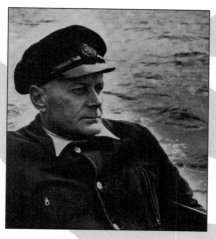

Ragnar Granit

It is not my intention to undervalue discoveries, but only to emphasize that it is really understanding that scientists are after, even when they are making discoveries. These are or can be of little interest as long as they are mere facts. They have to be understood, at least in a general way, and such understanding implies placing them into a structural whole where they illuminate a relevant step forward or solidify known ideas within it.

(Granit, 1972)

Granit's Life and Work

Ragnar Granit (1900-1991) received his medical degree in 1927 from Helsingfors University in Helsinki with the intention of pursuing a research career in the physiology of the visual system. He furthered his education in experimental physiology and electrophysiology at Oxford University with Sir Charles Sherrington and at the University of Pennsylvania at the invitation of Dr. D.W. Bronk. He then returned to Helsingfors University as professor of physiology. In 1940, he moved to the Royal Caroline Institute of Stockholm and eventually headed a department in the Medical Nobel Institute. He remained at the Royal Caroline Institute until his retirement in 1967.

Granit was awarded the Nobel Prize in physiology and medicine in 1967, with George Wald and Haldan Hartline, for his work on the visual system. Using electrophysiological methods, he showed that the eye of the frog has distributions of spectral sensitivities that can be explained only by assuming at least three cone pigments. This work foreshadowed later research demonstrating the existence of three distinct pigments. Granit was also cited for his early work on inhibitory processes in the retina. In the late 1940s, he switched from this work on the visual system to investigations of the spinal motor apparatus. The paper included in this chapter represents one of his earlier publications in this area.

Granit made many important contributions to the area of spinal mechanisms of motor control and laid the foundations for several contemporary lines of research. In the paper presented here (Granit, 1950), he provided an early study of inhibitory, force-dependent reflexes in the spinal cord and argued that these reflexes are mediated by Golgi tendon organs. This work appeared shortly after Lloyd's classic work defining the "myotatic unit" concept (Lloyd, 1946). According to this view, coordination of synergistic and antagonistic muscles of a joint is mediated by a network of spinal pathways arising from the primary receptors of the muscle spindle. The Ia afferents from these receptors project monosynaptic excitation to the motoneurons of the agonist and synergistic muscles and disynaptic inhibition to antagonistic muscles. Lloyd believed that this network is adequate to subserve identical and reciprocal innervation, two major patterns of activation of muscles that occur during natural movements. That is, these pathways would reinforce the coactivation of synergistic muscles and the reciprocal activation of antagonistic muscles. The myotatic unit represented the then-current model of the way the spinal network mediates coordinated motor behavior.

However, it was also clear that other spinal pathways must be important in motor coordination. The presence of force receptors, the Golgi tendon organs, was recognized, but the functions of these receptors were unknown. Furthermore, Sir Charles Sherrington (1909) had described a phenomenon known as the "lengthening reaction" (described in more detail later) that could not be explained by the myotatic unit concept. In addition, Denny-Brown (1928) had pointed out that the silent period (described later) could represent an apparent inhibition in response to a tendon-jerk reflex of that muscle. In the myotatic unit, each muscle receives only excitatory reflexes from itself, so the silent period required another explanation.

Granit reopened this question by investigating the possibility that receptors from a given muscle give rise to inhibitory pathways to the same muscle. Granit referred to this self-inhibition as "autogenetic inhibition." As explained in the notes to this chapter, Granit used the method of excitability testing to show that inhibition and excitation (facilitation) to a motoneuron pool are mediated by separate sensory receptors that are both associated with rapidly conducting afferent axons. He showed further that these pathways were both autogenic (or "autogenetic") and intermuscular. The additional evidence that the inhibitory component was strongly dependent on muscle tension allowed Granit to argue that this component was probably mediated by Golgi tendon organs.

This work provided a strong basis for further investigations of the properties and distribution of feedback from tension receptors. In a subsequent and widely quoted paper, Laporte and Lloyd (1952) reported on the synaptic organization of the system of pathways presumed to arise from Golgi tendon organs. The work of Laporte and Lloyd was extended by Sir John Eccles, Rosamond Eccles, and Anders Lundberg (1957) in terms of the synaptic distribution of afferents from Golgi tendon organs. However, Granit provided an early description of the force dependence of the inhibition, examined the differences in intermuscular distribution of reflexes arising from muscle spindles and Golgi tendon organs, and discussed the implications of these distributed pathways for coordination. Therefore, Granit was thinking about the functional implications of these pathways in terms of musculoskeletal mechanics as well as circuit organization.

During the 1960s and 1970s, the adequate stimulus of Golgi tendon organs was more precisely defined as active contractile force (Houk and Henneman, 1967). It was also proposed that autogenic inhibition is integrated with monosynaptic excitation from muscle spindle receptors to regulate muscular stiffness. This hypothesis has not been strongly supported, since attempts to demonstrate autogenic inhibition at the whole-muscle level have not generally met with success. However, rapid intermuscular inhibition such as that observed by Granit between the gastrocnemius and quadriceps muscles can be observed under a variety of circumstances and may serve to mediate interjoint coordination (Nichols, 1994; Nichols et al., 1999). Therefore, integrated force and length feedback is likely to be important in mediating coordination, but the integration occurs most likely at the network level rather than the single-muscle level. Granit's work stands as one of the earliest attempts to understand the functions and mechanisms of inhibitory limb reflexes in the spinal cord.

Following his work on reflex inhibition, Granit turned to the subject of muscle spindle receptors and their motor innervation through gamma motoneurons. In addition to investigations of the firing properties of muscle spindle receptors, Granit's work contained discussions of important functional issues. In the early 1950s, Merton (1953) had proposed the length servo hypothesis, in which he postulated that the stretch reflex constitutes a feedback system controlling muscle length. Merton also suggested that motor commands could be delivered through gamma motoneurons in addition to alpha motoneurons and that each of these two routes of excitation would have functional advantages for different motor tasks. Granit and his coworkers (Granit et al., 1955) provided experimental evidence that, in fact, muscle activation could be supported by both alpha and gamma routes. Granit is also associated with the concept that alpha and gamma motoneurons may be activated together. He termed this coactivation "α-γ linkage." This notion later developed into the concept of servo assistance (Matthews, 1970), in which both α and γ routes are used simultaneously. Although the hypothesis that the reflex apparatus functions as a length servo-mechanism is no longer tenable, this idea was important for the development of modern concepts of reflex action. Granit's work and influence provided a major driving force for the development of these ideas.

In 1958, Granit published a seminal paper that provided a synthesis of his work on reflex systems. To account for the contributions of the components of the stretch reflex, he measured muscle extension, discharge frequency of muscle spindle receptors, firing rates of active motoneurons, and muscle force. He found that motoneurons tended to fire at relatively constant rates, suggesting recruitment as a major mechanism for increasing force (see Cope and Pinter, 1995 for an update on mechanisms of orderly recruitment). Furthermore, both the firing rates of spindle receptors and muscle force were found to increase proportionately with muscle length. Granit also cut afferent and efferent connections between the muscle and spinal cord and stimulated the muscle electrically. The results showed that muscle force also increased with length due to the intrinsic mechanical properties of muscle. All of these results have provided the stimulus for many investigations over the past four decades. For example, Matthews

(1959) also investigated the relative contributions of intrinsic muscle mechanics and reflex action to the responses of muscles to stretch. In 1972, Grillner argued that the intrinsic properties were adequate to explain postural support and questioned the role of reflexes particularly during locomotion. Both reflex mechanisms and intrinsic properties have subsequently been shown to provide important contributions to mechanical properties of muscle under a wide variety of conditions (see Nichols et al., 1999).

During the 1960s, Granit and his coworkers utilized intracellular recording and current injection to study the firing properties of motoneurons. The behavior of the motoneuron could be described in terms of a "frequency-current" plot that documents the dependence of firing rate on the magnitude of injected current. This work led to the demonstration by Daniel Kernell (1965) that motoneurons tend to fire in two linear ranges, referred to as the primary and secondary ranges. The slope of the "F-I" relationship is higher in a range of larger injected currents known as the secondary range. This description of motoneuron firing remains a building block of contemporary spinal cord physiology.

Taken together, these examples illustrate Ragnar Granit's prescience in recognizing the central questions concerning the role of spinal mechanisms in motor coordination. He addressed these questions using state-of-the-art technology, continued to learn new techniques until the end of his career, and continually attempted a synthesis of his own results and those of others into a conceptual, structural whole.

Reflex Self-Regulation of Muscle Contraction and Autogenetic Inhibition*

Ragnar Granit
Nobel Institute for Neurophysiology, Karolinska Institutet, Stockholm, Sweden

(Received for publication December 5, 1949)

The development that followed upon Sherrington's original discovery of the lengthening reaction (45) and P. Hoffmann's demonstration of the silent period in the electromyogram accompanying the knee jerk (28) may be well known but so much time has now elapsed since these problems were the subject of active experimentation that it is necessary, in reopening the field, to begin by surveying the ground in the light of recent research in order to show where we stand and why again reasonably some progress may be expected.

*Reprinted from Granit 1950.

Sherrington pointed out that the lengthening reaction in the quadriceps muscle was accompanied by Philippson's reflex of crossed extension as well as by ipsilateral flexion, thereby giving autogenetic inhibition a functional status within the framework of reciprocal innervation. The silent period was held by Denny-Brown (9), on similar evidence, to be but an expression of autogenetic inhibition. It was hypothetically localized to the annulo-spiral afferent system and shown to require a strong synchronous efferent volley, set up by a tap on the tendon or by an electrical shock to the motor root. Hoff, *et al.* (27) found a silent period in one extensor after excitation of another only when the former had discharged owing to facilitation.

At the time it was necessary to preserve intact efferent supply in order to study the silent period by means of silver pins stuck into the muscle. We have since learned that strong synchronous stimuli—at least electrical ones—set up a centripetal 'back-response' due to electrical cross-excitation in the muscle (34,30) as well as back-responses from artificial synapses formed by severed nerves, especially in the unanaesthetized decerebrate preparation (23) used by Denny-Brown. Such back-responses are particularly strong in the afferents. If, as found by him, the silent period requires strong synchronous efferent volleys, we are entitled to conclude from his work that the motoneurones may have been tested by combined synchronous afferent and efferent (antidromic) back-responses, to which they responded by setting up positive after-potential and subnormal excitability. Of this the silent period would have been a consequence.

The last conclusion was, in fact, suggested by Gasser (18) who, having demonstrated the correlation between the late positive phase of the cord potential and inhibition (18,20,29) explained the silent period as the result of such subnormal excitability. My own work on the retina had at about the same time led to the conclusion that excitation and inhibition were associated with potential changes in the electroretinogram of opposite sign (see *e.g.* summary, 22). Then followed the demonstration by Eccles and Pritchard (14) that an antidromic volley delivered into a motor root elicits a root potential of the same general shape as that of the superior cervical ganglion (10), an initial negative phase accompanied by hyperexcitability followed by a positive phase and consequent subnormality. In 1939 (12) Eccles pointed out that orthodromic stimulation of dorsal roots sets up a similar type of potential change on the ventral side and finally (13) he published a very complete analysis of this ventral root potential (the well-known phenomenon discovered by Umrath (46) and studied by Barron and Matthews (2)). In this work it was ultimately proved that no internuncial excitation was required for the ventral root potential so that it legitimately could be called the synaptic potential of the motoneurones.

The general line of thinking, inaugurated by Gasser and followed by Bremer and Bonnet (4,5) in important work, would seem, indeed, to have settled, once and for all, the question of the silent period, the more so as Bernhard (3) showed that a shock to the afferent gastrocnemius nerves was followed by a depression of the ensuing monosynaptic volley to a second shock and accompanied by a positive change in the root potential. In this work, however, the conditioning shock was strong and therefore Lloyd's (35) high-threshold group II and group III fibres were not excluded. In addition, the positive component of the root potential was held to be something peculiar for extensor motoneurones whilst the silent period is seen in the flexors also (9).

Problem and principle of analysis

In coming to the conclusion that the silent period need be no more than an interesting physiological artefact due to a subnormal phase following a synchronous normal orthodromic volley in monosynaptic stretch-afferents, we have successfully done away with true autogenetic inhibition. We would then be compelled to explain Sherrington's lengthening reaction as an ordinary nociceptive response inducing the flexion reflex whilst inhibiting the extensors. This does not seem very likely in view of Cooper and Creed's (7,8) demonstration of highly complex facilitatory effects of synergistic and inhibitory effects of antagonistic muscles turning up in muscles subjected to stretch or induced to contract. Neither does it seem likely that the single-shock technique can uncover all the essential features in the normal interplay of reflexes to stretch and contraction which arise from a minimum of five sense organs in the muscle. In returning to the work of the Oxford school, to the papers mentioned as well as to those of Liddell and Sherrington (32) and of Fulton and Pi-Suner (17), we can take advantage of the fact that a great many questions today can be simplified by testing directly the state of excitability of a given set of well-defined motoneurones subjected to afferent influences from the muscle. It is no longer necessary to try the devious route over the silent period in the electromyogram and to keep the complicating efferent supply intact.

The method developed (26) is based on Lloyd's (36) important demonstration that the monosynaptic reflex of Eccles and Pritchard (14) runs in the largest afferents from the muscle and back again through the efferents of the same muscle. The monosynaptic response from the severed ventral root may therefore be used as a test of the excitability of a particular set of motoneurones destined for a given muscle. Since it is faster than any other reflex volley through the cord, it will gauge their level of excitability, as determined by any given amount of preceding afferent influx from stretch or contraction, without the complication of the additional impulses set up by the contraction initiated by the test volley itself (see Fig. 1 [*figure 6.1 here*]).

The full theoretical significance of the analysis by means of the monosynaptic volley should not be missed. If, for instance, the test shock

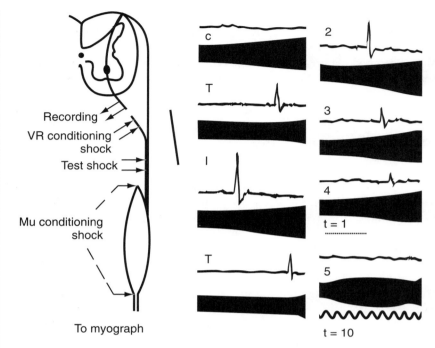

Figure 6.1
Excitability of gastrocnemius motoneurones during contraction of gastrocnemius. *Left.* Diagram illustrating experimental arrangement. *Right.* c, conditioning shock alone, its discharge above, its myogram below; T (upper) test shock with its myogram; 1-4, both together at different time intervals (t = 1 msec.); T (lower) test shock alone at t = 10 msec.; 5, together with conditioning shock at t = 10 msec. (Reprinted from Granit 1950.)

finds the motoneurones inhibited, then by whatever synergistic muscle this inhibition has been produced and independently of how many synapses it has traversed, this inhibition has ultimately by some central mechanism been applied on to the motoneurone itself. The monosynaptic test volley, running a non-stop course to the motoneurone, cannot itself have been held up by clashing with internuncial refractoriness or subnormality. An inhibition shown by the monosynaptic test will always be genuine and can be due to post-excitatory subnormality of the tested motoneurone, only when this has discharged, for instance, when stimulated from the muscle supply the afferents for the monosynaptic test volley itself. The internuncial mechanism can come in at a pre-motoneurone level only if the inhibitory impulses succeed in stopping a facilitatory background discharge which is assumed to be necessary for maintaining the excitability of the motoneurone.

Technique

Most animals were in light dial anaesthesia, 0.3-0.4 cc./kg. Some, in addition, were made spinal by a section at or just above Th12. Some decerebrate cats were used but the 'tonic' changes were found to be too much of a complication at this stage of the analysis. The ventral roots from L5 downwards were severed, the long L7 and S1 often in the middle, leaving a central stump for recording and a peripheral stump for neuromyal stimulation of the muscle by the conditioning shock (see Fig. 1 [*figure 6.1 here*]). The leg to be used was denervated, leaving only the medial and lateral gastrocnemius nerves for stimulating electrodes buried between the muscles in the closed wound. This stimulus, which below is usually referred to as the test shock (for the monosynaptic volley), was triggered about every 5 seconds by the synchronizing circuit of the electrical system. In some experiments the nerve to the quadriceps muscle was preserved also. In such experiments ileopsoas was cut, together with the muscles around the hip joint. In addition, the rectus component of the quadriceps was removed. The conditioning shock sometimes stimulated muscles around the spine to contract. Further sectioning of muscles was then carried out at the beginning of the experiment, the effect being checked by stimulation and gastrocnemius alone contracted. The muscle contracted isometrically and tension was recorded by the Brown-Shuster myograph to which were fitted two crossing coils, one fixed and fed by a high-frequency current, the other moveable with the myograph lever. The capacitative changes, caused by the slight myograph excursions, were amplified and transmitted to the lower beam of a double cathode-ray oscillograph. The monosynaptic volley was recorded on the upper beam (Fig. 1 [*figure 6.1 here*]). When the muscle afferents were to be stimulated by stretch the myograph was pulled upon by a string running over a pulley to the middle of a lever (on the floor), the free end of which was provided with a rotating circular disc. To the axis of a cogwheel driven by a motor was fixed a bar with a handle that pressed on the disc about every fifth second, triggering the sweep circuit by a microswitch. The myograph return to zero was speeded up by rubber bands. The onset of stretch, as recorded by the myograph, is not accurate to the millisecond. Two flip-flop stimulators, triggered by a delay circuit, and a condenser-coupled amplifier completed the electrical outfit. Time was recorded by a Philips sound generator.

Sources of error

The monosynaptic response often varies in size. This difficulty could be overcome by taking a sufficient number of readings, often up to 10, for each position of the test shock and checking less accurate experiments by more accurate ones. The points in the curves are averages of all the readings for a given position. The effects to be described are a very large order and the main findings confirmed by several modifications of the experimental conditions. In particular stretch can be—and actually was—used to confirm the findings obtained by setting up muscle contractions. This provided a check on sources of error such as stimulus escape to the spinal cord. Besides, the motor fibres are large and of low threshold so that strong stimulation of the roots is by no means necessary. The question of peripheral refractoriness in the nerve used for the test shock is another source of error which is dealt with in Section 6.

Results

1. Motoneurons excitability during contraction and stretch

To the right in Figure 1 [*figure 6.1 here*] are some records from an experiment in which the muscle is contracting in response to a shock to the peripheral stump of the ventral root, a fast time base being used for c (conditioning shock alone), for test shock alone (T, upper) and the combined responses 1-4 whilst a slow time base is used for record 5 which illustrates complete inhibition at a long interval between conditioning shock and test shock, the latter being placed as in the control (T, lower). Figure 2 [*figure 6.2 here*] is a complete analysis of the excitability changes in the same experiment, the size of the control being given by the line 1.0. It should be noted that the interval between conditioning and test shock is given in logarithmic units. The muscle contraction is fully developed within 25-30 msec. The illustrated sequence of changes—facilitation—inhibition is typical for most cats. Facilitation is rarely absent in a good preparation; the depth and extent of inhibition varies a great deal from animal to animal. The same result was obtained by stimulating the muscle directly.

In figure 3 [*figure 6.3 here*] a similar experiment has been performed with the root stimulated by a slowly rising current in order to exclude direct cross-excitation by a synchronous muscle action potential. The form of the stimulating current is shown in record 1, 2 is the muscle contraction set up by this stimulus by itself (conditioning stimulus), 3 the monosynaptic response of the test shock alone, and 4-9 the combined responses at increasing time intervals. The test shock is repeated in 10. Clearly the same sequence, early facilitation followed by inhibition, is obtained. Similarly, in some experiments with the flexor tib. ant. the same type of curve was obtained.

Finally, in figure 4 [*figure 6.4 here*], there is a complete analysis of the results obtained by triggering the sweep and stimulating the muscle under light tension by a 4 mm. stretch. Some actual records from another experiment are given in Figure 10 [*figure 6.10 here*]. The stretch is slow compared with the contractions, its maximum being reached within a time of 80-100 msec. The initial phase of facilitation accordingly is longer. The phase of inhibition in Figure 4 [*figure 6.4 here*] appears contracted on account of the logarithmic time scale. In this experiment it is succeeded by a second facilitation appearing before the final level of stretch has been reached. Sections 5 and 6 will be devoted to effects of stretch.

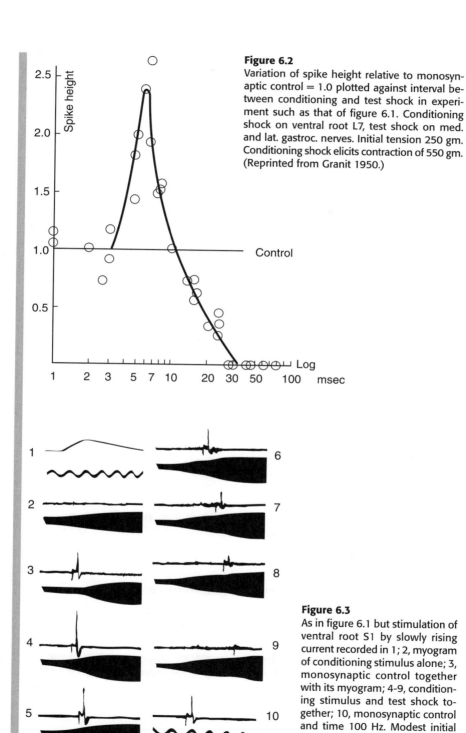

Figure 6.2
Variation of spike height relative to monosynaptic control = 1.0 plotted against interval between conditioning and test shock in experiment such as that of figure 6.1. Conditioning shock on ventral root L7, test shock on med. and lat. gastroc. nerves. Initial tension 250 gm. Conditioning shock elicits contraction of 550 gm. (Reprinted from Granit 1950.)

Figure 6.3
As in figure 6.1 but stimulation of ventral root S1 by slowly rising current recorded in 1; 2, myogram of conditioning stimulus alone; 3, monosynaptic control together with its myogram; 4-9, conditioning stimulus and test shock together; 10, monosynaptic control and time 100 Hz. Modest initial tension. (Reprinted from Granit 1950.)

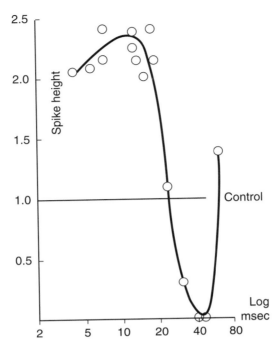

Figure 6.4
Spinal cat. Analysis of effect of stretch of gastrocnemius muscle on its monosynaptic re-sponse. Ordinates spike height in terms of control 1.0; abscissae, time from beginning of visible stretch of, in all, 4 mm. at modest initial tension. *Note*: Stretch increasing during the time shown. (Reprinted from Granit 1950.)

Conclusion. The muscle action is aided by a central reflex mechanism of self-regulation, first speeding up, then damping its activity. Primary governors are the end organs recording muscle tension. Autogenetic inhibition is thus no physiological artefact but, on the contrary, facilitation and inhibition are aspects of a physiological integration incorporated in the normal performance of the muscle machine.

2. Size of test shock and effect of initial tension

Maximal or supramaximal test shocks have generally been used for the monosynaptic volley in order to overcome refractory phenomena in the nerve and excessive fluctuation in the size of the monosynaptic response. Figure 5 [*figure 6.5 here*] shows that a diminution in the strength of the test shock (half maximum instead of maximum response) may deepen and expand the inhibitory trough in the curve. This is what one would expect.

Muscle tension is the most important factor in determining the form of the excitability curve of the motoneurones under proprioceptive firing. There are great differences from preparation to preparation. Some animals have

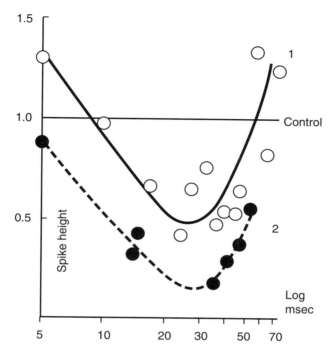

Figure 6.5
Experiment, plotted as in figure 6.2, to show effect of size of monosynaptic control on autogenetic inhibition. Initial tension 250 gm. Curve 1, maximal monosynaptic volley eliciting contraction of 275 gm. Curve 2, small monosynaptic volley eliciting contraction of only 50-75 gm. Conditioning shock to ventral root S1 elicits 150 gm. tension. (Reprinted from Granit 1950.)

actually given a definite phase of inhibition to stimulation of the root—as in Figure 2 [*figure 6.2 here*]—despite no initial tension whatever. This is perhaps not surprising in view of the fanlike organization of the gastrocnemius muscle fibres around longitudinal septa of fascicular tissue which makes it difficult to predict how and where tensile stress occurs. There may also be a low-threshold component of cross-excitation in some muscles with consequent subnormal phase of refractoriness in the motoneurones. Inhibition at zero initial tension is shown in Figure 6 [*figure 6.6 here*] (circles). At the other extreme, in the same figure, an initial tension of 700 gm. (black squares) produces a much heavier inhibition. In this experiment, at 700 gm. tension, stimulation was afterwards shifted to the muscle. The slightest contraction sufficed to give strong inhibition: indeed, it proved difficult to make the stimulus sufficiently weak so as to obtain the curve of Figure 7 [*figure 6.7 here*] with the phase of depressed excitability still above the zero line. The inhibitory phase was succeeded by a second facilitation. Secondary facilitations are very common (*cf.* Fig. 4 [*figure 6.4 here*], to stretch) but these phenomena will not be treated in the present paper.

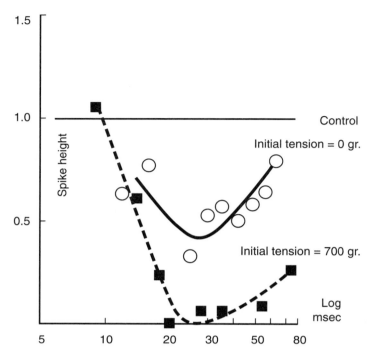

Figure 6.6
As in figure 6.2 to show effect of initial tension on autogenetic inhibition. Conditioning shock to ventral root S1 and maximum monosynaptic response. (Reprinted from Granit 1950.)

Whilst, in general, the greater the initial tension, the better marked the inhibition, there have been exceptions in the sense that certain preparations are prone to give facilitations alone or merely a relative depression in an excitability curve running entirely above the line of control in the figures (see below, Section 4, concealed inhibition). Drs. K. E. Hagbarth and K. Naess,[1] working with the same apparatus, have found it possible to obtain more inhibition by combining stretch with contraction. In one of their experiments stretch and contraction by themselves merely gave facilitation. A slight contraction added in the midst of a stretch set up inhibition.

Within narrow limits facilitation also is favoured by an increase of tension, but important receptors, setting up facilitation, must have very low thresholds. In favourable preparations it is sometimes quite easy to obtain facilitation alone at low initial tensions and inhibition succeeding it after a slight increase in tension. In order to demonstrate the effect of tension it is by no means necessary to use extremes as in Figure 6 [*figure 6.6 here*]. The full inhibitory effect is generally obtained below 300 gm. of initial tension. The facilitatory phase is hardly ever missing. When strong, it may occlude or greatly postpone inhibition. Initial tension has the same effect upon the response to stretch as on that to contraction. High initial tension should be

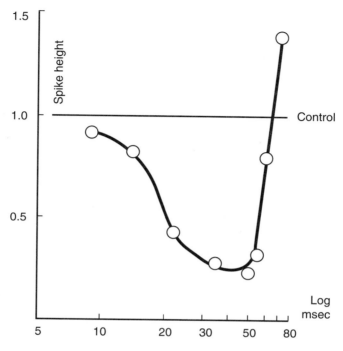

Figure 6.7
Same experiment as in figure 6.6 but conditioning shock shifted to gastrocnemius muscle, still at 700 gm. initial tension. Very weak conditioning shock. *Note:* rise after inhibition. (Reprinted from Granit 1950.)

used with great caution because the stretch reflex (32), as well as the afferent discharge (39), is known to suffer from it. This may explain why in Denny-Brown's work (9) the silent period was absent at very high initial tensions. Having investigated the effect of tension, I used modest or, whenever possible, low initial tension in the work that followed.

Conclusion. Increase of initial tension, within limits, may augment the excitatory phase of the excitability curve but has a fairly regular and relatively greater effect on the inhibitory trough which deepens and expands.

3. Effect of strength of stimulus eliciting contraction

This experiment introduces an interesting new aspect of the problem because of Leksell's (30) important observation that selective stimulation of the small efferent fibres in the ventral roots does not add to the muscle tension but discharges afferent fibres, provided that the muscle is under some initial tension. His so-called gamma efferents (cat) became activated at about three times the threshold for the motor alphas and the gamma maximum generally appeared around 15 times the alpha threshold. The alpha maximum as completed at about three times the threshold value. At this region of stimulus further increase does not add to the contraction of the muscle but introduces gamma activity with consequent increase of afferent input into the cord. On Leksell's evidence (to be compared with Barker's (1) recent histological work on the muscle spindles), the gamma efferents supply the muscle spindles in addition to larger motor fibres of the alpha class. It is thus clear that, on gradually increasing stimulus strength to the root, one is approaching a region, around thrice the threshold of the motor units, in which a second afferent outburst occurs owing to gamma activation of the muscle spindles. From this strength upwards the muscle contraction remains constant (until the shock is strong enough to excite repetitive firing or spread to the spinal cord) whilst the afferent input increases.

In order to study the effect of this afferent secondary discharge on inhibition it is necessary to place the test shock in such a position relative to the muscle contraction that the monosynaptic response remains well above zero in the inhibitory phase. Otherwise, on increasing stimulus strength, it soon disappears owing to complete inhibition, with the consequence that this inhibition itself cannot be gauged. Facilitation is less important in this connexion because it is maximal at such low stimulus strength that it is difficult to know whether the secondary contraction of the muscle spindles has added to it or not and, also, because we need hardly doubt that muscle spindles can originate it.

In Figure 8 [*figure 6.8 here*] a single shock to the peripheral stump of the ventral root was applied in the usual fashion and two positions, 15 and 32 msec., were chosen for the interval between conditioning and test shock. There is clearly a low-threshold inhibition, due to motor alphas; facilitation then gets the upper hand with further increase in the muscle contraction up to about thrice the threshold for the motor alphas. The 15 msec. curve is facilitated and passes above the control line; for the 32 msec. curve the excitability remains depressed, though less so than before. Beyond this strength of stimulus, inhibition increases in spite of the fact that the contraction did not alter. Facilitation, however, had not disappeared. Tests at shorter intervals between conditioning and test shock showed that facilitation still was present, even at maximum stimulus strength, but its duration had shortened so that it no longer extended to the 15 msec. shock interval. This experiment is interesting because both the motor alpha primary and the motor gamma secondary discharge from the afferents could be shown to have an inhibitory component. In many experiments the former low-threshold inhibition is completely absent or covered by facilitation, the latter high-threshold inhibition is present in most cases. When stimulus strength is gradually augmented, it is occasionally possible to show very clearly that inhibition continues to increase beyond the moment when the muscle contraction has reached its maximum. This effect, however, is not always demonstrable and the experiment suffers from the difficulty that the results cannot be checked by stretch.

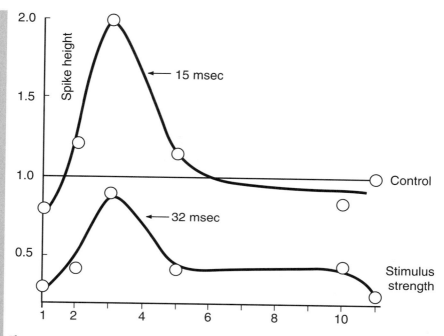

Figure 6.8
Effect of strength of conditioning shock for gastrocnemius muscle from ventral root S1 on size of monosynaptic response at intervals 15 (upper) and 32 (lower) msec. between conditioning and test shock. Abscissae, stimulus strength in multiples of threshold strength. Modest initial tension. (Reprinted from Granit 1950.)

Conclusion. The experiment suggests that gamma efferents going to the muscle spindle, by setting up a discharge from this organ, have initiated inhibition and thus indicates that autogenetic inhibition can be obtained from the muscle spindles.

4. Concealed inhibition

In preparations which, to all appearance, give pure facilitation there may nevertheless be concealed inhibition. Figure 9 [*figure 6.9 here*] is from an animal with a small monosynaptic response which increased a great deal when the muscle was stretched or made to contract. The stimulus was the slowly rising current of constant duration (*cf.* Fig. 3 [*figure 6.3 here*], record 1) applied to the peripheral stump of ventral root S1. The currents of relative plateau strength 1.0 and 4.0 gave the two lower curves whilst the large rise of facilitation was obtained with relative current strength 1.6.

It seems that, at plateau strength 4.0 for the stimulating current to the root, new end organs in the muscle must have been activated by the contraction and also that the new afferent fibres concerned cannot have had very much slower conduction rates than the excitatory fibres, previously activated, since otherwise there would have been an initial rise of facilitation

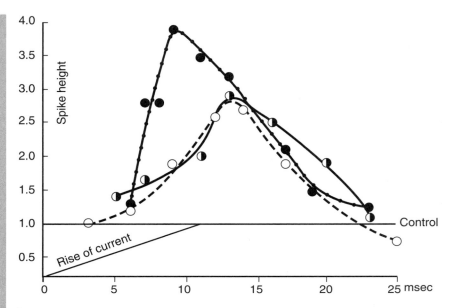

Figure 6.9
Concealed inhibition. Conditioning stimulus is the slowly rising current of record 1 in figure
6.3, stimulating gastrocnemius muscle to contract from motor roots S1 and L7. Plotted as
figure 6.2 but time linear. Part of sensory L7 cut across for control of test shock from the
gastrocnemius nerves. Plateau strength of current of constant rising time varied. Strength:
1.0, half-filled circles; 1.6, filled circles; 4.0, open circles. Good initial tension. (Reprinted from
Granit 1950.)

followed by a drop when the current increased from 1.6 to 4.0. As it is,
inhibition sets in early enough to suppress part of the initial facilitation to
current strength 1.6 without succeeding in doing away with it completely.
It is evident that, in rising to plateau strength 4.0, the current must have
traversed the value 1.6. End organs with considerable inhibitory effects,
represented among the fast fibres, must have been slightly excited at or
somewhat below current strength 1.6 to be able to come in so definitely
when, owing to a further increase in current strength, the muscle spindles
(or other muscle fibres) were induced to contract more strongly.

Conclusion. The phenomenon of concealed inhibition, when seen with
slowly rising currents, may be employed to show that there are some end
organs with greater inhibitory effects than others.

5. Observations on stretch

In a number of animals light stretch of the gastrocnemius muscle merely
induces facilitation; heavy stretch also induces inhibition. Thus the
threshold, in terms of tension caused by stretch, is higher for inhibition

than for excitation. In such preparations it is easy to see how, as the stretch increases, suddenly a point is reached where inhibition appears. If facilitation is very prominent it may be difficult to obtain good inhibition. On the hypothesis of motoneurone subnormality this is difficult to understand. Why do the motoneurones refuse to become sub-normal? The records of Figure 10 [*figure 6.10 here*] show the effect of stretch of the gastrocnemius on the monosynaptic volley from its own nerves. An analysis of another similar experiment was given in Figure 4 [*figure 6.4 here*].

Tension and length of stretch are interchangeable in the sense that good inhibition may be obtained by slight stretch at high tension or, alternatively, by heavy stretch in a muscle at low initial tension. A certain amount of tensile stress is therefore necessary for inhibition. It cannot be explained as a necessary consequence of preceding facilitation. The inhibition can increase without increase of facilitation. We have never gone beyond 6 mm. stretch which, after all, is less than a third of what muscles can do easily (32).

Conclusion. By increasing stretch or initial tension it can be shown that inhibition increases without an increase of facilitation, or even in spite of diminished facilitation, a fact very difficult to explain without assuming that there are separate inhibitory end organs.

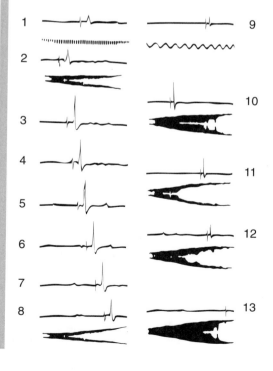

Figure 6.10
Spinal cat. Effect of stretch of gastrocnemius muscle on its own monosynaptic response, shown as control in 1 and 9 together with times 1000 and 100 Hz respectively; 2-8, test shock shifted in early phase of stretch of which myographic controls, to save space, have been left only in records 2 and 8; 10-13, same stretch of 3 mm. record 9. In record 13 complete inhibition. Modest initial tension. (With increased tension more inhibition was noted.) (Reprinted from Granit 1950.)

6. Effect of stretch of one extensor upon another

In several cases afferent control of the test shock was included in order to find out whether part of the inhibition might not be peripheral, due to refractoriness in the nerve which would diminish the size of the test volley. Such an effect was occasionally seen but not with good monosynaptic responses. In order to avoid this complication entirely but also in order to study the central distribution of autogenetic facilitation and inhibition, the stretch was set up in the quadriceps muscle or in one component of the divided gastrocnemius muscle whilst the monosynaptic volley was elicited from the gastrocnemius nerve—in the latter case not the half that was stretched. Thus the motoneurones tested were in the first case not at all, in the second perhaps only to some extent, identical with those receiving the impulses from tension organs in the muscle through the monosynaptic arc.

Figure 11 [*figure 6.11 here*] is an analysis of an experiment with the divided gastrocnemius muscle and the test shock on the severed lateral nerve to the gastrocnemius. There is the usual sequence of facilitation-inhibition in response to stretch of the medial component that had its afferent nerve intact. According to Lloyd (37) there should be monosynaptic direct facilitation across the two gastrocnemius nerves, tested by the single shock technique. Figure 12 [*figure 6.12 here*] shows the effect of stretch of quadriceps

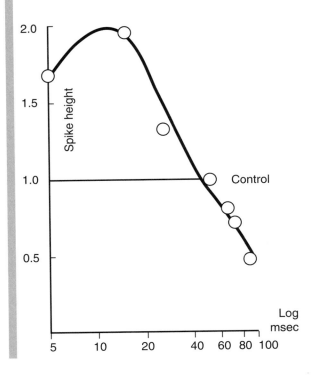

Figure 6.11
As figure 6.4, lateral and medial components of gastrocnemius muscle separated. Test shock for monosynaptic response to severed lat. nerve, medial component in good initial tension stretched 4-5 mm. (Reprinted from Granit 1950.)

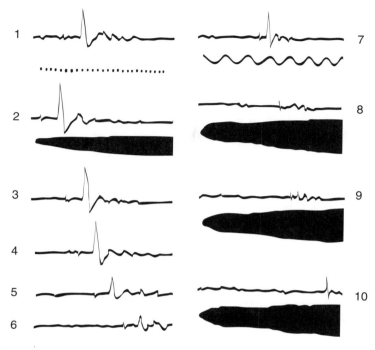

Figure 6.12
Spinal cat. Effect of 4 mm. stretch of quadriceps muscle at light initial tension on monosyn-aptic volley elicited from the severed gastrocnemius nerves. 1 and 7, monosynaptic controls at times 1000 and 100 Hz respectively. 2-6, early phase of stretch analyzed with faster sweep and stretch control included in 2; 8-10, later phase of stretch with slower sweep. *Note:* Recovery from full inhibition in 10. (Reprinted from Granit 1950.)

(in all experiments lacking the rectus component) on the gastrocnemius monosynaptic volley. The curve is of the characteristic type, facilitation succeeded by inhibition at a certain degree of stretch. Records of this type have been analysed in Figure 13 [*figure 6.13 here*], curve marked 37°.

There has been inhibition in all the experiments in which the effect of stretch of quadriceps was tested on the gastrocnemius monosynaptic volley. There has been facilitation also but not as marked as in the experiments kept within the gastrocnemius system. Thus, for instance, in the experiment of Figure 10 [*figure 6.10 here*] the gastrocnemius monosynaptic control was 5 times increased by stretching the gastrocnemius muscle. The stretch was then shifted to the quadriceps which gave an optimal facilitation of only 1.34 times the monosynaptic control. All facilitations from the quadriceps field upon the gastrocnemius motoneurones have remained below 50 per cent. In one of the experiments pure facilitation was obtained by slight stretch of a quadriceps at low initial tension, good inhibition as soon as the initial tension had been increased. However, all these differences are

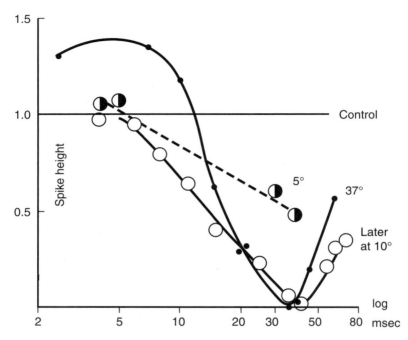

Figure 6.13
Quadriceps in light initial tension stretched 4 mm.; gastrocnemius motoneurones tested by volley from their severed motor axons. Thermode on quadriceps nerve. Plotted as in figure 6.4. Full explanation in text. (Reprinted from Granit 1950.)

differences of degree rather than of kind. This is evident when comparing Figures 4, 10, 11, 12, and 13 [*figures 6.4, 6.10, 6.11, 6.12, and 6.13 here*].

Conclusion. The autogenetic facilitation and inhibition from one extensor upon its own motoneurones is reflected in synergistic leg muscles. Hoff *et al.* (27) have shown that the effect of one extensor upon another led to a silent period only when it succeeded in discharging its motoneurones; it now remains to be investigated whether inhibition to stretch can occur without preceding facilitation of the inhibited motoneurones.

7. Independent fibres for excitation and inhibition

It is, of course, perfectly clear (see *e.g.* 45, 36, 6, 24) that there are inhibitory fibres in the muscles but what remains to be proved is that there are special inhibitory fibres from end organs responding to *stretch* or increase of tension. Warming of nerves is a method for selective activation of small fibres, as established by C. von Euler (15), and by this method it was shown (24) that warming of the gastrocnemius nerves in a decerebrate animal causes slight excitation succeeded by complete inhibition of the tension maintained by the static postural stretch reflex. However, these fibres may be the pain fibres (cf. 31,21) and they are at or below the delta range because these are the largest afferents stimulated by warming (15,24).

In order to find out whether there are special tension end organs for inhibition of synergistic muscles the following types of experiment were performed. (i) A U-shaped thermode was placed on the quadriceps nerve cooling a length of 1 cm. While the test shock to the gastrocnemius nerves was shifted between facilitatory and inhibitory positions during stretch of the quadriceps. In Figure 13 [figure 6.13 here] is shown the original excitability curve with the quadriceps nerve at 37°. Then water was passed through the thermode (the nerve and the thermode itself were covered with cotton pads soaked in paraffin) and it is seen that facilitation almost disappeared while part of the inhibition still was left. The nerve was cooled for some time until the supply of cold water in the tank had run out when the water temperature, measured by a thermo-couple just outside the animal, had risen to 10°. In this slightly damaged nerve there was only pure inhibition left. (ii) Pressure is known to attack the fibres of greatest diameter first (19). In the experiment of Figure 14 [figure 6.14 here] the quadriceps muscle was stretched while its nerve was compressed between thumb and forefinger of the experimenter. The monosynaptic test volley came from the severed popliteal nerve. Initially a position of facilitation (F-p) and one of inhibition (I-p) were chosen, as shown in the uppermost row of control records before pressure. Then pressure was applied and, when (vertical row, left) the facilitation had disappeared, the test shock was quickly shifted over into the inhibitory position. There was still strong inhibition. The test shock was shifted back into the facilitatory position. Facilitation was still absent (lowermost record). The nerve quickly recovered and the middle row of records was obtained in the same fashion. This time part of the inhibition disappeared, too. The nerve still recovered a couple of times from repeated exposures to pressure but ultimately a steady state was reached in which all facilitation was lost and only part of the inhibition remained, variable in amount and not as great as before (vertical row, right). In this, just as in the experiments on cooling, the excitatory fibres in the long run proved more sensitive to interference than the inhibitory ones, perhaps merely because the latter were better represented in the centre concerned. In other similar experiments the margin between disappearance of excitation and of inhibition was still narrower, if it was present at all.

The same nerve could not be used for both test shock and pressure because the slight pull, on touching it, augmented facilitation, sometimes to such an extent as to occlude inhibition, or, at any rate, so as to make the controls unreliable. Also, on pressing or cooling the nerve, artificial synapse tended to arise (23,25) as well as excitability changes spreading electronically to adjacent regions (23). These sources of error proved to be very disturbing. Accordingly this type of experiment was soon given up in favour of the one employed above.

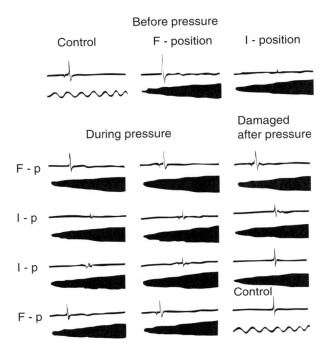

Figure 6.14
Quadriceps in light initial tension stretched 4 mm. and test shock on popliteal nerve. Effect of pressure upon quadriceps nerve, as fully explained in text. Time 100 Hz. (Reprinted from Granit 1950.)

Conclusion. Since the excitatory component of the excitability curve can be separately removed, without concomitant changes in the inhibitory component, inhibition cannot be due to post-excitatory subnormality in the tested motoneurones which show no signs of having been activated. Inhibition must arise in some other manner and in this sense the remaining fibres are true inhibitory fibres.

8. Relative size of excitatory and inhibitory fibres

There was so little facilitation from the large quadriceps field upon the smaller field of the gastrocnemius motoneurones that it seemed reasonable to expect that no facilitation would be left if the situation was reversed, *i.e.,* if the quadriceps motoneurones were tested by the monosynaptic volley and stimulated from the smaller gastrocnemius system. This proved to be true. Actually Brooks and Eccles (6), by the single shock technique, found no facilitation when conditioning and test shock were applied respectively to gastrocnemius and quadriceps nerves. (They do not mention ever having tried reversing conditioning and test shock).

In the experiment of Figure 15 [*figure 6.15 here*] contraction was used instead of stretch in order to obtain a better measure of time intervals. It is

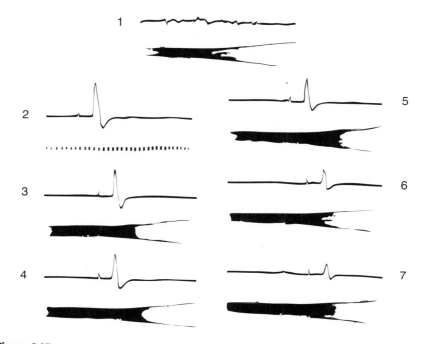

Figure 6.15
Effect of gastrocnemius contraction on quadriceps motoneurones. Contraction of gastrocnemius muscle elicited from ventral roots L7 and S1. Test shock for monosynaptic volley on
severed nerve to quadriceps 1, at high amplification, shows effect on recording leads (L6) of
gastrocnemius contracting to conditioning shock; 2, test shock and time 1000 Hz; 3-7, combined responses. Inhibition did not increase later in the contraction. Spinal cat. (Reprinted
from Granit 1950.)

thus a repetition of the experiment of Figure 1 [*figure 6.1 here*], but this time
with the monosynaptic test shock applied to the severed quadriceps nerve
instead of to the gastrocnemius nerves. The leads are on L6 and the
gastrocnemius muscle is made to contract by a shock to the severed motor
roots L7 and S1. No other muscle contracted in response to this stimulus.
Record 1, at higher amplification than the others, shows that the
conditioning shock to the root elicited a muscle contraction and, after 6
msec., a very small response in L6. This response should be compared with
the monosynaptic control at half maximum size and low amplification in
record 2. We can never know with absolute certainty whether the small
response of record 1 is from an artificial synapse, or is due to cross-excitation
in the gastrocnemius muscle or to mechanical stimulation of its tension
receptors. But, considering that the latent period of the monosynaptic test
response is of the order of 3 msec., it is clear that the conditioning volley
which perhaps has travelled about thrice this distance in 6 msec. must have
been conducted in very fast fibres. At the moment (6 msec.) when this volley
appeared at the leading-off electrodes the test shock was discharged into

the quadriceps nerve. When its volley arrived into the spinal cord it just escaped inhibition; when discharged between 0.5 and 1.0 msec. later it fell into the early phase of inhibition as shown by the complete analysis of the experiment in Figure 16 [*figure 6.16 here*]. If the receptors setting up inhibition from the gastrocnemius nerves had discharged through fibres very much smaller than those setting up the stretch reflex (and facilitation), a result like this would have been impossible. In this experiment, however, it is possible that direct and indirect inhibition are mixed. Brooks and Eccles (6) have found the inhibition of gastrocnemius upon quadriceps to be so early as to suggest that it is direct. We cannot ascertain the moment of initiation of the afferent discharge and therefore must be content with these approximations. They suggest, as did the previous experiments, that the conduction time of excitatory and inhibitory impulses is of much the same order of magnitude and therefore that the fibres are of much the same size. When inhibition survived excitation in the experiments of the last section the most probable interpretation would seem to be that the inhibitory fibres had a very much better peripheral or central representation than the excitatory ones.

The experiment was finally carried out with tetanic conditioning stimulus which gave a long-lasting complete inhibition to zero level. Figure 17 [*figure 6.17 here*] compares a single shock with tetanic stimulation.

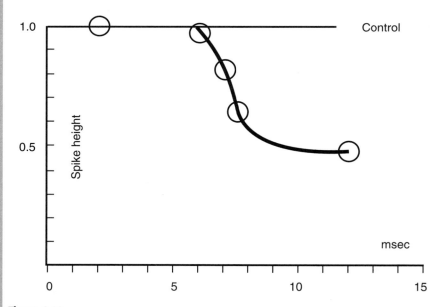

Figure 6.16
Experiment of figure 6.15 analyzed as in figure 6.2 but time between conditioning shock and test shock linear. (Reprinted from Granit 1950.)

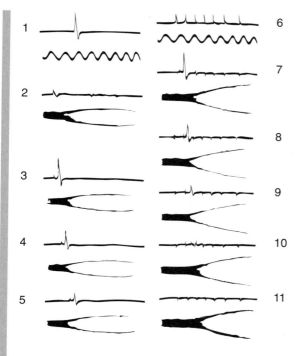

Figure 6.17
Same experiment as in figure 6.15 but recorded somewhat later and with slower sweep speed in order to compare single conditioning shock (left) and tetanic conditioning shock (right). 1, quadriceps monosynaptic control; 2, effect of conditioning shock alone at high amplification; 3-5, combined responses; 6, form of tetanic stimulus; 7-11, combined responses showing complete inhibition that lasted within the visible range of the tetanic gastrocnemius contraction, whilst with the single shock (left) inhibition nowhere in the contraction went below minimum illustrated in record 5. Time 100 Hz. (Reprinted from Granit 1950.)

Conclusion. Fibres from excitatory and inhibitory end organs in the muscle are both represented among the large and rapidly conducting fibres.

Discussion

Skeletal muscle is provided with nervous governors for facilitation and inhibition which are pitted against one another in the spinal centre. In the normal mode of operation of the muscle machine the contraction is first speeded up by facilitation, then damped by inhibition. The greater the initial tension or the more (in stretch) the muscle is stretched, the more important become the inhibitory brakes. Special sense organs exist in the muscle for excitation and for inhibition, both being represented among the large and rapidly conducting fibres (smaller ones not excluded). The effects of inhibitory sense organs is probably reinforced by motoneurone refractoriness following strong synchronous afferent excitation of the kind that plays a less important role in normal muscle activity. In the leg extensor system (analyzed in detail above) fibres are distributed from both excitatory and inhibitory end organs to allied muscles across one joint to the next joint. Excitatory end organs have a more restricted central distribution than inhibitory ones. Yet some facilitation and a great deal of inhibition are shared by extensors capable of synergistic co-operation—for instance, while maintaining posture of the limb. The inhibitory fibres are, of course, only inhibitory in the sense that they represent autogenetic inhibition. They may well be excitatory on antagonists (9,45).

On the evidence obtained, the self-regulation of the muscle contraction (stretch, also, would—if the ventral roots were intact—induce contraction) can be discussed from two points of view: (i) its central mechanism, (ii) nature of end organs concerned.

Central mechanism

Since the gastrocnemius motoneurones are inhibited by stretching the quadriceps muscle, and, since in this case monosynaptic transfer seems unlikely (37), the process is probably carried across internuncials. This process may be some kind of blocking of the facilitatory internuncial bombardment of the motoneurone (its so-called general background activity) leading to a drop of motoneurone excitability sufficient to prevent activation by the monosynaptic system. To be as efficient and fast as it is, the blocking process would have to be localized to the immediate neighbourhood of the motoneurones. Actually there is no reason whatever to assume that the mechanism for indirect autogenetic inhibition differs in the least from that of the direct immediate inhibition of Renshaw (40) and Lloyd (33). It is an unexplained effect at the level of the motoneurone. Brooks and Eccles (6) stress the significance of specific positive focal potentials. The question as to whether this process merely acts by removing facilitatory background or by active anodal polarisation of the cell membrane of the motoneurone is hardly ripe for discussion. The time relations of the autogenetic inhibition, as well as the fact that it attacks the motoneurones of synergistic muscle across a joint without evidence for preceding facilitation, seem to exclude the idea of motoneurone refractoriness. Motoneurone refractoriness and subnormality due to positive afterpotential must play a role with large synchronous afferent volleys (silent period).

Nature of end organs

Ruffini (42,43) and Sherrington (44) agreed in placing the fibre sizes at the level of the end organ in the following order: annulo-spirals, Golgi tendon organs both relatively large as compared with the flower spray endings. Barker's (1) recent work suggests the same conclusion. But there is a missing link in the histological evidence; the relative fibre sizes are not known in the nerve stem itself. On our evidence there could be inhibitory fibres smaller than the largest excitatory ones, provided that there are some very large inhibitory fibres too, and this view does not disagree with Lloyd's demonstration that the monosynaptic myotatic afferents would have to be the largest ones. These on Matthews' (39) evidence would have to be the A2 or the B endings, the former assumed by him to be the annulo-spirals, the latter the Golgi tendon organs. Either of the two would have to be inhibitory for synergistic muscles. The lower mechanical threshold of the

A2 endings is in favour of their being excitatory for their own muscle. The facilitation may be supported by A1 endings which run in smaller fibres and were assumed to be the flower spray endings (39). It is difficult to ascribe inhibition to them because they are of the "in parallel" type, first postulated by Fulton and Pi-Suner (17) and then found by Matthews. These are silenced in twitch, silenced in tetanic contraction, and the more effectively the greater the initial tension. They are thus silent under conditions when inhibition is at its very best.

When Matthews ascribed the silent period to the Golgi tendon organs, his B organs, he based his conclusion on experiments (9) which could be satisfactorily explained by motoneurone subnormality. For this no special inhibitory end organs are needed. Our results, as they stand at the moment, are best explained by assuming the annulo-spirals (A2) to be excitatory and the Golgi tendon organs (B) inhibitory. This presupposes that the latter have higher mechanical thresholds though not necessarily as high as one is led to assume from Matthews' results with a few selected samples. Our experiments with pressure applied to nerve cannot differentiate A2 from B endings because there are fibre properties which are not distributed in proportion to fibre size (see *e.g.* 16).

Inhibitory end organs, on our evidence, are likely to exist in the muscle spindles also. Actually Sherrington (44) pointed out that there are Golgi tendon organs also in the tendons of some muscle spindles. Barker (1) states that they "frequently occur in association with muscle spindles." These could be responsible for the low-threshold inhibition to contraction and the secondary inhibition in the experiments varying stimulus strength to the ventral roots (Section 3). Motoneurone refractoriness may also provide an alternative explanation of the low threshold inhibition in slack muscles which was demonstrated only in experiments on contraction. We also know from Ruffini's (42,43) work that the Golgi tendon organs often are associated with special types of Pacini corpuscles and, in addition, there are few nerve endings in the muscle spindles. The latter seem to represent small fibres (1) and may be pain receptors. Next to the ear, the eye, etc., the muscle spindle, according to Ruffini, is the most highly developed sense organ in the body and clearly more detailed information is needed about its physiology.

Rexed and Therman (41) as well as Lloyd and Chang (38) agree in finding three definite groups in the calibre spectra of muscle afferents. These have not yet been correlated with the types of endings in the muscle. It is obvious, too, that some development on the afferent side of the type of analysis used in this work still can add a great deal more to the specification of the properties of the end organs responsible for autogenetic inhibition.

Summary

In experiments on acutely de-efferented cats the monosynaptic reflex response from the gastrocnemius nerves has been used to test the excitability of the gastrocnemius motoneurones during contraction or stretch of the muscle. Whatever the mode of stimulating the tension end organs, by making the muscle contract by a conditioning shock or a slowly rising current from electrodes on the motor root, from electrodes in the muscle itself, or by merely stretching it, there is first an increase of excitability of its motoneurones followed by a depression, as gauged by the size of the monosynaptic test volley.

Contraction or stretch of the synergistic quadriceps muscle (deprived of its rectus component) causes the same sequence of excitability changes in the gastrocnemius motoneurones, first facilitation, then inhibition.

The facilitatory component can be selectively removed by cooling the quadriceps nerve or by compressing it gently, leaving the inhibitory component intact, and thus indicating that inhibition is initiated by separate tension receptors. These can also be isolated directly by testing with the quadriceps monosynaptic volley and making the gastrocnemius muscle contract. There are thus for synergistic extensors separate inhibitory fibres responding to stretch and they have been shown to conduct almost as rapidly as the fibres causing facilitation of the motoneurones.

Inhibition is favoured by an increase of initial tension of the muscle and it is found to possess a slightly higher mechanical threshold than facilitation.

In conclusion it is pointed out that the muscle machine is working under self-regulation from autogenetic governors, first aiding it to contract, then damping the discharge from its motoneurones; also that the inhibitory brakes are put on with greater efficiency, the more the damping becomes necessary owing to increase of tensile stress.

The results are discussed from the points of view of the central mechanisms concerned and the receptors engaged as governors.

Acknowledgment

I am indebted for support to the Rockefeller Foundation and the Medical Research Council of Sweden. In some of the experiments I have had valuable help from Drs. K. E. Hagbarth, K. Naess and V. Suursoet.

Endnote

[1] Private communication from work to be published in *Acta. Physical. Scand.* 1950.

References

1. BARKER, D. The innervation of the muscle spindle. *Quart. J. Micr. Sci.*, 1948, 89: 143-186.
2. BARRON, D. H. AND MATTHEWS, B. H. C. The interpretation of potential changes in the spinal cord. *J. Physiol.*, 1938, 92: 276-321.
3. BERNHARD, C. G. Slow cord potentials of opposite sign correlated to reciprocal function. *Acta Physiol. Scand.*, 1947, 14: Suppl. 47.
4. BREMER, F. AND BONNET, V. Contributions a l'etude de la physiologie generale des centres nerveux. II. L'inhibition reflexe. *Arch. Int. Physiol.*, 1942, 52: 153-194.
5. BREMER, F., BONNET V., AND MOLDAVER, J. Contributions a l'etude de la physiologie generale des centres nerveux. I. La sommation centrale. *Arch. Int. Physiol.*, 1942, 52: 1-56.

6. BROOKS, C. McC AND ECCLES, J.C. Inhibitory action on a motor nucleus and focal potentials generated therein. *J. Neurophysiol.*, 1948, *11*: 401-416.
7. COOPER, S. AND CREED, R.S. Reflex effects of active muscular contraction. *J. Physiol*, 1927, *62*: 273-279.
8. COOPER, S. AND CREED, R.S. More reflex effects of active muscular contraction. *J. Physiol.*, 1927, *64*: 199-214.
9. DENNY-BROWN, D. On inhibition as a reflex accompaniment of the tendon jerk and of other forms of active muscular response. *Proc. Roy. Soc.*, 1928, *103B*: 321-336.
10. ECCLES, J.C. Slow potential waves in the superior cervical ganglion. *J. Physiol.*, 1935, *85*: 464-501.
11. ECCLES, J.C. The interpretation of potentials led from the superior cervical ganglion. *J. Physiol.*, 1939, *87*: 41P-43P.
12. ECCLES, J.C. The spinal cord and reflex action. *Ann. Rev. Physiol.*, 1939, *1*: 363-384.
13. ECCLES, J.C. Synaptic potential of motoneurones. *J. Neurophysiol.*, 1946, *9*: 87-120.
14. ECCLES, J.C. AND PRITCHARD, J.J. The action potential of motoneurones. *J. Physiol.*, 1937, *89*: 43P-45P.
15. EULER, C.V. Selective responses to thermal stimulation of mammalian nerves. *Acta Physiol. Scand.*, 1947, *14*: Suppl. 45.
16. FRANKENHAEUSER, B. Ischaemic paralysis of a uniform nerve. *Acta Physiol. Scand.*, 1949, *18*: 1-24.
17. FULTON, J.F. AND PI-SUNER J. A note concerning the probable function of various afferent end-organs in skeletal muscle. *Amer. J. Physiol.*, 1927-28, *83*: 554-562.
18. GASSER, H.S. IN ERLANGER, J. AND GASSER, H.S. *Electrical signs of nervous activity.* Philadelphia, University of Pennsylvania Press, 1937, 221 pp.
19. GASSER, H.S. AND ERLANGER, J. The role of fibre size in the establishment of a nerve block by pressure or cocaine. *Amer. J. Physiol.*, 1929, *88*: 581-591.
20. GASSER, H.S. AND GRAHAM, H.T. Potentials produced in the spinal cord by stimulation of dorsal roots. *Amer. J. Physiol.*, 1933, *103*: 303-320.
21. GELLHORN, E. AND THOMPSON, M.B. The influence of excitation of muscle pain receptors on reflexes of the decerebrate cat. *Amer. J. Physiol.*, 1945, *144*: 259-269.
22. GRANIT, R. *Sensory mechanisms of the retina.* London, Oxford University Press, 1947. xxiii, 412 pp.
23. GRANIT, R., LEKSELL, L., AND SKOGLUND, C.R. Fibre interaction in injured or compressed region of nerve. *Brain*, 1944, *67*: 125-140.
24. GRANIT, R. AND LUNDBERG, A. Heat- and cold-sensitive mammalian nerve fibres. Some somatic reflexes to thermostimulation. *Acta Physiol. Scand.*, 1947, *13*: 334-346.
25. GRANIT, R. AND SKOGLUND, C.R. The effect of temperature on the artificial synapse formed by the cut end of the mammalian nerve. *J. Neurophysiol.*, 1945, *8*: 211-217.
26. GRANIT, R. AND SUURSOET, V. Self-regulation of the muscle contraction by facilitation and inhibition from its proprioceptors. *Nature*, 1949, *164*: 270-271.
27. HOFF, H.E., HOFF, E.C., BUCY, P.C., AND PI-SUNER, J. The production of the silent period by the synchronization of discharge of motor neurones. *Amer. J. Physiol.*, 1934, *109*: 123-132.
28. HOFFMANN, P. *Untersuchungen uber die Eigenreflexe (Sehnenreflexe) menschlicher Muskeln,* Berlin, Springer, 1922.
29. HUGHES, J. AND GASSER, H.S. Some properties of the cord potentials evoked by a single afferent volley. *Amer. J. Physiol.*, 1934, *108*: 295-306.
30. LEKSELL, L. The action potential and excitatory effects of the small ventral root fibres to skeletal muscle. *Acta Physiol. Scand.* 1945, *10*: Suppl. 31.
31. LEWIS, T.H. *Pain*, New York, Macmillan, 1942. xiv, 197 pp.
32. LIDDELL, E.G.T. AND SHERRINGTON, C.S. Reflexes in response to stretch (myotatic reflexes) *Proc. Roy. Soc.*, 1924, *96B*: 212-242.
33. LLOYD, D.P.C. A direct central inhibitory action of dromically conducted impulses. *J. Neurophysiol.*, 1941, *4*: 194-190.
34. LLOYD, D.P.C. Stimulation of peripheral nerve termination by active muscle. *J. Neurophysiol.*, 1942, *5*: 153-165.
35. LLOYD, D.P.C. Neuron patterns controlling transmission of ipsilateral hind limb reflexes in cat. *J. Neurophysiol.*, 1943, *6*: 293-315.
36. LLOYD, D.P.C. Conduction and synaptic transmission of reflex response to stretch in spinal cats. *J. Neurophysiol.*, 1943, *6*: 317-326.

37. LLOYD, D.P.C. Facilitation and inhibition of spinal motoneurones. *J. Neurophysiol.*, 1946, 9: 421-438.
38. LLOYD, D.P.C. AND CHANG, H.-T. Afferent fibres in muscle nerves. *J. Neurophysiol.*, 1948, 11: 199-207.
39. MATTHEWS, B.H.C. Nerve endings in mammalian muscle. *J. Physiol.*, 1933, 78: 1-53.
40. RENSHAW, B. Influence of the discharge of motoneurones upon excitation of neighboring motoneurones. *J. Neurophysiol.*, 1941, 4: 167-183.
41. REXED, B. AND THERMAN, P.O. Calibre spectra of motor and sensory nerve fibres to flexor and extensor muscle. *J. Neurophysiol.*, 1948, 11: 133-139.
42. RUFFINI, A. Observations on sensory nerve-endings in voluntary muscles. *Brain*, 1897, 20: 368-374.
43. RUFFINI, A. On the minute anatomy of the neuro-muscular spindles of the cat, and on their physiological significance. *J. Physiol.*, 1898-99, 23: 190-208.
44. SHERRINGTON, C.S. On the anatomical constitution of nerves of skeletal muscles with remarks on recurrent fibres in the ventral spinal nerve-root. *J. Physiol.*, 1894, 17: 211-258.
45. SHERRINGTON, C.S. On plastic tonus and proprioceptive reflexes. *Quart. J. Exp. Physiol.*, 1909, 2: 109-156.
46. UMRATH, K. Der Erregungsvorgang in den Motoneuronen von Rana esculenta. *Pflug. Arch. Ges. Physiol.*, 1933, 233: 357-370.

Notes on the Text

The following comments provide additional historical background for some of the phenomena described by Granit. The notes also attempt to trace the current status of several of the ideas that arose from this work.

Introduction: The Lengthening Reaction

The lengthening reaction is a phenomenon described by Sir Charles Sherrington (1909) that has become particularly important in a clinical context. As originally described, the lengthening reaction is the second of two sequential responses to external manipulation of the limb of an animal with a spinal injury. Sherrington reported that if the knee joint of the animal were to be extended by the experimenter, the joint would tend to remain in the extended posture even without continued support from the experimenter. This reaction was named the "shortening reaction." If the knee were then to be forcibly flexed, an initially strong resistance would be felt followed by a sudden release of the quadriceps muscles and relaxation of the knee. The knee would then remain in the flexed posture. This sudden relaxation was termed the "lengthening reaction." This reaction is similar to what is now referred to as the "clasp-knife reflex" that can be elicited from patients with spinal cord injury. In this paper, the lengthening reaction is considered to constitute evidence for "autogenetic inhibition" from tension receptors, such as the Golgi tendon organs. In fact, it has been widely believed that feedback from Golgi tendon organs is responsible for the clasp-knife reflex. More recent studies, however, have shown that the clasp-knife reflex, which can be obtained in spinal animals but only rarely in decerebrate animals, is due to feedback from group III and IV (lightly myelinated and unmyelinated) sensory fibers from the muscle. Therefore, the lengthening reaction appears to be due to autogenic (or autogenetic) inhibition as suggested by Granit, but the receptors responsible for this reflex are likely to be free nerve endings rather than Golgi tendon organs.

Introduction: The Silent Period

When a muscle is stretched using a rapid, transient lengthening, an initial burst of activity due to the stretch reflex occurs and is followed by a brief period of reduced activity. This period of depression is known as the silent period. As described by Granit, the silent period was originally thought to result from an inhibitory, autogenic reflex. However, as further explained by Granit, Erlanger and Gasser (1937) had suggested that the synchronous discharge of motoneurons evoked by the stretch reflex would necessarily be followed by reduced activity because the refractory periods of these motoneurons would then temporally correspond. Here, Granit brings up the difficulty produced by arguing from indirect results. The silent period could be evidence for autogenic inhibition, but it could equally well be explained by the synchronized bursting of motoneurons.

Paragraph 2: Philippson's Reflex of Crossed Extension

Another reaction due to spinal circuitry is the crossed-extension reflex. When a flexion-withdrawal reflex is elicited by a noxious stimulus applied to one limb, the extensor muscles of the opposite limb are activated. This pattern of response is intrinsic to the spinal cord; it may be observed after some kinds of damage to the central nervous system and may also be a part of normal postural regulation. Sherrington (1906) observed that all four limbs of a quadruped are in fact involved. If the stimulus is applied to the left hindlimb, for example, the right hindlimb exhibits crossed extension. In addition, the left forelimb exhibits flexion and the right forelimb extension. This pattern was called the "reflex figure" by Sherrington and apparently constitutes a primitive postural system to maintain weight bearing and stabilization of the center of mass of the animal.

Problem and Principle of Analysis: Paragraph 1

Here Granit is referring to the complexities of using indirect methods such as the silent period to investigate reflex mechanisms. He refers to the evaluation of motoneuron excitability as a more direct way of evaluating afferent or central inputs to motoneurons.

Paragraph 2

Granit then introduces the use of what is known as monosynaptic testing to evaluate motoneuron excitability. This method was introduced by Renshaw (1940) and used by Lloyd (1941), and it has become widespread for both clinical and experimental uses in human and animal subjects in a form known as the Hoffman reflex, or H-reflex. This method is based on Lloyd's demonstration that the most rapidly conducting and therefore lowest-threshold afferents arise from muscle spindle receptors. The largest fibers are recruited at the lowest thresholds by an electrical stimulus because these fibers have the lowest axial resistance to current flow. Therefore, an appropriately small electrical stimulus (or "shock") delivered to a muscle nerve excites the corresponding motoneurons through the monosynaptic pathway formed by the synapses of group Ia fibers onto motoneurons. The response to this stimulus can then be obtained using electromyographic (EMG) recordings in the muscle. As the excitability of the motoneurons changes, the number of motoneurons recruited by the stimulus changes; and the EMG signal, or H-reflex, varies in a corresponding way. The activation of the Ia fibers is known as the test stimulus. Another stimulus, the conditioning stimulus, can then be delivered at a given time interval before or after the test stimulus. If the conditioning stimulus alters the excitability of the motoneurons, then the H-reflex will vary accordingly. This method can then be used to investigate the influence of the inputs to the motoneurons that are activated by the conditioning stimuli.

Paragraph 3

Granit points out that this method can unambiguously detect changes in motoneuron excitability and therefore indicates changing synaptic inputs to the motoneurons. Since the test stimulus consists of a single volley of action potentials, the confounding effects of motoneuron refractoriness are avoided. Therefore, the H-reflex can be used to investigate various reflex and central inputs to the motoneurons.

Technique

The animals were anesthetized using a barbiturate known as Dial (allobarbitol). This drug has been replaced for both experimental and clinical uses by a number of newer barbiturate drugs. The test input consisted of an electrical stimulus applied to the nerves of the medial and lateral gastrocnemius muscles (see figure 6.1). The response was recorded electrically from the ventral root filaments, containing only the motor output of the spinal cord. The ventral roots were cut distal to the recording electrodes to avoid the complication of antidromic activation of the motoneurons from the test stimulus. Conditioning stimuli were delivered either to the distal ventral roots going to the gastrocnemius muscles or to the muscles themselves (intramuscular stimulation). The object here was to activate tension receptors (Golgi tendon organs) in the muscles using the conditioning stimuli and to test whether the sensory feedback from these receptors caused increases or decreases in motoneuron excitability. These effects would then be interpreted as excitatory or inhibitory synaptic influences, respectively, on the motoneurons. In addition, stretch of the gastrocnemius muscles was also used to provide a natural conditioning stimulus. In this case, muscle spindles, Golgi tendon organs, and perhaps other receptors would be activated. Similarity of the patterns of response using either electrical or natural conditioning stimuli would indicate that the observed patterns were most likely due to the activation of specific pathways rather than an artifactual effect of the electrical stimulus directly on the spinal cord.

Results: Section 1, Pages 190–192

Granit used the measurement of excitability to demonstrate that the conditioning stimuli caused excitatory and inhibitory effects on the motoneuron pool, and that the inhibitory effect outlasted the excitatory. During muscle stretch, muscle spindles and Golgi tendon organs would be activated, giving the mixed effect shown in figure 6.4. In the case of a conditioning ventral root stimulation (figure 6.1), excitatory and inhibitory effects were observed as well. The internal force input resulting from ventral root stimulation would have activated the Golgi tendon organs. The excitatory effect is, however, more difficult to explain since activation of the muscle would produce at least a small internal shortening of the muscle fibers and of the muscle spindles. However, the primary (annulospiral) ending of the muscle spindle is extremely sensitive to small, rapid changes in length. Therefore, the initial movement of the muscle upon ventral root stimulation probably causes a rapid burst that accounts for the excitatory effect in the motoneurons. Granit notes that the inhibitory response is more variable than the excitatory, evidence suggesting that the two effects arise from different receptors.

Section 2, Pages 192–195

Granit found that increasing the initial tension in the muscle by initially stretching it out led to substantial increases in the inhibition of excitability. It is now known that Golgi tendon organs are activated by active contractions in muscle (Houk and Henneman, 1967). Because the force of contraction is increased at longer lengths, the increase in initial tension would have resulted in larger contractions due to the conditioning stimuli. More vigorous responses of Golgi tendon organs would therefore have been the result. Inhibition was found to increase more than excitation at longer lengths, providing additional evidence that the two effects were mediated by different receptors. In a later section (section 5, page 198), Granit expands on the dependence of inhibition on either muscle stretch or muscle tension, and states that inhibition depended mainly on tension. Since the extent of inhibition did not covary with the magnitude of excitation, the likelihood of a common mechanism such as motoneuron refractoriness became even less.

Section 3, Pages 195–197

When he increased the strength of the conditioning stimulus, Granit found that the early excitatory effect passed through a maximum and began to decline in a range of strengths where gamma motor axons were believed to become active. Granit proposed that the activation of gamma motor axons evoked a response from muscle spindle receptors that produced an inhibitory effect on motoneurons. Another interpretation is that the gamma stimulation reduced or foreshortened the excitatory response of muscle spindles to the internal muscular stimulation. The reduced excitation would have opposed the early increase in motoneuron excitability. Since activation of some types of gamma motor axons can cause a decrease in the dynamic responsiveness of the primary spindle receptor, a reduction of the initial, rapid activation of the spindle receptor on the initiation of muscular contraction would have resulted.

Section 6, Pages 200–202

To rule out the possibility that the conditioning stimulus produced an apparent inhibition by rendering the nerve refractory for the subsequent test stimulus, Granit used the stretch of a different muscle as the conditioning stimulus. The results of this experiment could then be used to determine how feedback is distributed to motoneurons of different muscles in the spinal cord. This work predated the extensive studies of Sir John Eccles and his coworkers (Eccles et al., 1957; Eccles and Lundberg, 1958) on the distribution of excitatory and inhibitory synaptic effects from muscle spindle receptors and Golgi tendon organs among motoneurons controlling the hindlimb of the cat.

By separating the two gastrocnemius muscles and applying stretch to only one, or by stretching the quadriceps muscles and testing the excitability due to a test volley in the gastrocnemius nerve, Granit found the same pattern of facilitation followed by inhibition that was observed when both conditioning and test stimuli were confined to the gastrocnemius nerves or muscles. These results anticipated later findings that both excitatory and inhibitory effects could be obtained within a single muscle and also between antigravity muscles. In a complementary experiment (section 8, page 205) in which the test stimulus was applied to the quadriceps nerves and the gastrocnemius nerves were used to provide the conditioning stimulus, only inhibitory effects were noted in the recording from the L6 ventral roots. This result is reasonable in the light of more recent evidence since the excitatory connections from receptors in the gastrocnemius muscles are weak. The inhibition was detectable for conditioning-test intervals as short as 6 ms, indicating that the afferent fibers responsible must have been rapidly conducting. This evidence would be consistent with the Golgi tendon organ as the responsible receptor since the corresponding group Ib afferent fibers have conduction velocities in the same range as those of the primary receptors of muscle spindles. Granit also brought up the notion of direct inhibition in reference to the short latency of the inhibition. It had been originally believed that inhibition from the periphery could be direct without any interposed interneurons. In the early 1950s, Eccles and his colleagues demonstrated that reciprocal inhibition involved an interneuron, thereby helping to demolish the notion of direct inhibition.

Section 7, Pages 202–204

By cooling or applying pressure to the nerve, Granit tried to obtain more direct evidence that the facilitation and inhibition were mediated by separate receptors. Cooling removed all facilitation, and pressure removed all facilitation and some inhibition as well. These experiments indicated that the sensory afferents responsible for the facilitatory effects were damaged independently of those responsible for the inhibitory effects. All of the evidence taken together indicated that the facilitation and inhibition were mediated by separate, rapidly conducting afferent pathways.

Discussion

Granit's interpretation of these data was that the feedback confined to a given muscle ("autogenetic feedback") consists of rapid facilitation followed by inhibition. In addition, antigravity muscles crossing different joints appear to be linked by similar facilitatory and inhibitory pathways. He speculated that these pathways function first to speed and enhance and then to dampen the contraction. As initial tension or stretch is increased, the inhibition or dampening effect becomes greater. During the 1950s, ideas concerning stability and control of the motor system began to gain influence in the interpretation of reflex function. Granit's is an early example of such an argument. More recent ideas concerning the stabilizing influences of autogenic reflexes have focused on reductions in the gain of the stretch reflex resulting from an initial movement (Lin and Rymer, 1997) rather than contributions of autogenic inhibition. The potentially stabilizing influences of force-related inhibition have been discussed recently (Nichols, 1999). However, since inhibitory force feedback is distributed primarily to muscles crossing different joints, these stabilizing influences occur at the level of the intact limb rather than single muscle.

The lack of facilitation of the quadriceps monosynaptic reflex in response to conditioning stimuli from the gastrocnemius nerve supported the generalization that excitatory pathways are less widely distributed among muscles crossing different joints than inhibitory pathways. Granit refers to this fact with reference to the synergistic activity of the muscles in maintaining posture. The functional significance of the differences in distribution between excitatory length feedback and inhibitory force feedback has been reevaluated recently. It has been proposed that inhibitory feedback links muscles crossing different joints in order to promote interjoint coordination (Nichols, 1994) and stability of the limb. That is, the feedback exists not to dampen the activity of a set of extensor muscles independent of their musculoskeletal arrangement but instead to promote the distribution of mechanical disturbances across the joints of the limb. Granit clearly recognized the importance of the spatial distribution of proprioceptive feedback in addition to its dynamic properties in determining the functions of the underlying pathways.

References

Cope, T.C. and Pinter, M.J. The Size Principle: Still working after all these years. *N.I.P.S.* 1995; 10:280-286.

Denny-Brown, D. On inhibition as a reflex accompaniment of the tendon jerk and of other forms of active muscular response. *Proc. Roy. Soc.* 1928; 103B:321-336.

Eccles, J.C., Eccles, R.M., and Lundberg, A. The convergence of monosynaptic excitatory afferents on to many different species of alpha motoneurons. *J. Physiol.* 1957; 137:22-50.

Eccles, R.M. and Lundberg, A. Integrative pattern of Ia synaptic actions on motoneurons of hip and knee muscles. *J. Physiol.* 1958; 144:271-298.

Erlanger, J. and Gasser, H.S. *Electrical Signs of Nervous Activity.* Philadelphia: University of Pennsylvania Press. 1937.

Granit, R. Reflex self-regulation of muscle contraction and autogenetic inhibition. *J. Neurophysiol.* 1950; 13:351-372.

Granit, R. Neuromuscular interaction in postural tone of the cat's isometric soleus muscle. *J. Physiol.* 1958; 143:387-402.

Granit, R. Discovery and understanding. *Ann. Rev. Physiol.* 1972; 34:1-11.

Granit, R., Holmgren, B., and Merton, P.A. The two routes for excitation of the muscle and their subservience to the cerebellum. *J. Physiol.* 1955; 130:213-224.

Grillner, S. The role of muscle stiffness in meeting the changing postural and locomotor requirements force development by the ankle extensors. *Acta Physiol. Scand.* 1972; 86:92-108.

Houk, J. and Henneman, E. Responses of Golgi tendon organs to active contractions of the soleus muscle of the cat. *J. Neurophysiol.* 1967; 30:466-481.

Kernell, D. High-frequency repetitive firing of cat lumbosacral motoneurones stimulated by long-lasting injected currents. *Acta Physiol. Scand.* 1965; 65:74-86.

Laporte, Y. and Lloyd, D.P.C. Nature and significance of the reflex connections established by large afferent fibers of muscular origin. *Am. J. Physiol.* 1952; 169:609-621.

Lin, D.C. and Rymer, W.Z. Nonlinear damping properties of the human muscle/reflex system with inertial loads. *Soc. Neurosci. Abstr.* 1997; 23: 763.

Lloyd, D.P.C. A direct central inhibitory action of chronically conducted impulses. *J. Neurophysiol.* 1941; 4:184-190.

Lloyd, D.P.C. Integrative pattern of excitation and inhibition in two-neuron reflex arcs. *J. Neurophysiol.* 1946; 9: 439-444.

Matthews, P.B.C. The dependence of tension upon extension in the stretch reflex of the soleus muscle of the decerebrate cat. *J. Physiol.* 1959; 147:521-546.

Matthews, P.B.C. The origin and functional significance of the stretch reflex. Oslo: Universitetsforlaget; 1970, pp. 302-315. Ed.: Andersen, P. and Jansen, J.K.S., *Excitatory Synaptic Mechanisms.*

Merton, P.A. Speculations on the servo-control of movement. London: Churchill; 1953, pp. 247-255. Ed.: Wolstenholme, G.E.W., *The Spinal Cord.*

Nichols, T.R. A biomechanical perspective on spinal mechanisms of coordinated muscular action: An architecture principle. *Acta Anat.* 1994; 151:1-13.

Nichols, T.R. Receptor mechanisms underlying heterogenic reflexes among the triceps surae muscles of the cat. *J. Neurophysiol.* 1999; 81: 467-478 .

Nichols, T.R., Cope, T., and Abelew, T.A. Rapid spinal mechanisms of motor coordination. *Exerc. Sports Sci. Rev.* 1999; 27: 255-284.

Renshaw, B. Activity in the simplest spinal reflex pathways. *J. Neurophysiol.* 1940; 3:374-387.

Sherrington, C.S. On plastic tonus and proprioceptive reflexes. *Quarterly J. Exp. Physiol.* 1909; 2:109-156.

Sherrington, C.S. *The Integrative Action of the Nervous System.* Charles Scribner's Sons, 1906.

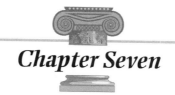
Helmholtz: Founder of the Action-Perception Theory

Stan Gielen

University of Nijmegen, The Netherlands

Revisiting the work of Hermann Ludwig Ferdinand (von) Helmholtz

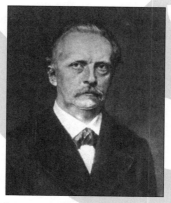

Hermann (von) Helmholtz

Hermann Ludwig Ferdinand (von) Helmholtz was born in 1821 and died in 1894. He was one of those exceptional scientists who was active at the front of science in several disciplines. He can be equally well regarded as a physicist, physiologist, physician, biologist, mathematician, philosopher, or engineer/inventor. His multidisciplinary training, approach, and interests, as well as his cross-fertilization of research fields, reflect the activities of this true scientific giant of the 19th century.

About Helmholtz

Helmholtz started his scientific career with medicine. For financial reasons he had to choose training as a medical doctor in the German army, receiving his degree in 1843. Studying medicine in the army was the best way for him to combine his scientific interests with his military duties in Germany, even though his heart was more with physics and mathematics. After his military service, he became a teacher of anatomy in 1848 (Berlin) and a professor of physiology in Königsberg (1849), Bonn (1855), and Heidelberg (1858) in succession. In 1871 he was appointed professor of physics in Berlin (1871), and from 1889 he served as president of the Physikalisch-Technische Reichsanstalt (the Physical-Technical Institute) in Charlottenburg (Germany). At birth, he received the names Hermann Ludwig Ferdinand Helmholtz. The honorary prefix "von" was granted in 1882 in recognition of his great scientific contributions at that time.

Helmholtz advocated a multidisciplinary approach, which led him to study a large variety of topics. For example, in his mathematical work he addressed the foundations of geometry (Helmholtz, 1968). In physiology he designed special techniques to study the conduction velocity of action potentials along the axon. He also tried to develop and confirm experimentally the phenomenological laws for the perception of music. As part of these activities he developed a theory about the role of timbre in auditory perception that would later be frequently used. His work on special topics like music theory, tone perception (Helmholtz, 1954), color vision, binocular vision (Helmholtz, 1867a), eye movements, and eye optics (Helmholtz, 1867b) also brought him much fame and is still highly relevant today. With his invention of the ophthalmoscope, Helmholtz initiated a rapid development of ophthalmology (see Helmholtz, 1910). The Helmholtz resonator, which he employed to analyze sound, is still used in studies of sound absorption.

In physics Helmholtz paved the way for many theoretical and experimental studies. For example, he proposed a new way to consider the well-known law of energy conservation. His name was given to "Helmholtz free energy," which provides the pressure and entropy for a system at equilibrium with volume and temperature as the independent variables (i.e., at minimum energy). He also contributed to hydrodynamics (including vortices and instabilities), optics, and electricity. In philosophy he worked on many epistemological problems. In summary, he studied complex systems with a mastery of all available conceptual and empirical research tools.

Although motor control was not the primary topic of his research, Helmholtz's scientific work in physiology, mathematics, and physics had a deep impact on motor control research in the last century. At the conceptual level, Helmholtz contributed greatly to motor control. In fact, by stressing the natural link between perception and action, Helmholtz was one of the founders "avant la lettre" of the action-perception theory, which states that perception and action cannot be studied in isolation since one affects the other. Although it may seem trivial to say that perception is a necessary step preceding action, we have fully understood only in the last two decades that movements are an indispensable mechanism for perception for many reasons. Another issue that Helmholtz discussed at great length was the fact that subjects do not perceive two different visual worlds although the images on the left and right retina are clearly different. This touches a very deep problem concerning the sensory interpretation of neuronal activity.

In this chapter we will consider some aspects of the work of Helmholtz and the impact of his work on studies of motor control today. Since it is impossible to give a full account of all his ideas and contributions, a selection of ideas and experiments had to be made. This selection is undoubtedly subjectively biased. I hope that it provides a representative sample of the wealth of rich ideas developed by Helmholtz and that it will stimulate readers to further familiarize themselves with his work.

Principles for an Empirical Theory of Perception

Helmholtz was one of the first to try to define a scientific way to study perception and action. The problem at that time was that contrary to the situation in physics, where the results of an experiment can be measured objectively, the results of perception were considered to be subjective and variable in time due to learning processes. These aspects made scientists reluctant to approach the field. Helmholtz demonstrated that experiments could be designed to give reproducible and accurate results that could be used to verify or disprove theoretical hypotheses. He spent considerable time explaining what the scientific approach to studying perceptual processes should be:

> The fundamental thesis of the empirical theory is: The sensations of the senses are tokens of our consciousness, it being left to our intelligence to learn how to comprehend their meaning. The tokens, which we get by the sense of sight, may vary in intensity and in quality, that is, in luminosity and in color. There may also be some other difference between them depending on the place on the retina that is stimulated, a so-called local sign. The local signs of the sensations in one eye are entirely different from those in the other eye. (1925, p. 533)

Helmholtz's ideas about the fundamental thesis of the empirical theory are further outlined in the text presented in the next section of this chapter.

On the Nature of the Causal Linkage Between Action and Perception

One of the fundamental problems of action and perception relates to the fact that perception without action on the one hand, and action without perception on the other hand, would be completely useless. It is because we have both that they both become meaningful. There are several arguments for this rather bold statement.

The first argument says that motor commands have to be adjusted all the time to generate movements in the proper direction and amplitude and with the proper timing. Various reasons (for example, fatigue, interaction with objects of variable size and weight, changes in the effector system during growth to adulthood) require that the effect of motor commands be monitored to adjust for errors in motor commands. Obviously, sensory systems like the visual system, but also the proprioceptive system, the vestibular system, and cutaneous receptors, are perfect mechanisms to provide feedback about the effect of motor commands.

A second argument for the important role of movements for perceptual processes tells us that movements are important since they can actively induce new sensory inputs. For example, head movements generate new retinal images, which among others can be used to estimate the distance of objects relative to each other. Also, head movements can reveal objects that were previously occluded by other objects along the line of sight. This argument explains that perception is not a passive process but rather an active process of gathering new information about the environment.

There is a third argument, less well known than the other two but much more compelling from a theoretical point of view. This argument relates to self-organization within the central nervous system. It is a much deeper argument, and I will illustrate it with an example. Everyone has seen a telephone-company cable with its large number of thin wires. In order to enable one to make sense of the large number of wires, each wire is labeled by means of a particular color of insulating material. The color labels the function of each wire and the significance of the signals in that wire such that an engineer who has to repair a fault in the system can easily find the wire responsible. Now imagine the optic nerve, which has a number of nerve fibers exceeding the number of wires in a telephone cable by at least a million. None of these nerve cells has an explicit label, like a color or chemical label. Although there is clearly some structure in the visual system (for example, topographical maps have been found in the lateral geniculate nucleus, visual cortex, and many other brain structures), it is also capable of a great deal of flexibility and recalibration. The self-organization and recalibration can take place only when the nervous system has knowledge of the meaning of the signals in each of the various nerve fibers and nerve cells. Without such meaning, there is no need for recalibration. Various suggestions have been made as to the mechanisms that may attribute a functional significance to the signals in nerve cells. Koenderink (1984) proposes that the central nervous system can make sense out of the huge number of incoming sensory fibers because of the overlap between receptive fields. The overlap in receptive fields causes a correlation of the activity of cells with neighboring receptive fields. The larger the overlap between receptive fields, the larger the correlation of activity of the cells. Therefore, the correlation of activity provides a measure for the overlap of the receptive fields. Through this it induces a functional ordering that allows the central nervous system to assign a "local sign" to each neuron, and to reconstruct a topological ordering in the receptive fields of the afferent sensory nerve fibers and therefore also in the functional meaning of the activity in these fibers. Obviously, this notion is not valid for only sensory afferent activity but is equally applicable to all neurons in the central nervous system since many neurons do have common input that causes a correlation of activity of various neurons.

In fact, the suggestion to use a correlation of activity to assign "local sign" to neurons is related to Hebb's notion (see Hebb, 1949) that the connectivity between neurons may be proportional to the correlation in activity between two cells. As such, the Hebb learning rule can be considered a neural implementation of a mechanism to establish functional order in a large number of neurons, based on their neural activity.

The arguments in the previous paragraphs explain how sensory information by itself is able to provide an ordering when receptive fields overlap. However, a functional order alone is not sufficient for successful sensorimotor behavior since it must be complemented by a metric that gives the position of objects in some frame of reference. Such a metric is necessary since it is not sufficient to know that one object is behind another object to grasp it. For a successful grasp we have to know the position of that object relative to, for example, the body, or relative to the present position of the hand. Such a metric is indispensable for navigating in any environment and for grasping objects in a cluttered environment. It is well known that visual cortex has a retinotopic organization and that many neurons in visual cortex have the same receptive-field position in retinal coordinates but with a different disparity sensitivity. The latter means that when the eyes fixate on a target in a particular direction and at a particular distance, there are many cells that respond to targets along the same gaze direction. However, these cells differ in the sense that they respond differently to targets in front or behind the fixation point. These cells are sensitive to depth. When we mature, the distance between the eyes increases, and therefore the retinal disparity of targets at the same distance increases. There is no way the central nervous system can "detect" changes in disparity due to changes in the distance between the eyes unless the central nervous system can generate head movements. Head movements generate changes in sensory afferent input, which are causally related to the head movements. By relating changes in sensory signals to motor commands, the central nervous system is able to induce a metric for the sensory signals that is sufficient for normal perception and motor behavior. Notice that this metric does not necessarily imply a metric in terms of extrinsic coordinates (for example, distance in meters) but rather a distance in terms of intrinsic sensorimotor command signals. Basically, this mechanism of using causal relations for self-organization and recalibration is the same mechanism that is used by experimental sciences like physics, chemistry, and psychology: If two phenomena (like thunder and lightning) are frequently observed simultaneously, they must have a causal relationship. Helmholtz was well aware of the usefulness of the causal relation between sensory signals and motor commands, as will become evident from the following passage.

Finally, the tests we employ using voluntary movements of the body are of the greatest importance in strengthening our conviction of the correctness of the perceptions of our senses. And thus, as contrasted with purely passive observations, the same sort of firmer conviction arises as is derived by the process of experiment in scientific investigations. The particular ultimate basis, which gives convincing power to all our conscious inductions, is the law of causation. If two natural phenomena have frequently been observed together, such as thunder and lightning, they seem to be regularly connected together, and we infer that there must be a common basis for both of them. And if this causal connection has invariably acted heretofore, so that thunder and lightning accompany each other, then in the future too like causes must produce like effects, and the result must be the same in the future. However, as long as we are limited to mere observations of such phenomena as occur by themselves without our help, and without our being able to make experiments so as to vary the complexity of causes, it is difficult to be sure that we really ascertained all the factors that may have some influence on the result. (1925, p. 29)

In addition to the functional role of correlation between the activity of neurons with regard to self-organization, correlation of activity has recently been recognized as an important feature of the coding of information by the nervous system. Until recently, information was thought to be coded by two mechanisms: the number of neurons that are active (recruitment) and the firing rate of active neurons. If these mechanisms are the only ones available, the question arises how the brain is able to code multiple features (for example visual and auditory features) that belong to the same object. It is well known that visual information is processed in various parallel channels (Desimone and Ungerleider, 1989). For example, visual information in cortex is processed along parallel channels, which separate channels for color, motion, and location of an object (the *where channel*) and identification of the nature of objects *(what channel)*. If different features of the same object are represented in various channels, and if one considers that we usually see multiple objects simultaneously, how does the brain label features in various channels as features belonging to the same object? This problem has been referred to as the "binding problem." It has been suggested that synchrony of firing is the label used to label features of identical objects. This coding principle is found not only in the visual system but also in motor cortex, where synchrony labels ensembles of neurons involved in movement of the same limb segment (see Singer and Gray, 1995).

The notion that correlation of activity is used to learn input-output relations has deep implications for perception and action. For example, we usually look at the world with two eyes, and head movements induce similar changes in the retinal images. This may explain why we frequently are not aware whether an object is being viewed by one eye or by both eyes. Or even more interestingly, since the two eyes view the world from different positions, the images on the two retinas are different. This raises the question why we do not perceive two different views, but a single three-dimensional world. This issue was discussed at great length by Helmholtz. As he pointed out:

Lastly, there is another question which comes up here, and which likewise is of some theoretical importance: that is, whether we can distinguish the impressions of one eye from those of the other. In this connection, it is well to remember that when groups of lines are seen stereoscopically the intervals of depth are always seen correctly, even by instantaneous electric illumination, but the relief is never reversed. Even when I tried to imagine as well as I could the reversal of the relief, in order to produce an intentional illusion (as I could do very quickly in reversing the relief of medals in the case of monocular vision), I found it simply impossible to alter the stereoscopic relief. And yet such reversal of the relief would be bound to take place if the impression of the two retinal images could be confused with that impression which would be obtained by interchanging the retinal images with each other. Hence, it follows, in the first place, that the instantaneous impression made by two retinal images must be distinctly and definitely different from that which the same retinal images would make if they were transferred to the corresponding points of the other eye.

The fact that ordinarily one is not clearly aware which eye it is with which he sees this image or the other, is a somewhat different thing. We cannot be certain about it, or at least not perfectly certain, and our judgement will depend on secondary considerations; for we cannot decipher anything from our sensations except those interpretations we have learned to make by oft-repeated observations. Thus we may have learned to tell perfectly that two double images of a certain sort, which are closely adjacent, and which have certain signs, signify an object that is farther from us than the point of fixation, and not one that is nearer to us; and still we may not be sufficiently well trained in interpreting the local signs of the images to tell which of the two half-images belongs to one eye, and which to the other eye. To be sure about this, one must close one eye or cover it; although this is not what one does in ordinary vision, where, as has been stated, the double images are usually not heeded at all. Therefore, as a rule, without making a special experiment for that very purpose, we are ignorant as to which image belongs to one eye; and which image to the other eye. Nor do the movements of the eye aid us much here, because when the eyes are convergent (as they will be in this case) we do not have any clear idea of the direction in which each eye by itself is shifted.

On the other hand, the extreme portions of the common field of view over on the right will be seen constantly by the right eye only, being concealed from the other eye by the nose. And, similarly, objects far over to the left will be visible to the left eye only. Consequently, when a region of the field is completely hidden from one eye, we naturally infer that the objects perceived there must be seen with the other eye. A striking experiment described by Rogers should be mentioned here. Make a tube about two inches in diameter with a piece of black paper, and, holding it up to the right eye, point it toward the far corner of the room over on the left. At the same time hold a sheet of paper several inches for the other eye, so as to screen this eye from the part of the room seen through the tube. Then you will have a very decided illusion as though you were looking at the corner of the room with your left eye through a hole in the paper; whereas there is no hole in it, and it is the other eye, and not the left eye, that is looking through the tube. (1925, pp. 458-459)

Helmholtz thought that one of the mechanisms, which is indispensable for the self-organizing process in mapping two different two-dimensional retinal images into a three-dimensional view of the world, was the use of efferent or outflow activity. In his view, the afferent information and neural effort or motor commands are used to teach the subject how to interpret sensory signals:

The direction of observed objects with respect to the observer is ascertained by the help of the feeling of innervation in the nerves of the ocular muscles. This feeling, however, is continually regulated by the result, that is by the shifting of the images produced by the innervations. When a person gazes through a prism and executes movements of his body and hands as they appear in his field of view, he soon learns to see through the prism correctly, notwithstanding the wrong directions of the incident rays. The phenomena of giddiness also indicates a change in the adjustment of the effect of certain innervations. (1925, p. 243)

Since saccadic eye movements have a rather short duration (about 50 ms), reflex activity would be useless for bringing the eye on target. However, although eye muscles do not have stretch reflexes, they do have muscle spindles, which may be used in learning to handle visual information and in the process of creating a three-dimensional world from two images that are two-dimensional. Although it is well known that efference copies and afferent information play a role in these processes, their precise role is still not known today.

In the text so far, we have discussed the importance of correlations in the process of learning to interpret incoming sensory information. The notion of correlation of activity to learn input-output relations is also relevant for the motor system. For example, everyone is able to make very accurate movements. Yet almost no one knows which muscles are involved in these movements. For example, five muscles contribute to flexion of the arm. This provides a redundancy with respect to flexion of the elbow. Yet everyone uses the same activation pattern when flexing the arm (see, e.g., van Zuylen et al., 1988). Sometimes medical treatment for trauma requires that the insertion or origin of a tendon be attached at a new location. After such surgery, subjects are very well able to use the muscle with its new mechanical action. This indicates that the stereotyped muscle activation patterns observed in many studies are not fixed at birth but can be modified as the result of some adaptive process.

Autonomous and Cognitive Aspects of Action and Perception

Action and perception require interaction with the environment. This environment also includes the effector system, which enables the organism to interact with the external world. This interaction, a very complex process, requires knowledge about the physical properties of the effector system and the external world. Since the properties of the effector system are not constant but can vary due to fatigue or during growth to adulthood, the interaction with the external world has to be learned and recalibrated all the time. As a result we can interact with the external world most of the time in a more or less automatic way. For example, when we flex the arm, we do not consciously think about which muscles to activate. Rather, activation of the appropriate muscles follows directly from the intention to flex the elbow. This is true for most perceptual and motor acts. Helmholtz wrote about this issue:

And this brings us, finally, to a last essential difficulty from which no intuition theory of space-perception has ever escaped yet, unless it confined itself to entirely general propositions; and that is, these theories are always obliged to assume that actually existing sensations can be squelched by an experience showing them to be unfounded. But there is not one single authentic instance of it. In case of all illusions of the senses produced by sensations that were stimulated abnormally, the illusory sensation is never abolished by the better knowledge we have to the contrary or by our insight into the cause of the illusion. The pressure images, the luminous streamers at the place where the optic nerve enters the eye, the after-images, etc., remain where they appear to be in the field of view, just as the image in a mirror continues to be seen behind the mirror, although in the case of all these phenomena we are well aware that they have no real existence. Of course, the attention can be distracted permanently, if desired, from sensations that have no relation whatever to external objects; for example, from the sensations of the fainter after-images or of the entoptical or other objects. Moreover, in estimating their intensity, fairly large errors are liable to occur on account of contrast; or we may make a mistake in apportioning them between two objects of which they are supposed to be the common effect, as is sometimes the case with contrast phenomena. In fact, as long as the distinction between conscious conclusions and inductive conclusions was not quite clear, one of the main objections of the senses were not destroyed by an insight into their mechanism nor by experience to the contrary. What would become of our sense-perceptions, if we had the power not only of not noticing a part of them that did not fit exactly into the chain of our experiences, but of converting it into its opposite? (1925, p. 556)

Frames of Reference for Perception and Action

In many sensorimotor tasks, various frames of reference are involved. Initially, visual information is encoded in a retinal coordinate system when it enters the brain. For the process of translating the visual information about target position and arm position into appropriate motor commands, several hypotheses have been put forward stating that end-point position for reaching is specified in shoulder-centered coordinates (Soechting and Flanders, 1989a,b; Flanders et al., 1992), hand-centered coordinates (Flanders et al., 1992; Gordon et al., 1994), or viewer-centered (McIntyre et al., 1997) frames of reference or a world frame of reference, depending on the instruction to the subject (Desmurget et al., 1997). Helmholtz addressed the question of which frame of reference is used in normal sensorimotor tasks. In particular he focused on the visual aspects of object localization. Which aspects contribute to the localization of a visual object? Obviously, not only retinal information is involved since the position of the eyes and the head is relevant too. According to Helmholtz:

Ordinarily, we see with both eyes at the same time, turning them in the head first one way and then the other, and likewise from time to time changing the position in space not of the head only but of the whole body. Thus, we are in the habit of letting our eyes roam about, fixating first one point and then another of the object in front of us; that is, both eyes are turned so as to get the image of the point of fixation on the centers of the two retinas simultaneously. By thus using the eyes, we are enabled to obtain correct perceptions of the location of the visible object whose rays pursue rectilinear paths and enter the eye without having been deflected.

In fact, according to the laws by which the light is refracted by the ocular media, as explained in §10, it is easy to see that when we know the position of the body and head, together with the positions of the two eyes in the head, including, therefore, the positions of their nodal points, and when we know also the locations of the two retinas on which the images of the luminous point are formed, theoretically we should be able to determine uniquely the place where the luminous point really is. For then all that is necessary is to draw a straight line from the retinal image in each eye through the corresponding nodal point and prolong it. The two lines of direction can meet only in one point, and the luminous object must be at this place.

Incidentally, the accuracy of the determination of the actual location of the visual object in space will depend on how accurate the various data are which have been enumerated above as being necessary.

Thus suppose we have given:

1. The requisite sensations for supplying correct information as to the position of body and head with respect to some base chosen for making the measurements, for example, the floor on which we happen to be standing.

2. The requisite sensations for enabling us to estimate correctly the positions of the eyes in the head; and

3. Factors in the sensation (so-called local signs), whereby the stimulations of the retinal areas, where the light acts which comes from the object-point A, can be discriminated from the stimulations of all other places on the retina (We know nothing whatever as to the nature of these latter stimulations; and we infer that they must be of the same kind there just because we have the faculty of distinguishing luminous impressions on different parts of the retina); then we have the requisite data for finding the unique location in space of the point A. If the data were anywhere else, another aggregate of sensations would have to be excited by it. We know by experience too that as a rule we do actually learn to judge correctly by sight the place where the point of the object is. It is true, the accuracy of this determination is variable and depends especially on how near the images of the point A in the two eyes are to the fovea centralis.

Accordingly, we shall have to inquire now how much the factors of the sensation above mentioned contribute by themselves to the accurate perception of the location of the object. There will be no need here of investigating further what sensations are concerned in judging of the position of the body with respect to the floor and of the head with respect to the body, as these are questions that belong to the physiology of the perceptions of the senses in general rather than to that of the sense of light. Let us assume, therefore, that the position of the head with reference to the base used for the measurements in space is accurately known in each instance. Then all that remains to be ascertained is how much is contributed to our recognition of the location of the object, (1) by movements of the head, (2) by movements of the eyes in the head, (3) by vision with one eye, and (4) by vision with both eyes. (1925, pp. 154-156)

It is amazing that many questions with regard to frames of reference used for sensorimotor control tasks are still unanswered, as the following examples suggest.

It is well known that subjects make consistent errors when asked to point to visual targets in space (Soechting and Flanders, 1989a). Both undershoot (Soechting and Flanders, 1989a; Darling and Miller, 1993; Gentillucci and Negrotti, 1996; McIntyre et al., 1997) and overshoot (Foley, 1975; Berkinblit et al., 1995; McIntyre et al., 1997) of reaching movements have been reported in the literature. These errors are different in conditions in which the visual target is visible throughout the movement and conditions in which subjects are asked to point to a remembered target position, that is, when the target disappears before the subject points. As already noted by Helmholtz, these errors in pointing depend critically on visual feedback (Berkinblit et al., 1995), on proprioceptive information (Soechting and Flanders, 1989a,b; Hocherman, 1993), and on eye orientation (Enright, 1995). However, the precise contribution of each of these is not known yet.

Usually when subjects point or move to a target, there is some time between the percept and localization of the target and the time of movement onset. In between, subjects do not stand still completely, but move. As a consequence, the initial target position has to be updated for movements made in the period between target localization and movement. In a recent study Medendorp et al. (1999) demonstrated that finger position systematically fell short of the target. Moreover, pointing errors after movements were considerably larger than pointing movements without any movement between target presentation and pointing movement. These findings demonstrated that subjects systematically underestimated self-made movements and that any movements contribute quite considerably to errors in pointing.

Perception and Navigation

Perception does provide us with information about the shape and position of objects. Suppose we look at a flat, concave, or convex surface that has a checkerboard pattern. When we view each of these objects frontally, the different curvatures of the surfaces cause a different projection of the check-erboard pattern on the retina. Experience, in which head movements asso-ciate a particular retinal image to a particular curvature of the object, gives rise to the percept of a flat, concave, or convex surface, even if no head movements are made. Recent experiments (Cornilleau-Peres and Gielen, 1996; Dijkstra et al., 1995) have shown that self-made movements assist in the percept of shape of objects. However, these studies showed that it is not the effect of self-motion per se that contributes to a better percept of the object shape but rather the improved retinal stabilization of retinal images (see Dijkstra et al., 1995 for a more detailed discussion on this topic). Helmholtz was well aware of the complex relationship between retinal image, head movements, and perceptual images:

Accordingly, I have made a plane chart showing the projections of the direction-circles in the field of fixation which have the same directions as the vertical and horizontal lines going through the point of fixation. The projections are found to be hyperbolas in this case. In order to bring them out as distinctly as possible, even where they are seen indirectly, I have exhibited the field of the pattern formed by the curves in black and white like the squares of a chess-board; as represented in Fig. 1 [*figure 7.1 here*] on a scale of three-sixteenths. The line A, reduced to the same scale, indicates the distance of the observer's eye, which must be placed directly opposite the center of the chart. He is supposed to gaze steadily at the center. The original chart was hung on the wall of the room with its center on a level

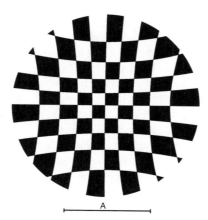

Figure 7.1
Drawing of texture that gives a perfect checkerboard pattern on the retina (with equally sized squares) when fixated in frontal view. The drawing has been made smaller. For reference, the line A should correspond to the distance between the eyes (taken from Fig. 22 on p. 181 of Helmholtz, 1925).

with my eyes. A draughts-man's forty-five degree right-triangle, the two sides of which were of the same length (20 cm) as the desired distance of the eye, was used for measuring. The distance was regulated by placing one of the legs of this triangle on the chart, while the vertex of the opposite angle rested against the outside angle of the eye.

Now, indeed under these circumstances, the direction-circles in the field of fixation projected as hyperbolas will appear as straight lines, or at least as being uncurved lines on the surface of the visual globe. The several vertical and horizontal rows of black and white blocks will appear to be straight from one end to the other, and of equal width, as long as the center of the figure is the steady point of fixation. But, of course, the curvature of the outer rows can be perceived by looking out toward them. In this case a peculiar illusion takes place. Thus when I let my eye wander, I see the drawing curved like a flat bowl, the curvature of the hyperbolas seeming to be a curvature of the surface, and the lines in this curved surface being apparently great circles (or shortest lines). To some extent the distinction between direct and indirect vision is made to disappear by the conception we get in this way. Along the directions in the field of view itself the hyperbolas are apparently not curved, but the field itself appears curved. (1925, pp. 180-181)

Perception also helps us with localizing the position of objects relative to our body and with navigating in a cluttered environment. This is easily understood. Suppose we are facing a wall with a checkerboard pattern and approach the wall. When we come closer to the wall, the square just in front of us becomes larger. The squares viewed in the periphery tend to be squeezed together in the radial direction. The particular retinal flow of an image due to movements of the head is a rich source of information about movement of objects relative to the body.

A quantitative interpretation of visual information on relative motion of an observer relative to an object can be obtained by analyzing the optic flow field. The optic flow field carries information about displacements of objects and about movements of the observer relative to an environment. Building on the work by Helmholtz, Koenderink and van Doorn (1976) showed that any optic flow field can be locally decomposed into four mathematically orthogonal components: a translation, an isotropic expansion or contraction, a rigid rotation, and a pure shear. The translation component does not provide much information about relative movement since any eye movement will induce a translation of the retinal image. The other three optic flow components are necessary and sufficient to allow a unique reconstruction of relative motion. Later experiments have shown that visual control of posture is largely affected by the optic flow field (van Asten et al., 1988a,b). This is another spin-off of the work by Helmholtz on action and perception.

Movements in Joints With Multiple Degrees of Freedom

Helmholtz did not actively investigate motor control of limb movements. However, he studied eye movements in great detail, and the results of these studies are highly relevant for motor control in general, even today. The main reason is that eye movements and limb movements share several properties although there are also some qualitative differences. Like the shoulder and the head, the eye has three rotational degrees of freedom, which allow the eye to fixate in any direction with the eye taking any orientation. Yet, as Helmholtz noticed, not all degrees of freedom are used in normal movements:

There is nothing in the mode of fastening the eyeball to prevent every sort of rotation of moderate amplitude. There are muscles also by which the eye can be turned about any axis. [Figure 7.2 shows a schematic mechanical model, which was built by Hemholtz to illustrate the mechanical action of the eye muscle.] However, careful investigation has shown that, under the

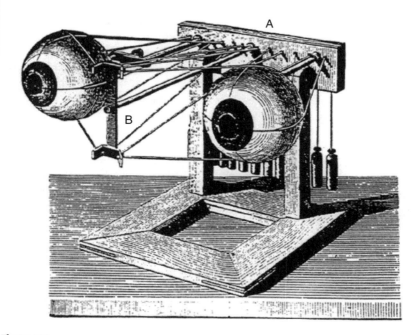

Figure 7.2
Schematic model, built by Helmholtz, illustrating the pulling actions of the six muscles of each eye. The model clearly shows that the muscles can rotate the eye about any axis in three dimensions (taken from Fig. 15 on p. 119 of Helmholtz, 1925).

ordinary conditions of normal vision, the human eye does not actually perform all the movements by any means that it is capable of executing, so far as its mechanical contrivances are concerned. Accordingly, the next question for us to investigate is, What motions are actually made by the human eye? (1925, p. 40)

First one must stress that all available degrees of freedom are accessible to stabilize gaze. For example, we can make eye movements in any direction, and in addition, the eye can rotate about the gaze direction (torsion). One can verify this easily by watching the eyes in a mirror while rotating the head. This illustrates that the eye can move along any axis in three dimensions. However, during saccadic eye movements, the amount of torsion is uniquely defined by the direction of gaze—a principle that has become known as Donders' law. As Helmholtz said, "[T]he angle of torsion in the case of the eye is a function simply of the angle of elevation and the angle of azimuth" (1867b, p. 44). Since the amount of torsion is uniquely defined by gaze direction, this implies a reduction of the number of degrees of freedom from three to two.

The problem with joints that have three rotational degrees of freedom is that rotations along non-colinear axes do not commute: The orientation of an object after two rotations along different axes depends on the order of the rotations. The consequence of using all rotation axes would be that the orientation of the eye would depend on all previous rotations in the past. In addition, the orientation of the eye could approach extreme values out of the normal physiological range. These problems can be solved by reducing the number of degrees of freedom from three to two as pointed out by several authors in the past (see Carpenter, 1988).

A more detailed description of eye position was given by Listing (see Carpenter, 1988). He noticed that the amount of torsion of the eye at a given gaze direction is the same as would be observed if the eye moved to that gaze direction from a particular reference position (the so-called primary position) by a rotation about a single axis in a plane perpendicular to the primary position. The particular reference position just mentioned is (in good approximation) the eye position in the skull when the head is held in natural erect position and when the line of sight is horizontal and straight ahead. Listing's law says that all rotation vectors, which describe the measured eye positions, lie in a flat plane, which is described by the equation $r_x = 0$. Here, r_x is the x-component of the rotation vector $\mathbf{r}$ (see Haustein, 1989 for more details), which is proportional to the amount of torsion of the eye. The r_y and r_z components refer to eye movements with a vertical or horizontal component, respectively.

In the last decade, a similar reduction of the number of degrees of freedom was reported by other authors for head movements and shoulder movements (Tweed and Vilis, 1987; Hore et al., 1992; Miller et al., 1992; Theeuwen et al., 1993). This shows that the findings for the eye are not specific for the eye but rather reflect a basic principle for dealing with rotations in joints with three degrees of freedom. However, there are also some differences—which need to be discussed to appreciate the various arguments—that have been proposed to explain the particular reduction of the number of degrees of freedom for joints with multiple degrees of freedom.

When subjects are instructed to make head movements to look at targets in various directions, the rotation vectors, which represent the postures of the head relative to a particular reference position, lie in a curved plane. In contrast to the equation $r_x = 0$, which defines a flat plane for the rotation vectors for the eye, the surface with rotation vectors for the head is given by the equation $r_x = -\alpha r_y r_z$, where α varies between 0.3 and 0.6 for various subjects (Theeuwen et al., 1993). Since the head has three rotational degrees of freedom, there is a reduction of the number of degrees of freedom for the head as for the eye. However, since the rotation vectors are in a curved rather than a flat plane as for the eye, there is a clear difference in the way the reduction of the number of degrees of freedom is realized for the eye and the head.

Similarly, when subjects are instructed to point to targets in various directions by shoulder movements with the fully extended arm, a reduction of the number of degrees of freedom becomes evident by the fact that the rotation vectors, which describe postures of the upper arm relative to some reference position, lie in a curved plane. This plane is mathematically represented by the equation $r_x = \alpha + \beta r_y + \gamma r_z + \delta r_y^2 + \epsilon r_y r_z + \zeta r_z^2$, where α, β, γ, δ, ϵ, and ζ are constants that vary within a small range for different subjects (see Gielen et al., 1997). This equation illustrates that the curvature is different for head movements and shoulder movements.

Normal movements to targets usually require movements in the shoulder and elbow. When the orientation of the forearm is plotted using rotation vectors, the rotation vectors fall in a curved plane as was found for the upper arm. However, the coefficients of the fits are slightly different (Gielen et al., 1997).

To summarize, these findings reveal a consistent reduction of the number of degrees of freedom from three to two for eye movements, head movements, and arm movements. However, there are some quantitative differences between eye, head, and arm movements in that the two-dimensional plane with rotation vectors has a somewhat different shape.

Underlying Mechanisms for the Reduction of Degrees of Freedom

Helmholtz seriously questioned the mechanisms that may underlie the reduction of the number of degrees of freedom. One possibility might have been the anatomy of the eye, including the origin and insertion of the muscles that move the eye. Although the rotation vectors of normal eye movements lie in the plane $r_x = 0$ (which means that there is no torsion of the eye), the eyes can rotate, as can be demonstrated easily by rotating the head. This illustrates that the reduction of the number of degrees of freedom is not constrained by the anatomy. Helmholtz was aware of this fact:

Lastly, we must see how the separate ocular muscles contribute to the individual normal ocular movements. As has been stated [see Helmholtz 1867a] the internal and external recti, acting by themselves, tend to turn the eye around a vertical axis. According to Ruette's findings, the axis about which the eye is turned by the superior and inferior recti is horizontal and makes an angle of about 70 deg with the line of fixation; its inner end being toward the front eye. The axis of the oblique muscles is likewise horizontal and makes an angle of about 35 deg with the line of fixation; its outer end being toward the front. Rotations about the vertical axis produced by the internal and external recti are in accordance with Listing's law, and hence this pair of muscles may act alone. But rotations around the other two axes are not in accordance with this law. In order to produce an upward motion of the eye by rotation around an horizontal axis extending from right to left, there must be a combination of a rotation produced by the superior rectus with one produced by the inferior oblique muscle; and for a downward movement the inferior rectus and the superior oblique muscle must act together. (1867b, pp. 52)

Several explanations other than ones that are anatomically based have been proposed to explain the reduction of the number of rotational degrees of freedom. A first rather general explanation was provided by postulating that movements are made with maximum comfort. This hypothesis implies that of the many possible configurations of the eye, head, or shoulder, the central nervous system chooses the particular configuration that is most comfortable to the subject (see Rosenbaum et al., 1995). The problem with this hypothesis is that it is hard to define the concept of "comfort" in terms of motor control effort. One could define minimal comfort in various ways, for example by choosing the posture that corresponds to minimal muscle activation or minimal fatigue, to name just two possibilities. Moreover, it might well be that several criteria for "comfort" might lead to the same predictions about optimal postures (see van Bolhuis and Gielen, 1999). Helmholtz was well aware of these problems when he wrote:

In regard to the theory of the ocular movements, there is one matter which I should like to mention, by way of supplement to the above, as it is, perhaps, not altogether unimportant. The mode of attachment of the eye to the conjunctiva and even in the connective tissue and fatty part of the socket is such that relatively the least tension is produced in these places by any movement of the eye that is in accordance with Listing's law. If the eye were to execute a rather large rolling movement which departed from this law, it would certainly result in tearing some parts of the conjunctiva and partial folding of individual pieces. Thus also from this point of view there would seem to be some connection between obeying Listing's law and having the least exertion and inconvenience, in analogy with the conclusions which Fick and Wundt reached as to the muscles of the eye. (1925, p. 123)

Helmholtz brought forward a second hypothesis, proposing that the reduction of the number of degrees of freedom serves a perceptual purpose. To appreciate the argument completely, we have to make a small detour. Imagine a cross affixed to a bar that can rotate along a vertical axis, nested in a frame that can rotate about a horizontal axis. Such a cardanic system is called a "Helmholtz system" (see figure 7.3). Now imagine what happens to the cross when it rotates along the vertical and horizontal axes. The orientation of the cross is not fixed; rather it changes as a function of the rotation along the vertical and horizontal axes. Obviously there is no real torsion. Yet the orientation of the axis changes. This phenomenon is referred to as "false torsion." It is easy to demonstrate that any convention using two rotation axes to rotate the cross will lead somehow to "false torsion." Similarly, the eye will also have some false torsion.

Now imagine a vertical line that is viewed by the eye in the primary position. When the eye rotates using two degrees of freedom, the eye will reveal some false torsion too. As a consequence, the orientation of the vertical line changes as a function of gaze direction of the eye. For a line at finite distance, the eyes have a vergence component, and as a consequence the false torsion of the two eyes is in opposite directions. Therefore, the vertical line will rotate in opposite directions on the two retinas. Now

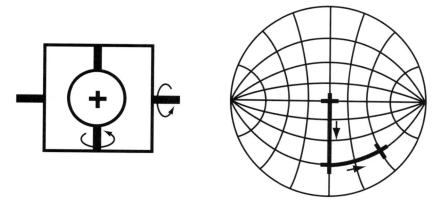

Figure 7.3
Helmholtz gimbal to adjust the gaze direction for the eye (left). The right-hand side shows how the orientation of the eye changes for different gaze directions using the Helmholtz gimbal.

Helmholtz proposed that any deviations of the projection of a vertical line on the retina from the projection of that line with the eye in the primary position should be as small as possible. A detailed mathematical analysis to solve this minimization principle resulted in eye movements close to that described by Listing's law. Both Helmholtz (1867a) and Hering (1865) argued that a consequence of Listing's law is that of the self-congruence of retinal images of oblique lines when gaze changes along these lines. This implies that no matter which point on the oblique line is fixated, the retinal image always stimulates the same set of retinal receptors. Whether or not this hypothesis is correct is not yet settled. However, the fact that the orientation of the flat plane with rotation vectors for the eye changes relative to the head—as a function of the orientation of the head relative to the gravity vector (Misslisch et al., 1994)—suggests that the perceptual hypothesis of Helmholtz cannot provide a full explanation.

A third hypothesis proposes arguments based on motor control to explain the reduction of the number of degrees of freedom in joints with three degrees of freedom. As shown before, the order of two rotations along non-collinear axes has an effect on the orientation of an object. The consequence of this non-commutative character of rotations is that the orientation of an object depends on previous rotations and that the amount of torsion can accumulate out of the physiological range. These problems can be solved by selecting a two-dimensional subset of the three-dimensional space with rotation vectors. This argument explains the reduction of the number of degrees of freedom from three to two. However, it does not explain why the rotation vectors lie in a flat plane (Listing's plane) for the eye and in a curved surface for the head and the eye. Also, the fact that the rotation vectors lie in different surfaces for the eye, head, and shoulder seems to complicate various visual-motor tasks in which the hands manipulate objects under visual control. A possibility could be that the different musculoskeletal systems are responsible for the different nature of the surfaces with rotation vectors. However, that hypothesis falls back on the anatomy of the muscles and of the origin and insertion of the tendons, which was discarded as the single factor explaining the observations.

Helmholtz's work on eye movements (as is true of the work reviewed here) dealt with kinematics only. Recently, several studies have appeared on the problem of reducing the number of degrees of freedom in dynamic conditions. The results suggest that inertia of the limb plays an important role in defining the trajectory of aiming movements. Sabes et al. (1998) have shown that particular features of arm movement trajectories can be well predicted when the sensitivity of the arm to perturbations as determined by its inertial stability is taken into account. To understand this, we have to realize that the same perturbation to the hand will have a different effect on hand position depending on the direction of the perturbation. For some directions, the inertia of the arm is small, giving rise to relatively large displacements, whereas in other directions the inertia is larger, leading to smaller hand displacements. Although dynamics is in general more difficult to understand than kinematics, it may well be that we have a better understanding of the constraints imposed on trajectory planning for the dynamics of aiming movements than for the kinematics determining arm postures. This is in line with other studies (Lacquaniti and Maioli, 1994) presenting evidence in favor of separate neural control of geometric and kinetic parameters.

In the literature to date, there are no compelling arguments in favor or against one or the other hypothesis. Many of the arguments and ideas presented by Helmholtz are along the same lines as those outlined by Bernstein (1967). In my view, discovering the basic principles that underlie the reduction of degrees of freedom is one of the major challenges of the near future.

References

Berkinblit B., Fookson O., Smetanin B., Adamovich S., Poizner H. (1995) The interaction of visual and proprioceptive inputs in pointing to actual and remembered targets. *Experimental Brain Research* 107:326-330.

Bernstein N. (1967) The problem of co-ordination and localization. In: *The coordination and regulation of movements*, pp. 15-69. New York: Pergamon.

Carpenter R.H.S. (1988) *Movements of the eyes*. London: Pion.

Cornilleau-Peres V., Gielen C.C.A.M. (1996) Interactions between self-motion and depth perception in the processing of optic flow. *Trends in Neuroscience* 19:196-201.

Darling W.G., Miller G.F. (1993) Transformations between visual and kinesthetic coordinate systems in reaches to remembered object locations and orientations. *Experimental Brain Research* 93:534-547.

Desimone R., Ungerleider L.G. (1989) Neural mechanisms of visual processing in monkeys. In: *Handbook of neuropsychology,* Vol. 2, Ed. F. Boller and J. Grafman, Amsterdam: Elsevier, 273-290.

Desmurget M., Jordan M., Prablanc C., Jeannerod M. (1997) Constrained and unconstrained movements involve different control strategies. *Journal of Neurophysiology* 77:1644-1650.

Dijkstra T.M.H., Cornilleau-Peres V., Gielen C.C.A.M., Droulez J. (1995) Perception of three-dimensional shape from ego- and object-motion: Comparison between small- and large-field stimuli. *Vision Research* 35:435-462.

Enright J. (1995) The non-visual impact of eye orientation on eye-hand coordination. *Vision Research* 11:1611-1618.

Flanders M., Tillery S.I.H., Soechting J.F. (1992) Early stages in a sensorimotor transformation. *The Behavioral and Brain Sciences* 15:309-362.

Foley J.M. (1975) Error in visually directed manual pointing. *Perception and Psychophysics* 17:69-74.

Gentilucci M., Negrotti A. (1996) Mechanisms for distance reproduction in perceptual and motor tasks. *Experimental Brain Research* 108:140-146.

Gielen C.C.A.M., Vrijenhoek E.J., Flash T., Neggers S.F.W. (1997) Arm position constraints during pointing and reaching in 3-D space. *Journal of Neurophysiology* 78:660-673.

Gordon J., Ghilardi M., Ghez C. (1994) Accuracy of planar reaching movements: I. Independence of direction and extent variability. *Experimental Brain Research* 99:97-111.

Haustein W. (1989) Considerations on Listing's law and the primary position by means of a matrix description of eye position control. *Biological Cybernetics* 60:411-420.

Hebb D.O. (1949) *The organization of behavior*. New York: Wiley.

Helmholtz H. von (1867a). *Handbuch der Physiologischen Optik* (1st ed.). Hamburg, Germany: Voss, vols. I and II. Translated into English by J.P.C. Southall as *Treatise on physiological optics*. New York: Dover, 1924.

Helmholtz H. von (1867b). *Handbuch der Physiologischen Optik* (1st ed.). Hamburg, Germany: Voss, vol. 3. Third edition translated into English by J.P.C. Southall as *Treatise on physiological optics*. New York: Dover, 1925.

Helmholtz H. von (1910) *Beschreibung eines Augenspiegels zur Untersuchung der Netzhaut im lebenden Auge*. Leipzig: Barth.

Helmholtz H. von (1954) *Die Lehre von den Tonempfindungen als physiologische Grundlage fuer die Theorie der Musik*. Translated into English by A.J. Ellis as *On the sensations of tone as a physiological basis for the theory of music*. New York: Dover.

Helmholtz H. von (1968) *Ueber Geometrie*. Darmstadt, Germany: Wissenschaftliche Buchgesellschaft.

Hering, H.E. (1865) Beitrag zur Frage der gleichzeitigen Tätigkeit antagonistisch wirkender Muskeln. *Zeitschrift für Heilkunde* 16: 129.

Hocherman S. (1993) Proprioceptive guidance and motor planning of reaching movements to unseen targets. *Experimental Brain Research* 95:439-458.

Hore J., Watts S., Vilis T. (1992) Constraints on arm position when pointing in three dimensions: Donders' law and the Fick gimbal strategy. *Journal of Neurophysiology* 68:374-383.

Koenderink J.J. (1984) Simultaneous order in nervous nets from a functional standpoint. *Biological Cybernetics* 50:35-41.

Koenderink J.J., van Doorn A.J. (1976) Local structure of movement parallax of the plane. *Journal of the Optical Society of America* 66:717-723.

Lacquaniti F., Maioli C. (1994) Independent control of limb position and contact forces in cat posture. *Journal of Neurophysiology* 72:1476-1495.

McIntyre J., Stratta F., Lacquaniti F. (1997) Viewer-centered frame of reference for pointing to memorized targets in three-dimensional space. *Journal of Neurophysiology* 78:1601-1618.

Medendorp W.P., van Asselt S., Gielen C.C.A.M. (1999) Pointing to remembered visual targets after active one-step self-displacements within reaching space. *Experimental Brain Research* 125: 50-60.

Miller L.E., Theeuwen M., Gielen C.C.A.M. (1992) The control of arm pointing movements in three dimensions. *Experimental Brain Research* 42:223-227.

Misslisch H., Tweed D., Fetter M., Vilis T. (1994) The influence of gravity on Donders' law for head movements. *Vision Research* 34:3017-3025.

Rosenbaum D.A., Loukopoulos L.D., Meulenbroek R.G.J., Vaughan J., Engelbrecht S.E. (1995) Planning reaches by evaluating stored postures. *Psychological Review* 1:28-67.

Sabes P.N., Jordan M.I., Wolpert D.M. (1998) The role of inertial sensitivity in motor planning. *Journal of Neuroscience* 18:5948-5957.

Singer W., Gray C.M. (1995) Visual feature integration and the temporal correlation hypothesis. *Annual Review of Neuroscience* 18:555-586.

Soechting J., Flanders M. (1989a) Sensorimotor representations for pointing to targets in three-dimensional space. *Journal of Neurophysiology* 62:582-594.

Soechting J., Flanders M. (1989b) Errors in pointing are due to approximations in sensorimotor transformations. *Journal of Neurophysiology* 62:595-608.

Theeuwen M., Miller L.E., Gielen C.C.A.M. (1993) Are orientations of the head and arm related during pointing movements. *Journal of Motor Behavior* 25:242-250.

Tweed D., Vilis T. (1987) Implications of rotational kinematics for the oculomotor system in three dimensions. *Journal of Neurophysiology* 58:832-849.

van Asten W.N.J.C., Gielen C.C.A.M., Denier van der Gon J.J. (1988a) Postural movements induced by rotations of visual scenes. *Journal of the Optical Society of America* A5:1781-1789.

van Asten W.N.J.C., Gielen C.C.A.M., Denier van der Gon J.J. (1988b) Postural adjustments induced by stimulated motion of differently structured environments. *Experimental Brain Research* 73:371-383.

van Bolhuis B.M., Gielen C.C.A.M. (1999) A comparison of models explaining muscle activation patterns for isometric contractions. *Biological Cybernetics* 81: 249-262.

van Zuylen E.J., Gielen C.C.A.M., Denier van der Gon J.J. (1988) Coordination and inhomogeneous activation of human arm muscles during isometric torques. *Journal of Neurophysiology* 60:1523-1548.

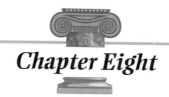

Chapter Eight

A.V. Hill and First Estimates of Maximum Muscle Performance in Humans

B.I. Prilutsky

Center for Human Movement Studies, Georgia Institute of Technology

Revisiting the work of A.V. Hill

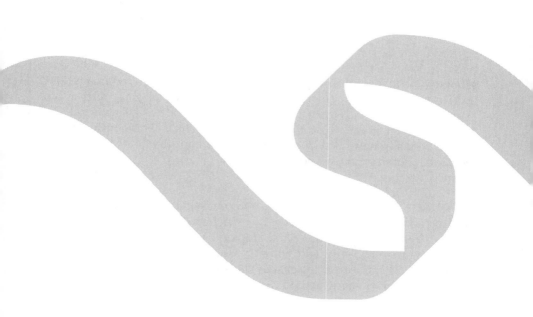

The paper that you are about to read was published by British physiologist and biophysicist Archibald Vivian Hill in 1922. This was one of the first papers in which the relationship among muscle force, work, efficiency, and velocity was studied in humans. Today the topic of this paper sounds as modern as it did almost 80 years ago. In fact, the questions the paper deals with ("How much work do muscles do in vivo?" "What is efficiency of human muscles in natural movements?" and "What are force-velocity relationships for specific human muscles?") are far from being settled (for recent reviews of these topics, see Aleshinsky, 1986; Josephson, 1993; van Ingen Schenau et al., 1997; Zajac, 1989).

In the years preceding the publication of the paper, as well as during a number of years afterward, Hill, according to his own account (Hill, 1965), was obsessed by the false idea that an activated muscle releases elastic potential energy that can be used to do external work, and that the velocity of shortening against different loads is primarily regulated by the internal resistance due to muscle "viscosity." More than 40 years later he wrote, "The simplicity of the visco-elastic theory, and the accuracy with which it fitted many of the facts, bewitched me (and several of my colleagues) too long" (1965, p. 84). Hill's background, his teachers and colleagues, and developments in muscle physiology at the time definitely affected his research interests and biases and the choice of experimental and theoretical methods.

A.V. Hill was born in Bristol on September 26, 1886, into a family that had been in the lumber business for several generations. His father, Jonathan Hill, deserted the family when Hill was 3 years old, and Hill's mother, Ada Priscilla Rumney Hill, raised him and his younger sister Muriel alone. Hill was educated at home by his mother until at the age of 7 he was placed in a preparatory school. In 1899 the family moved to Tiverton, Devonshire, where Hill attended Blundell's School. As a student he demonstrated exceptional abilities in mathematics, joined the debating team, and participated in long-distance running races (Richman, 1995). In 1905 Hill won scholarships to Trinity College, Cambridge, where he studied mathematics. He completed a three-year course in two years, placing third in his class. Following the advice of his teacher, physiologist W.M. Fletcher (1873-1933), he began advanced studies of physiology. In 1909 he completed his examinations in natural sciences with honors and then joined the Physiological Laboratory at Cambridge.

In November 1909, J.N. Langley (1852-1925), the head of the Department of Physiology at Cambridge and director of the laboratory, proposed in a letter to Hill that he "settle down to investigate the efficiency of cut-out frog's muscle as a thermodynamic machine. . . . There is an especial problem suggested by Fletcher and Hopkins' work, as to the efficiency of the muscle working with and without oxygen" (Hill, 1965, pp. 3-4). According to Hill, this idea fitted exactly the atmosphere of the Cambridge at that time and his own inclinations and, as became clear several years later, would bring important discoveries. Hill became involved in research on the heat production in muscle contraction and stimulated nerve, and studied drug and enzyme kinetics. He received a fellowship from Trinity College and spent the winter of 1910-1911 in Germany learning from several researchers including K. Burker (1872-1957) and F. Paschen (1867-1947) about myothermic equipment and observations. For the next three and a half years until the outbreak of World War I in 1914, he used a galvanometer bought from Paschen for his heat production measurements. In 1913 Hill married Margaret Neville Keynes, who was a social worker. They would have two sons, David and Maurice, and two daughters, Mary and Janet.

During the war Hill served as captain and brevet-major, and also as director of the Anti-Aircraft Experimental Section, Munitions Investigations Department (Nobel Lectures, 1999). For his service during the war he was knighted in 1918. In the same year he was elected into the Royal Society. He returned to his studies of muscle physiology in 1919 and started a cooperative effort with German physiologist O.F. Meyerhof (1884-1951) from Kiel. The two scientists studied the problem of muscle contraction independently using different methods. Hill analyzed heat production dynamics during muscle contraction, while Meyerhof employed chemical methods to investigate the oxygen consumption and the conversion of carbohydrates and lactic acid in the muscle (Johansson, 1922). In 1920 Hill was appointed Brackenburg Professor of Physiology at Manchester University. There he expanded his studies on muscle physiology and carried out first studies on muscular exercise in humans. These studies led to the introduction of the terms "oxygen debt" and the "steady state of exercise" (Hill and Lupton, 1922; Hill et al., 1924b) widely used in modern exercise physiology. The 1922 work included in this book was done during this period. In 1922 Hill and Meyerhof shared the Nobel Prize in physiology or medicine for their discoveries relating to the production of heat and the relationship between the consumption of oxygen and the metabolism of lactic acid in the muscle.

From 1923 to 1925, Hill was a Jodrell Professor of Physiology at University College, London. In 1926 he became the Royal Society's Foulerton Research Professor and directed the biophysics laboratory at University College. During the period from 1940 to 1945, he served as a member of Parliament representing Cambridge University. In the same period he served on a number of commissions dealing with issues related to World War II. In particular, he was a member of the War Cabinet Scientific Advisory Committee and participated in establishing the Academic Assistance Council to help refugee scientists (Katch, 1997). After World War II Hill returned to his research at age 59 and continued experimental work long after his retirement in December 1951. During this period he published many influential works, including three books (Hill, 1960, 1965, 1970). Sir Archibald Vivian Hill died on June 3, 1977.

In his 1922 paper, Hill measured work done by human subjects in maximum elbow flexion at different speeds. On the basis of obtained measurements he estimated the maximum work and efficiency of human muscles and the shortening speed at which the efficiency is maximal. At the time preceding the publication, Hill used thermodynamic methods to explain heat produced by the isolated muscle and the role of lactic acid and oxygen in muscle contraction. It seems natural for him to have expanded his research from measurements of heat produced by the muscle to analysis of muscle work and efficiency.

Interpreting the relation between heat production and the duration of stimulus in one of his early works, Hill concluded that muscle contraction results from elastic potential energy produced in the muscle from chemical energy (Hill, 1911). The fact that the estimated hypothetical elastic energy in a short contraction was approximately equal to the heat produced by the muscle convinced Hill of the correctness of the idea (Hill, 1913). Interestingly, long before W.O. Fenn (1923, 1924) challenged Hill's idea, Heidenhain in 1864 correctly concluded on the basis of his measurements that processes underlying shortening of the active muscle are different from those in a stretched rubber band (cited in Hill, 1965, p. 9). Hill thought that the maximum external work a muscle can do was equal to the potential elastic energy produced in the muscle, or to the product Tl (where T is the maximal muscle force developed in isometric conditions at the muscle length l). The facts that the amount of external work obtained from the muscle by letting it shorten was much smaller than Tl, and that the measured external work was inversely proportional to the average speed of muscle shortening, led Hill to suggest that muscle internal resistance due to viscosity was responsible for dissipating part of the elastic energy produced in the muscle. The theory of muscle viscosity allowed Hill to predict mechanical efficiency of the muscle and average speed of contraction at which the efficiency is maximal. In several subsequent studies, Hill and his colleagues verified the predictions of the viscosity theory in human subjects (Lupton, 1922, 1923; Hill et al., 1924a; Dickinson, 1928; and others).

A good correspondence between predictions of a theory and many experimental facts does not, of course, guarantee that the theory is correct since there may exist other theories with similar predictions. Several facts did not fit the viscosity theory. For example, Fenn (1923, 1924) demonstrated that the heat produced by the contracting muscle does not depend on shortening velocity and that the liberated energy during muscle shortening (lengthening) is higher (lower) than during isometric development of force. Fenn's conclusion from these and later works (Fenn and Marsh, 1935) was that the liberation of energy from the muscle and the decrease in force with increasing shortening speed are governed by chemical rather than mechanical (viscous) factors. In his famous 1938 paper, Hill confirmed Fenn's results and rejected the viscosity theory.

In Hill's 1922 study the inertia wheel was employed for the first time, allowing the subject to do nearly maximum work at a given speed of movement. This instrument was designed and made by Hill's technician, A.C. Downing. The idea of the apparatus was so good that it has been used for many years in research and student practical courses (Hill, 1965, p. 86). As an undergraduate student in the 1970s and later as a lecturer in the Department of Biomechanics of Central Institute of Physical Culture in Moscow, Russia, I myself worked with a similar device.

Another important contribution of Hill's 1922 paper was the attempt to estimate the mechanical efficiency of human muscles. Hill showed, in particular, that the efficiency defined as the ratio of work done to the total amount of liberated energy *(W/H)* has its optimum at a certain speed. This fact was confirmed later in many more-accurate experiments (see, for example, Woledge et al., 1985). Hill realized that a fundamental difficulty existed in determining the mechanical efficiency of human natural movements such as level walking at a constant speed. In such movements the net sum of positive and negative work done, or the net external work, is negligibly small (1927, p. 22). Hill avoided this difficulty in his 1922 paper, however, by studying a movement in which only positive work was done. The problem of mechanical efficiency in natural movements (in particular, those including the stretch-shortening cycle) is still unsettled and intensely debated almost 80 years later (van Ingen Schenau et al., 1997).

It would take a great deal of space to describe all of Hill's important contributions to muscle physiology and movement science in general. Some of the contributions of Hill and his colleagues include the following:

1. Development of what is known as Hill's equation, which describes aggregation of the molecules of hemoglobin in the blood (Hill, 1910)

2. Discovery of the mechanisms of heat production in the muscle and explanation of the role of oxygen in the combustion of lactic acid in muscle contraction (Nobel Lectures, 1999)

3. Introduction of the terms "oxygen debt" and "steady state exercise" (Hill and Lupton, 1922)

4. Introduction of the concepts of the active state and series elastic component of the muscle (Gasser and Hill, 1924; Hill, 1949), which are important components of modern models simulating muscle behavior in vivo (Hatze, 1977; Zajac, 1989)

5. The first estimation of air resistance of a runner using runner's physical model and a wind tunnel (Hill, 1928)

6. Development of what is known as Hill's equation to describe the relation between muscle force and velocity of shortening (Hill, 1938), which is widely used today for simulation of in vivo muscle actions (Hatze, 1977; Zajac, 1989)

7. Extending the analysis of the relationship between the dimensions of animals and their performance (Hill, 1950)

Hill was against separating teaching from research (Hill, 1960, p. 49). More than 100 students who worked with Hill and whom he advised were an important part of his contribution to movement science. Hill's advice may be of interest to students today. He counseled young physicists or chemists working with him to study at least one biological subject "to soak in some biology through their skin . . . so a study of biology may make a physicist or a chemist less inclined to be too certain of the objective existence of all he sees, or thinks he sees, perhaps more humble and more liberal in the face of the mysteries of the universe" (Hill, 1960, pp. 18 and 23). On the other hand, Hill urged young physiologists and biologists to study exact sciences: "The principles of biology are as certain as those of physics, . . . and the study of the exact sciences may make a biologist less 'woolly-headed'" (pp. 17-18). Hill encouraged young students first to learn to do one thing well, and only then add other skills. Looking back at the careers of many his students, Hill noted with satisfaction that his advice had been correct. Hill taught his students to continually question what they were told. At the same time, he warned that "those who disbelieve from ignorance and meanness are as many as those who believe from stupidity and laziness" (Hill, 1960, p. 38). Who knows?—perhaps this advice encouraged Fenn (see Fenn, 1923, 1924), who was working in Hill's laboratory at the time, to challenge the theory of muscle viscosity proposed by Hill in his 1922 paper.

The Maximum Work and Mechanical Efficiency of Human Muscles, and Their Most Economical Speed

A.V. Hill, F.R.S.[1]

(From the Physiological Laboratory, Manchester.)

This paper deals (i) with experiments by which the maximum work performed by human muscles in a single voluntary contraction may be determined, and (ii) with the various factors affecting the work done in, and the mechanical efficiency of, muscular movement in man.

Previous work on the isolated muscle has made it clear (1 & 9) that in an isometric twitch the force developed (T) is a measure of the mechanical energy liberated, and that T is related to H, the total energy set free, by certain comparatively simple relations when the temperature, strength of shock, and initial length are varied (2). In a twitch there is evidence (1, p.

151) that the theoretical maximum work of a muscle (*i.e.* the potential energy set free) is some constant fraction of Tl, l being the length of the muscle; and in the case of the frog's sartorius, this fraction was found (9) to be about $1/6$.[2] The proportion existing between the mechanical energy available, and the quantity Tl, has been confirmed by Doi (5, p. 340), employing a "maximum work" device described by myself (3 & 4); Doi showed that W, the maximum work performed when a frog's sartorius is allowed to shorten, bears a constant ratio to T, the force developed when the muscle carries out all isometric contraction in response to the same shock, and under the same initial conditions. In actual practice however the maximum realisable work was much less than $Tl/6$, viz. at 15° about $0.043Tl$. The difference would seem to be due to the phenomenon described by Hartree and Hill (6) who found that when the length of a muscle is altered passively a considerable quantity of heat is evolved, which is greater the more sudden the change of length; this degradation of mechanical energy they ascribed to viscous resistance to a change of form, and it is obvious that any agency which degrades mechanical energy into heat when a muscle changes its form passively must work equally when the change of form is caused by the activity of the muscle itself.[3] The response therefore of a frog's muscle to a single shock is so rapid that only about $1/4$ of the total mechanical energy set free, at 15° C, can be realised experimentally as work; the remaining $3/4$ is degraded into heat, owing to the viscous resistance of the muscle to a rapid change of form. If the twitch could be made to last longer the change of form by which the work is obtained would not need to be so rapid, and more work would be done, provided that the viscous resistance of the muscle to change of form were not increased at the same time. A fall of temperature increases the duration of a twitch, and Doi's results at 5° give an average value of 0.051 for W/Tl, which is some 20 % greater than his average 0.043 for 15° C; the reason why the difference is not greater is presumably that a fall of temperature has simultaneously increased the viscosity of the muscle.[4] The contraction however can be, and in ordinary life is, increased in duration by another means, viz. by increasing the duration of the stimulus, and we should expect that the realisable maximum work would become a larger fraction of the theoretical maximum as the duration of the contraction is increased. This deduction has not yet been verified on isolated muscle, but the experiments described below show that it is true in the case of human muscle. In order to make the argument clearer, it is proposed to adopt the terms "realisable maximum work," and the symbol W, to mean the maximum work obtainable by any actual experimental means, from a contraction of any given duration; and the term "theoretical maximum work," and the symbol W_o, to mean the mechanical potential energy set free, *i.e.* the maximum work which would be obtained were the resistance of the muscle to rapid change of form to be abolished, or in other words $W_o = W +$ (the mechanical energy degraded in the rapid change of form).

In a single twitch there is evidence (1 & 9) that the mechanical potential energy set free, *i.e.* W_o, is a large fraction, nearly 100 % of the total initial heat-production. In the oxidative recovery process (10) about as much heat is liberated as in the combined initial processes of contraction and relaxation, a fact which has been confirmed more exactly by recent, hitherto unpublished, experiments. Thus the total energy liberated in, or as a result of, a twitch is equal approximately to $2W_o$, so that the theoretical efficiency is about 50 %. In a prolonged contraction the "initial" heat-production (1) made up of two parts, one representing and equal to W_o, the potential energy set free, the other proportional to t, the duration of the stimulus; thus in all cases we may write the total heat, $H = 2 (W_o + bt)$ where b is some constant. Thus the theoretical efficiency W_o / H has its maximum value of 50 % when $t = 0$, and diminishes continually as t is increased. The actual efficiency W/H behaves in a different manner, and passes through a maximum value as t is increased; this we shall show below.

In order to obtain the maximum work from a contracting muscle it is necessary to oppose its contraction at every stage by a force which it is only just able to overcome. The use of a smaller opposing force wastes some of the mechanical energy, of a larger opposing force stops the contraction altogether. The "isotonic" system possesses both disadvantages; at the commencement of the contraction, work is wasted because the "load" is too small, at the end the shortening cannot continue because the "load" is too great. Apart from the use of complicated cams, or of complicated electromagnetic devices, the only practicable means of securing the right-at-all-stages load would appear to be to oppose the muscle to the inertia of a mass whose "reaction" (in the Newtonian sense) would always be equal to the force applied to it by the muscle. It is not convenient experimentally to oppose the contraction of a human muscle directly by the reaction of a suspended mass, the mass required being far too large (up to half a ton or more) and incapable of variation. It is necessary therefore to employ gearing, using a smaller mass but "gearing up" its reaction to the muscle. In the case of a frog's muscle the system suggested by myself (3) and employed by Doi (5) consisted of an arm balanced on knife-edges, and carrying two balanced masses, the "reaction" being "geared up" by allowing the muscle to pull at a point on the arm much closer to the knife-edges than the balanced masses.[5] As a matter of fact, the design of this instrument was anticipated by A. Fick, who describes a similar device in a book (7) which I had never previously seen, but which has been sent to me very kindly by Professor Meyerhof of Kiel.[6] The rate at which the contraction takes place can be varied by varying the "gearing," in this case by varying the point of attachment of the muscle, or the distance of the balanced masses, in other words by varying the "equivalent mass" of the system. The "equivalent mass," which is measured by Mk^2/a^2, Mk^2 being the moment of inertia of the system about the knife-edges, and a the distance therefrom of the point of attachment of the muscle, is defined as that mass which, suspended freely and pulled directly by the muscle, would oppose the contraction by the same reaction as does the actual system considered; in other words the muscle, as regards the rate and force of its contraction, would be incapable of distinguishing between the actual system and its "equivalent mass." It is found that as the "equivalent mass" of the system is increased the work done in a twitch increases up to a certain maximum, and then decreases again; this maximum is the "realisable maximum work" W. The reason why the maximum occurs is as follows; for a small equivalent mass the shortening of the muscle is too rapid, and much of its mechanical energy is dissipated in overcoming its viscous resistance to the rapid change of form[3]; for too large an equivalent mass the shortening is too slow, and is not complete before relaxation has begun, so that some of the mechanical energy is never realised at all. Apart from the onset of relaxation there is no doubt that the work done would increase continually with the equivalent mass, until it finally attained asymptotically the theoretical maximum W_o.

In the case of human muscles it is not practicable to use a maximum work device of the kind referred to above, as it would be inconvenient and unwieldy. It was decided therefore to employ a heavy fly-wheel, shown in Fig. 1 [*figure 8.1 here*], to provide the inertia against which the muscle has to work. A string is wound round one of the pulleys, and the subject of the experiment pulls the end of the string, employing only the biceps and brachialis anticus muscles as described below, and producing rotation in the fly-wheel. The speed of rotation is measured by a hand tachometer of the type D. 31 supplied by Messrs Moul & Co. of Westminster, and the

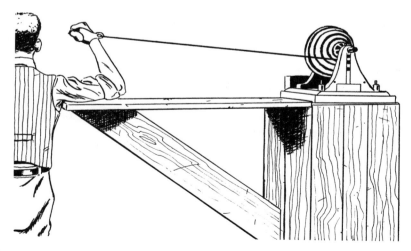

Figure 8.1
Apparatus employed.

energy developed calculated, after preliminary calibration, from the reading of the tachometer. Variation of the "equivalent mass" of the fly-wheel is obtained by winding the string round one or other of the different sized pulleys of the fly-wheel. The fly-wheel itself, with spindle, weighs about 35 kg,[7] and was made from an iron casting. The shaft on which it runs is of mild steel, and the wheel was accurately turned up between centres on its own shaft. The shaft runs in 3/4-inch[8] ball-bearings, mounted in the cast-iron standards shown in the figure. It has altogether (counting the shaft itself) eight different sizes of pulley on which to wind the string. Each pulley is provided with a short steel peg, projecting some 4 mm, over which a loop at the end of the string is dropped before it is wound round the pulley. When the string unwinds the loop drops off the peg and leaves the fly-wheel free to revolve. The effects of friction are negligible during the time required to obtain a reading with the tachometer. After each reading the fly-wheel is stopped by pressing a block of wood against it. The kinetic energy in kilogram-metres[9] corresponding to a given reading of the tachometer is obtained, and the instrument calibrated, as follows. A mass of about 16 kg is hung on a string, which is wound round one of the pulleys (preferably the smallest one) and the fly-wheel twisted till the mass has been raised through a measured height. It is then allowed to drop, the speed of the wheel so produced being measured by the tachometer. Allowance being made for the small amount of kinetic energy developed in the falling mass itself, it is then found experimentally that the work done by the mass is (as is necessary theoretically) proportional to the square of the angular velocity generated, and the constant c of this proportion enables W, the work done (in kilogram-metres[9]), to be calculated from the reading r (in revs. per min.) of the tachometer by means of the formula, $W = cr^2$. The "equivalent mass" of the fly-wheel is determined as follows. Suppose the moment of inertia about the shaft to be Mk^2, and the string to be pulling with a force F on a pulley of radius a. If ω be the angular velocity of the wheel, $Mk^2 d\omega/dt = aF$, or $(Mk^2/a^2)(ad\omega/dt) = F$. But $ad\omega/dt$ is the linear acceleration of the edge of the wheel, so that the string (and the hand of the subject) are accelerating at the same rate as they would if pulling horizontally at a large mass Mk^2/a^2 hung upon a long string. Thus Mk^2/a^2 is the "equivalent mass" of the system, and so far as the muscle is concerned the contraction is precisely similar to one taking place against the inertia of a mass Mk^2/a^2 suspended freely. By making a sufficiently small, Mk^2/a^2 can be made sufficiently large. The equivalent masses of the system employed, using the eight different pulleys, are respectively in kilograms:

$$579, \ 308, \ 189, \ 66.4, \ 35.1, \ 21.8, \ 13.55, \ 11.3.$$

This is a wide enough variation for most purposes. The value of Mk^2 is obtained from the calibration described above, and the value of (a) from the total length of string making two or three circumferences of the pulley.

It is necessary, in making experiments of this type, to ensure that only certain definite muscles are used, that no appreciable kinetic energy is developed in the limb employed, and that the experiment is reasonably simple for an untrained person to undertake. For these reasons it was decided to employ the flexion of the arm, in such a position that the biceps and brachialis anticus muscles were the only muscles involved. The subject stands upright, with his (or her) arm stretched sideways horizontally, and resting on the flat support shown in the figure, with the side of the body pressed firmly against the support, and facing straight forward. It is necessary to provide boards to raise the subject to the height required, to enable the stretched horizontal arm to rest on the support. He then grips the handle attached to the string firmly in his hand, palm upwards, and the string is wound round the pulley by the observer until the arm is just fully extended. The length of the string is so adjusted that a full contraction of the arm leaves a few centimetres of the string still on the pulley, which falls off freely as the fly-wheel continues its revolution. In this way the full tale of work may be done by the contracting muscles. A warning is given and then, at a signal, the arm is flexed, as powerfully as possible, care being taken to maintain it in the lateral vertical plane, and so to avoid the use of other and more powerful muscles, and to ensure that the elbow never rises from the support.[10] The movement should be treated as a piece of "drill," the body being held rigidly square, as at "attention," and no subsidiary movements of any kind allowed, either of the head, the trunk, or the legs. With a little practice, and by insisting on the subject following the routine, the movement is carried out with regularity and precision, successive readings on the same pulley agreeing accurately with one another. Professor J. S. B. Stopford, who has kindly advised me, agrees that when the movement is properly performed none of the work is done by muscles other than the biceps and the brachialis anticus.[11] Without precautions, of course, serious errors may result, especially if the powerful pectoral muscles be employed.

The Relation Between the Total Work Done in a Contraction, and the Equivalent Mass.

The experiments were made on a variety of different individuals, and mean curves were constructed as shown in Fig. 2 [*figure 8.2 here*]. In addition, one careful standard curve (Fig. 3 [*figure 8.3 here*]) was made on the subject shown in Fig. 1 [*figure 8.1 here*], a powerful active man of 24 in good physical condition, by means of repeated observations extending over three weeks; this curve will be used as the basis of calculation, as it is very accurate. The experiments shown in Fig. 5 [*figure 8.5 here*] were all made on the subject shown in Fig. 1 [*figure 8.1 here*]. To determine the relation between the total work and the equivalent mass, the subject, after preliminary practice, makes a series of maximal pulls, starting usually on the smallest pulley (*i.e.* on the one corresponding to the greatest equivalent mass) and proceeding step

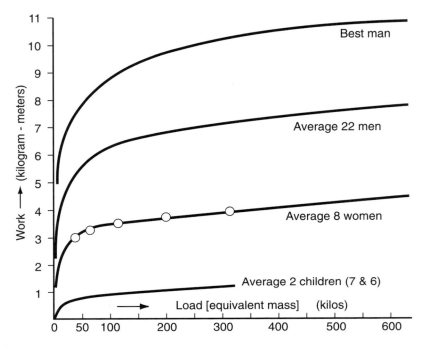

Figure 8.2
Relation between maximum work *W* and equivalent mass *M*, in various individuals.

by step to the largest (the least equivalent mass), then repeating the complete series in the reverse order. In this way two observations are obtained with each equivalent mass, and by taking the mean of these one eliminates the effects of fatigue (which are in any case small). Thus a series of readings is made relating the work done to the equivalent mass of the load, which when plotted give the curves shown in Fig. 2 [*figure 8.2 here*]. Moreover, it is obvious that the work done against zero equivalent mass must be zero, so that the origin also lies upon the curve. In this way nine points are obtained on each curve. In Fig. 2 [*figure 8.2 here*] the curves represent (i) the mean of 22 men students in this laboratory, (ii) the mean of eight women students, (iii) the strongest student, and (iv) the mean of two children aged 7 and 6 years. The curves are easy to draw, the actual means for (i) and (ii) all lying accurately upon them. From these curves we see that, in all subjects, the greater the equivalent mass the greater the work done, the work increasing rapidly at first with equivalent mass and then more slowly, but continuing to increase up to an equivalent mass of over half a ton. The explanation, as pointed out above, is probably a simple one. The more rapidly a muscle shortens, the more the potential energy developed in it on stimulation is wasted in the passive and viscous processes associated

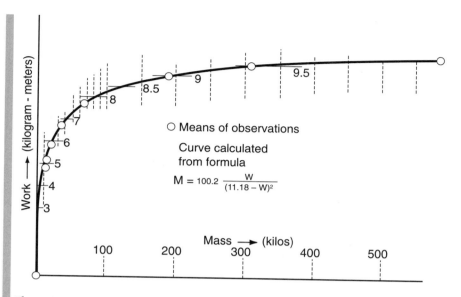

Figure 8.3
"Standard" relation between maximum work *W* and equivalent mass *M*, obtained by repeating observation on one individual.

with the change of form. Only by allowing a passively stretched muscle to shorten infinitely slowly can the full tale of potential energy be obtained from it, and what is true of the inactive muscle under a tension of external origin is almost certainly true of the active muscle under the tension of its own contraction.[3] A quantitative confirmation of this view will be given below, in connection with the standard curve of Fig. 3 [*figure 8.3 here*].

The curves shown in Fig. 2 [*figure 8.2 here*] are instructive in themselves. The strongest man in 22 was able to do some 40 % more work than the average of the remainder, and it is of interest that the three men giving the largest readings were all fast bowlers at cricket. Moreover, the average work of 22 normal young men is some 80 % greater than that of eight normal young women. The curves shown in Fig. 2 [*figure 8.2 here*] are, in a general way, similar, the curves for women and children being like those for men but on a reduced scale; for a given equivalent mass the women did about 4/7 as much work as the men, and the children 1/7 as much. The curves however are not exactly similar; if they were their final slopes would not, as in Fig. 2 [*figure 8.2 here*], be approximately the same. For a given equivalent mass the work done by the average man does not bear a constant ratio to that done by the average woman; the ratio decreases as the load is increased. The meaning of this, suggested by the theory of dimensions, is as follows. If we assume that the woman is able to impart to one kilogram exactly the same velocity as the man to two kilograms, then the men's and the women's curves become identical. We have merely changed the unit of mass, it being purely a matter of chance that the ratio is exactly two to one. Taking the men's curve, it is possible then to construct the women's curve as follows. With an equivalent mass of 50 kg a man can do just as many kilogram-metres of work, as a woman with 50 half-kg can do half-kilogram-metres of work; with 100 kg a man can do as many kilogram-metres as a woman with 100 half-kg can do half-kilogram-metres; and so on. Working with this rule the points shown with circles on the women's curve have been calculated from the men's curve. The agreement is perfect. Thus to a healthy normal individual, and for a given type of response, we may allot a "strength constant" λ, such that he can impart to any mass $M\lambda$ the same velocity as some standard individual can impart to the mass M. Expressed in terms of the average man of Fig. 2 [*figure 8.2 here*], the "strength constant" of the average woman, for this particular movement, is 0.5.

Another striking fact is the large amount of work done by the muscles. The "average man" on the smallest pulley does some 8 kilogram-metres of work.[12] By the kindness of Dr G. E. Birkett of the Manchester Royal Infirmary I have been able to obtain an estimate of the mass of the muscles involved; the biceps and brachialis anticus together of a fairly muscular man weighed about 250 g. Assuming this to be the mass of the muscles, in the case of the average man, each kg of muscle is able to do some 32 kilogram-metres[13] of work in one contraction, an amount sufficient to raise its own weight through 32 m. If the whole of this mechanical energy were degraded into heat the rise of temperature of the muscle would be about 0.076° C. Actually the rise of temperature of the muscle is much greater than this, partly because the oxidative recovery process gives another 0.076° C, partly because the energy dissipated in maintaining the contraction is considerable. The time occupied in the pull against the greatest equivalent mass is some 2.5 sec,[14] and if the heat-production of a man's muscle, exerting a maximal response at 37° C, could be extrapolated from that of a frog at lower temperatures (1, p. 138) the total rise of temperature of the human muscle should be about 2° C. This estimate is probably excessive, but the fact that the rise of temperature is large agrees with the subjective impression that considerable energy is expended by the muscles in these movements.

In a recent paper Hartree and A. V. Hill (8, p. 119) gave experiments, in which the maximum work of frog's muscles in a prolonged contraction was recorded. A pair of sartorius muscles weighing 0.33 g did 95 g·cm[15] of work in response to 0.4 s tetanus at 21° C. With a greater equivalent mass, and a more prolonged contraction, the work might conceivably have become as great as 200 g·cm[16], a quantity sufficient to raise the muscle through 6 m. This is less than 1/5 of the 32 m attained by the human muscle.

It is possible, with certain simple assumptions as to the viscous resistance of the muscle to change of form, to calculate from first principles the shape of the curve in Fig. 3 [*figure 8.3 here*]. The pressure required to drive a fluid through a capillary tube of given dimensions, is proportional to the coefficient of viscosity of the fluid and to the volume forced through per second. If we wish to increase the velocity with which the fluid flows through we must increase the pressure in the same ratio. Thus the work done in the transference of a. given amount of fluid through the capillary, which is equal to the pressure multiplied by the volume, is proportional to the velocity with which the process is carried out. The change of form of a muscle involves the flow of fluid through the protoplasmic or colloidal network and the visible structures of the cells, and a given change of form is similar, in general character, to the flow of a given amount of fluid through a set of capillary tubes. Thus the mechanical energy degraded into heat should be proportional to the rate at which the given change of form is caused. Suppose a muscle, when undertaking a maximal contraction, to possess mechanical potential energy W_o; then if the shortening be against the reaction of an almost infinitely great mass, it will be very slow, and practically the whole of the mechanical energy will be realised as work; if however the mass providing the reaction be finite, the change of form will proceed at a finite rate, and a finite proportion of the mechanical energy will be degraded into beat; only the remainder, W, say, being realised as work. Thus $(W_o - W)$ is equal to the energy dissipated in the shortening, which, from above, we should expect to be proportional to the velocity with which the shortening is carried out. Now it is shown experimentally below that the external force actually exerted by the arm in pulling a given mass may be taken as constant throughout the pull, varying however with the mass. Let P be the average force exerted on mass M, and l the length of the pull. Then $W = Pl$, and the time t occupied in the pull is given, according to the simple laws of mechanics, by the formula, $l = 1/2Pt^2/M$. Now the energy degraded, being directly proportional to the average speed of the change, is inversely proportional to t, so that $W_o - W = k/t$ where k is some constant varying as the coefficient of viscosity. Substituting $\sqrt{2lM/P}$ for t, $W_o - W = k\sqrt{(P/2lM)}$. Putting W/l for P from above, squaring and rearranging, we then find, $M = KW/(W_o - W)^2$, where K is another constant equal to $k^2/2l^2$. Suppose that $K = 100.2$ and $W_o = 11.18$. Then the equation becomes $M = 100.2W/(11.18 - W)^2$, from which the curve shown in Fig. 3 [*figure 8.3 here*] has been constructed. The actual mean observed points are shown with circles, and the agreement between calculated and observed is very good, so good as to provide strong evidence for the accuracy of the theory. We may assume therefore that we are correct in ascribing the shape of the curves of Figs. 2 and 3 [*figures 8.2 and 8.3 here*] to the viscous resistance of the muscle to a change of form, and in supposing that the function of a stimulated muscle is to develop potential energy, which is then transformed into work to a degree depending on purely physical factors.[17]

In this equation the quantity W_o has been taken as 11.18. W_o is determinable within 1 % from the observations, so that by plotting the latter and fitting a curve to them the potential energy developed can be measured. Thus in the subject employed the potential energy developed is 11.8 kilogram-metres.[18] If this be equated to $Tl/6$, and if l be put equal to 0.15 m, we find $T = 450$ kg—about half a ton.[19] It is difficult to realise the enormous force developed by comparatively small muscles. The quantity K is proportional to the square of the coefficient of viscosity of the fluids in the muscle, and inversely proportional to the square of the muscle's length. In a given subject, K can change only as the result of a change in the coefficient of viscosity of the muscle fluids, and it would be interesting to see how far alterations of K can be associated with alterations of bodily condition, or with treatment such as massage. Other things being equal, the muscle wasting less of its energy in the rapid change of form will carry out its movements with greater power and speed.

Assuming that the force exerted on the wheel by the arm of the subject is constant throughout any given contraction, an assumption shown to be true with sufficient accuracy by the curves of Fig. 5 [*figure 8.5 here*], the time taken in the shortening can be calculated from the relations given above, viz. $W = Pl$ and $l = 1/2t^2P/M$. These give $t = l\sqrt{2M/W}$. In the subject employed in the observations of Fig. 3 [*figure 8.3 here*], l was about 60 cm. Thus $t = 85\sqrt{M/W}$. In this formula it is necessary to express M and W in absolute C.G.S.[20] units, so that if M be expressed in kilograms and W in kilogram-metres it is necessary to multiply M by 1000, and W by $981 \cdot 10^5$. Thus the time of the shortening is given in seconds by $t = 85\sqrt{M/98100W} = 0.27\sqrt{M/W}$. From this formula we may calculate the time occupied in any of the contractions recorded by circles in Fig. 3 [*figure 8.3 here*]; and in Fig. 4 [*figure 8.4 here*] W, the work actually done in a contraction, is plotted against t its duration. W increases with t, attaining the theoretical value W_o asymptotically as t is increased. The energy wasted in overcoming viscous resistance is given, as shown above, by the formula, $W_o - W = k/t$. Thus

$$W = W_o - k/t.$$

Here W_o and k are the same quantities as are referred to above. W_o has been found to be 11.18 kilogram-metres, or in absolute units $11.18 \cdot 10^5 \cdot 981$ erg; K, which is equal to $k^2/2l^2$, was found to be 100.2, or in absolute units 110.2 $\cdot 10^8 \cdot 981$. From this k may be calculated, and found to be $2.66 \cdot 10^8$ absolute units. If we employ kilogram-metres as units we must divide by $981 \cdot 10^5$, which gives a value of k of 2.71; the curve in Fig. 4 [*figure 8.4 here*] is constructed with $W_o = 11.18$ and $k = 2.70$, *i.e.* from the equation $W = 11.18 - 2.7/t$. There is practically perfect agreement between calculated and observed. The curve, of course, is little but another manner of expressing the facts of Fig. 3 [*figure 8.3 here*], so that we should expect to find the same good agreement as we found there. The result however in Fig. 4 [*figure 8.4 here*] is put in a more directly useful and intelligible form, and we shall use

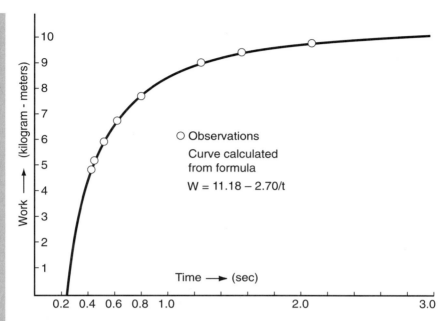

Figure 8.4
Relation between maximum work W and duration of contraction t, plotted from the same data as figure 8.3.

the expression for W as a function of t in the discussion of the mechanical efficiency given below.

It should be noted, of course, that the constants in the equation $W = 11.18 - 2.7/t$ are not absolute constants, but depend upon the size, shape, character and condition of the muscle. Writing the equation more generally as $W = W_0 - k/t$, W_0 will vary in direct proportion to the mass of the muscle employed, and will increase with training and decrease with fatigue; while k also will vary in direct proportion to the mass of the muscle, but will depend upon the viscosity of the muscle fluids, and upon the channels which they follow when the shape of the muscle is changed.[3]

The following rough calculation shows that viscous resistance to a change of form is quite large enough to cause a very considerable dissipation of energy. Poiseuille's formula for flow in a capillary tube is $\mu = \pi p r^4 t / 8 l V$, where μ is the coefficient of viscosity, p is the pressure difference, r is the radius, l the length, and V the volume of fluid forced through in time t. The work done being pV may he put equal to $8 l V^2 \mu / \pi r^4 t$; this may be equated, in absolute units, to k/t where k is the quantity used above, so that $8 l V^2 \mu / \pi r^4 = 2.66 \cdot 10^8$. We will assume, in order to obtain some idea of the dimensions of the network through which fluid is forced when the muscle shortens, that the viscosity of the fluid is the same as that of serum, and that one-third of the whole volume of the fluid in the muscle, say 100 cm³, is involved in the flow. We will assume also that $l = r$, *i.e.* that the length of each capillary is equal to its radius; this simplification is introduced to allow roughly for the fact that the set of capillaries considered is really an indefinite network of membranes. We then have

$$r^2 = 8 \, (100)^2 \, \mu/3.14 \cdot 2.66 \cdot 10^8 = 9.6 \cdot 10^{-5} \, \mu.$$

Holker (12) has given values for the viscosity of normal serum relative to water at 25° C. This appears to be about 1.6. Assuming it to be the same relative to water at 37° C, its absolute value is about 0.01. Putting $\mu=0.01$ we then find $r = 0.01$ cm $= 0.1$ mm approximately. Thus the flow of only 1/3 of the volume of fluid in the muscle, through a network as large as 0.1 mm, would provide a wastage of energy, through viscosity, sufficient to account for that actually observed. The wonder is not that viscosity can dissipate so much energy, but that it actually wastes so little.

It should be noted that no error of serious importance is introduced into the experiments recorded here by neglecting the kinetic energy developed in the forearm of the subject. Even in the case of the smallest equivalent mass used, the velocity of the hand does not exceed, at the end of the contraction, (say) 300 cm per s, so that the kinetic energy of a forearm, of mass (say) 1.5 kg, and supposed (for the sake of calculation)[21] to be of uniform section, does not exceed $1/6 \cdot 1500 \cdot 300^2$ erg. This is equal, approximately to 0.23 kilogram-metres and is an extreme value, introducing in the worst case an error of not more than 5 or 6 % in the observed result. In the case of the slower movements associated with the higher values of the equivalent mass, the kinetic energy developed in the subject's forearm is quite negligible. Had observations been made at still smaller values of the equivalent mass (say 5 kg or less) the kinetic energy produced in the forearm would have become an appreciable fraction of the whole kinetic energy obtained, and a correction would have been necessary. Over the range considered however the kinetic energy produced in the fly-wheel may be regarded as the only external mechanical effect of the potential energy developed by the muscle.

When employing a very small equivalent mass (say one kg or less) the kinetic energy of the forearm becomes a large fraction of the whole mechanical energy set free. In the case of ordinary voluntary maximal muscular movements, carried out against the reactions of small masses, this loss of energy is to some degree avoided (as in throwing a cricket ball) by the use of a jerk, by means of which the kinetic energy of the moving limb is concentrated at the critical moment in the part immediately in contact with the object. Success in any form of sport or athletics involving rapid movement must depend upon the development of nervous and muscular co-ordination enabling such concentrations of kinetic energy to be produced inexpensively at the right time and place.

The Relation Between the Work Done and the Time in a Single Contraction.

To determine this relation it was necessary to make all instantaneous and continuous record of the velocity of the fly-wheel throughout a contraction. The first method tried was to connect to the fly-wheel by a belt a small dynamo, and to record on a string galvanometer the current produced by the dynamo. Had a suitable instrument been available, this method would doubtless have proved satisfactory. In lack however of a good small dynamo another method was used. A circular ebonite ring mounted on a brass bush was furnished with eight brass pins driven into radial holes uniformly spaced in the ebonite, and making electrical contact with the bush. The pins were cut off flush with the circumference of the ring, the bush was then driven on to the spindle of the fly-wheel, which was mounted between centres and the ebonite ring with the brass pins in it turned accurately in a lathe. A phosphor-bronze spring, with a sharp V-shaped contact, rubbed upon the circumference of the ebonite ring, and another similar spring upon the spindle of the wheel. Each time that the surface of one of the eight pins came in contact with the V-shaped portion of the first spring an electrical connection was established between the two springs, and by introducing a battery and an electromagnet into the circuit it was possible to record accurately on a drum the moment at which each pin passed under the V. The electromagnet was of the small light type made by the Harvard Apparatus Co., and was capable of carrying out well over 100 complete movements per second; this is more than twice the number required in any actual experiment. The magnet was caused to write upon a rapidly moving drum revolving at a determined speed, so that the times between successive 1/8's of a complete revolution of the wheel could be read off on the record. The initial position of the V-contact (as a fraction of the interval between two pins) was noted, so that after measurement the relation between the angle through which the wheel had revolved and the time could be plotted. From the curve so obtained it is possible to calculate the angular velocity, and therefore the kinetic energy of the wheel, and to express it as a function either (a) of the time, or (b) of the distance through which the string pulled by the subject has moved. The former does not appear to be of much interest, and the results have been expressed as shown in Fig. 5 [*figure 8.5 here*], in terms of the relation between work done and distance pulled. It is seen that in all cases the work done increases, not exactly but more or less uniformly with the distance, showing that the force exerted on the wheel is approximately constant throughout a given pull, until the limit of the contraction is reached. The pull of an isolated muscle falls off rapidly as the muscle shortens, and the relative constancy of the force exerted by a man's arm is due to the increasing mechanical advantage of the lever system as the contraction proceeds. Since work is equal to the product of force and distance, the slope of the curves of Fig. 5 [*figure 8.5 here*] gives the external force exerted by the arm at any particular degree of contraction; the slope of any curve does decrease somewhat as the shortening proceeds, and this falling off is no doubt due to the more rapid movement at the end than at the beginning of the process, more of the total available force being required in the later stages to overcome the intrinsic resistance of the muscle itself to its more rapid change of form. The same fact is brought out by the different curves; at any given degree of shortening the slope of the curve for the greater mass is steeper than that for the smaller mass—showing that at every stage of contraction the force exerted is greater the less the rate of movement, and *vice versa*.[22] The curves of Fig. 5 [*figure 8.5 here*] can be used for the calculation, by the simple rules of mechanics, of other factors in muscular contraction; it is unnecessary however to give such further calculation here.

It has been shown above that the slower the contraction the greater the work done. This does not mean however that the slower the contraction the more efficiently it is carried out, using the word "efficiency" as denoting mechanical efficiency, the ratio of work done to energy degraded in doing it. The more prolonged contraction necessarily involves a greater degradation of energy in the *physiological* processes necessary to maintain the contraction, and this factor rapidly neutralises the advantage of obtaining more work from the more prolonged contraction. The relation established, for maximal isometric contractions, between the total heat-production H and the duration of the stimulus t, may be written as shown above,

$$H = 2(W_o + bt),$$

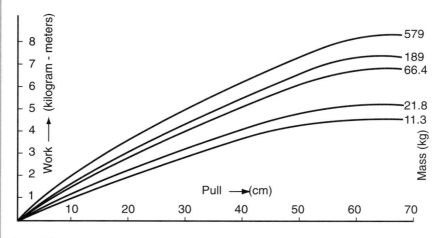

Figure 8.5
Relation between work done and distance pulled in a single contraction; various loads.

where b is some constant. It is clearly impossible to determine b by the direct thermoelectric method employed with the sartorius of the frog; it might however be possible to obtain an approximate estimate of it by experiments on the oxygen consumption of a man sustaining a maximal isometric effort. In the case of the experiments shown in Figs. 3 and 4 [*figures 8.3 and 8.4 here*], $W_o = 11.18$ kilogram-metres; b is not known, but for the sake of calculation it has been assumed to be 5 in the following calculation. There is strong indirect evidence given below that this value is not far wrong; in any case the chief points in the argument are independent of the actual value of b, it being necessary to allot a number only for the sake of drawing an actual curve (Fig. 5 [*figure 8.5 here*]).

The work done also increases with the duration of the stimulus, following the equation $W = W_o - k/t$. Here $W_o = 11.18$ and $k = 2.7$. The mechanical efficiency therefore is

$$E = W/H = (W_o - k/t) / 2 (W_o + bt).$$

One conclusion can be drawn at once from this experiment: the efficiency E passes through a definite maximum value as the duration of the contraction is increased. The numerator $(W_o - k/t)$ increases at a decreasing rate, starting from zero when $t = k/W_o$, and finally attains a value W_o. The denominator increases indefinitely at a constant rate from the finite value $2W_o$. Thus E starts at 0 and finishes at 0, as t increases, and must therefore pass through a maximum value. This maximum value of the efficiency corresponds to the most economical speed of working, the size of the pulley determining what we may call the "optimum gear-ratio." Putting $W_o = 11.18$, $k = 2.7$, $b = 5$, the mechanical efficiency E may be calculated and plotted, as in Fig. 6 [*figure 8.6 here*]. It is seen that the efficiency starts from zero (at a time equal to that occupied in the flexion of the unloaded arm), rises rapidly to a maximum of about 26 % and then slowly falls again, as the duration of the contraction is increased. The actual height and position of this maximum depend upon the value of b, all the other constants being known. This maximum can be shown mathematically to occur at a time given by

$$t = k/W_o [1 + \sqrt{1 + W_o^2/kb}]$$

and for different values of b these "optimum times," and the corresponding maximum efficiencies, are as shown below.

Table 8.1

b	0	1	2	3	4	5	6	7	8	10	12
Optimum t	∞	1.91	1.43	1.22	1.10	1.02	0.95	0.90	0.87	0.81	0.77
Maximum E	0.5	0.374	0.330	0.303	0.281	0.263	0.248	0.234	0.223	0.204	0.188

There is evidence from the work of Douglas (11) that the mechanical efficiency of human muscular movement may rise to 25 or 26 %. Benedict and Cathcart (13), in observations controlled by no-load experiments with a motor-driven ergometer, found that the *average* efficiency in all experiments was not far from 27 %, but they state that owing to extraneous muscular movements in the control experiments this value is probably too high. They obtained still higher values for the efficiency by taking as a "base-line" an experiment with a lower rate of work, but in view of the conclusions reached below as to the lower efficiency of a submaximal effort these values would seem to be unreliable and we are probably justified in assuming that the maximum efficiency of human muscular movement lies round about 25 %. It is striking that Benedict and Cathcart expressly emphasize that the efficiency decreases with a high rate of pedalling. This entirely agrees with the deduction given above, and with the curve of Fig. 6 [*figure 8.6 here*].

Assuming that 25 to 26 % is the maximum mechanical efficiency attainable we are able, from the above table, to make an approximate estimate of the quantity b in the expression for the heat produced. This would seem to be about 5.5, in the movement and with the subject investigated here, in which case the curve of Fig. 6 [*figure 8.6 here*] is approximately the correct one. The time occupied in the most efficient contraction, *i.e.* the "optimum time," would be about 1 sec. Benedict and

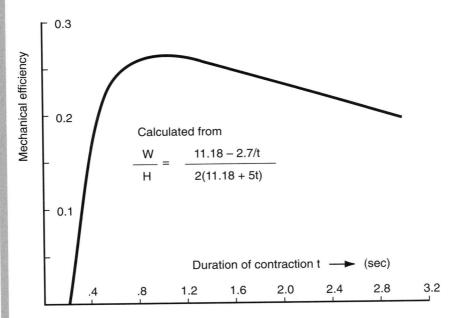

Figure 8.6
Calculated relation between mechanical efficiency and duration of contraction.

Cathcart found the maximum efficiency of a subject pedalling a bicycle ergometer to occur at about 70 revolutions per min, *i.e.* each contraction occupied just under 1 sec. This is in striking agreement with the deduction given above and confirms the general validity of the theory. Assuming the value of b to be about 5.5, the equation for the total energy set free in a maximal effort becomes approximately $22.36(1+1/2t)$. This depends upon the mass of the muscles involved, and upon their condition and training, but—for a given condition and degree of training—we may assume that the same relation holds for other muscles, in the form

$$H = 2W_o (1 + 1/2t).$$

Moreover the work done in a maximal effort, $W = 11.18 - 2.7/t$, also depends upon the mass of muscles and upon their condition and training, and again—for a given condition and degree of training—this may be written, for any muscle,

$$W = W_o(1 - 0.24/t).$$

Thus the efficiency of any maximal muscular movement may be expressed approximately by the relation

$$E = W/H = (1 - 0.24/t)/(2 + t).$$

This relation between E and t is very nearly the same as that shown in Fig. 6 [*figure 8.6 here*].

The rapid rise and the slow fall of the curve relating E to t is of fundamental interest. It shows (i) that by *decreasing* comparatively slightly the time occupied in a muscular movement a serious loss of efficiency may be caused, but (ii) that a comparatively large *increase* in the time may cause only a small loss of efficiency. Moreover the maximum is shown to be a very "blunt" one; over a wide range of speeds the efficiency remains more or less constant. This is doubtless the reason why all observers working on the mechanical efficiency of the body have obtained values round about 20 % to 26 %; their subjects have instinctively worked within the wide limits giving something near the maximum efficiency.

Hitherto we have dealt entirely with maximal muscular efforts. A submaximal effort is probably nothing but a maximal effort of some of the muscle fibres, the inactive fibres having their form changed passively by the activity of their neighbors. Thus the potential energy set free, or the maximum theoretical work, is proportional to the fraction n of the fibres taking part in the contraction, and may be called nW_o. The heat-production also, $2(W_o + bt)$, is reduced in the same ratio, and becomes $2n(W_o + bt)$. The energy wasted however in the change of form has not been altered by the submaximal nature of the effort, since the change of form has been the same, and has (we assume) occupied the same time. We may write the energy wasted therefore as k/t, as before. The mechanical efficiency then becomes,

$$E = (nW_o - k/t)/2n(W_o + bt) = (W_o - k/nt)/2(W_o + bt).$$

This is always less than the quantity $(W_o - k/t)/2(W_o + bt)$ since n is less than 1, and for weak efforts may become very considerably less. Thus a submaximal effort is always less efficient than a maximal effort occupying the same time, and, in general, the weaker effort is the less efficient.[23] Moreover, the formula for the "optimum time,"

$$t = k/W_o [1 + \sqrt{1 + W_o^2/kb}]$$

clearly shows that if k is increased to k/n, as in the submaximal effort, the optimum time is increased. The highest efficiency of a submaximal effort is obtained in a slower contraction than that of a maximal effort.

These facts are of importance in relation to methods of observing the mechanical efficiency in man. In such observations, in order to eliminate the error in the heat-production introduced by the basal metabolism B, the work done W, and the heat-production H (calculated from respiratory measurements), have been measured at two different levels of the power exerted, the efficiency being calculated then from the formula, $E = (W_1 - W_2)/(H_1 - H_2)$. It has been assumed that in this way the constant "basal" heat-production B has been eliminated by subtraction. This might be correct. The assumption however has been made implicitly that the efficiency of the less powerful effort, viz. $E_2 = W_2/(H_2 - B)$, is the same as that of the more powerful effort, viz. $E_1 = W_1/(H_1 - B)$. Only if this assumption be made do both E_1 and E_2 become equal to $(W_1 - W_2)/(H_1 - H_2)$. Now we have shown that the efficiency of a weaker effort is necessarily less than that of a stronger effort, so that E_2 *is* less than E_1. Hence the efficiency determined in this manner is liable to a serious error, and results obtained by it must be discarded. It can be shown moreover that efficiencies thus measured will be too high, and it is striking in Benedict and Cathcart's paper that the highest values (up to nearly 50 %) were so determined. The most reliable method would appear to be another they adopted, viz. the use of a "base line" in which the ergometer is driven artificially, by a motor, at the same speed as in the actual working experiment.[24]

All these facts have their importance in ordinary and industrial life. It is not contended that the purely muscular factor discussed here is the only important, or the most important, of the many factors which determine the optimum conditions of work: it is one factor however, and the simplest one, and a scientific study of it may at any rate help us to understand the optimum conditions and so to apply them in our ordinary life.

The results obtained here have a possible application to heart muscle. It is shown that the more slowly a muscle contracts the more of its potential energy W_o is liberated as work W. In a heart, the beat corresponds to a single twitch of a skeletal muscle, and it would seem likely that no more energy is used up in a long beat than in a short one; hence if the theoretical maximum efficiency W_o/H be constant, the realisable efficiency W/H is greater in a slow beat than in a rapid one, and this may be one reason for the fact that athletic individuals tend to show a very slow beat. It should be possible to investigate the matter on the isolated heart, either by purely mechanical experiments on a dead heart or by observations on a surviving one.

My sincere thanks are due to Mr A. C. Downing of this laboratory, who not only constructed the special instruments employed, but was responsible for their detailed design, and assisted me continually in the observations recorded here.

Summary

(1) An instrument is described by means of which the maximum work of human muscles (biceps and brachialis anticus) can be determined. This instrument employs the inertial reaction of a fly-wheel to take up the pull of the muscle, the work done being calculated from the speed of revolution of the fly-wheel, as measured by a hand tachometer of standard pattern.

(2) Experiments are given relating the maximal work W in a maximal contraction to the "equivalent mass" M of the load. As M increases W increases also, at first rapidly and then more slowly, tending to reach a definite final value W_o, equal to the potential energy set free. It is shown experimentally that M and W are connected by the relation $M = KW/(W_o - W)^2$ where K is a constant.

(3) In a maximal effort the duration of the shortening may be changed by changing the load. The greater the duration t the greater will be the work done W. It is shown experimentally that W and t are connected by the relation $W = W_o - k/t$, where k is a constant. In this equation t is not less than the time occupied in a maximal contraction without load.

(4) These facts and relations can be deduced quantitatively from the hypothesis that a muscle, when stimulated, produces potential energy W_o, which in any actual contraction is employed partly in doing external work W and partly in overcoming the viscous resistance of the muscle to its change of form. The energy dissipated $(W_o - W)$ in overcoming viscous resistance to a given change of form should be proportional to the speed $(1/t)$ with which the change is carried out, and to the coefficient of viscosity (k) of the muscle fluids. This hypothesis leads to the preceding mathematical relations, and is in keeping with what is known as to the "thermo-elastic" properties of muscle.

(5) An instrument is described enabling a continuous record to be deduced of the relation between the work done and the distance pulled,

in the course of a single contraction. Curves are given showing this relation for a variety of loads.

(6) The mechanical efficiency of human voluntary movement is discussed. It is shown that the total energy H set free in a maximal contraction of duration t is given approximately by the relation $H = 2W_o(1 + bt)$, where W_o has the same meaning as before, and b has a value about equal to $1/2$. From this the mechanical efficiency W/H may be calculated as a function of the duration of the contraction, and it is shown that there is a certain optimum speed of movement below which the efficiency falls slowly, and above which it falls rapidly.

(7) The mechanical efficiency of a submaximal effort is always less than that of a maximal effort occupying the same time, and in general the stronger effort is the more efficient. Moreover the stronger effort has the greater optimum speed.

(8) The bearing of these conclusions upon results obtained by the use of a bicycle ergometer, as well as upon human muscular movement in general, is discussed.

The expenses of this research have been borne in part by a grant from the Governments Grants Committee of the Royal Society.

References

(1) Hartree and A. V. Hill. This Journal, 55, p. 151. 1921.
(2) Hartree and A. V. Hill. Ibid. p. 389. 1921.
(3) A. V. Hill. Proc. Physiol. Soc. This Journal, 53, p. lxxxviii. 1920.
(4) A. V. Hill. Ibid. p. xc.
(5) Doi. This Journal, 54, p. 335. 1921.
(6) Hartree and A. V. Hill. Phil. Trans. B. 210, p. 153. 1920.
(7) A. Fick. Mechan. Arbeit. u. Wärmeentwickelung b. d. Muskelthätigkeit. Leipzig. p. 63. 1882.
(8) Hartree and A. V. Hill. This Journal, 54, p. 84. 1920.
(9) A. V. Hill. Ibid. 46, p. 453. 1913.
(10) A.V. Hill. Ibid. 46, p. 28. 1913.
(11) Campell, Douglas and Hobson. Phil. Trans. B. 210, p. 122. 1920.
(12) Holker. Journ. of Path. and Bact. 24, p. 416. 1921.
(13) Benedict and Cathcart. "Muscular Work." Publication No. 187, Carnegie Institute of Washington. 1913.

Addendum

It may be objected that the diminution of work with increased rate of shortening is due, at least in part, to the fact that with a small equivalent mass, an appreciable amount of the shortening has occurred before the full force of the contraction has had time to develop. This is not so. Experiments, which will be described in a later paper, have been made on the rate of development of an isometric contraction in the biceps and brachialis anticus muscles of the subject of the observations described above. These experiments have shown that the development of the contraction is so rapid that, even in an extreme case, not more than 0.5 % of the total work is lost by this cause, while in the more prolonged contractions, the loss is entirely negligible. The loss is due to the actual process of shortening, not to the fact that the shortening occurs before the maximum force has been developed.

Acknowledgment

The preparation of the introduction and "Endnotes" was supported in part by a grant to the Center for Human Movement Studies (Director Dr. Robert J. Gregor) from the Office of Interdisciplinary Programs at Georgia Institute of Technology.

Endnotes

[1] F.R.S. stands for Fellow of the Royal Society. A.V. Hill was elected a Fellow of the Royal Society in 1918, served as secretary from 1935 to 1945, and served as foreign secretary in 1946 (Nobel Lectures, 1999).

[2] The theoretical maximum work of a muscle must be smaller than Tl because (i) muscle cannot shorten to zero length; (ii) at given stimulation and muscle length, force developed during shortening is smaller than during isometric force development (this fact was not clearly recognized at the time of publication of the paper; Hill, 1970, p. 23); and (iii) if $l < l_o$ (l_o is muscle length at which T is maximum), T should decrease with muscle shortening according to the force-length relationship (Blix, 1894).

[3] Here Hill refers to muscle viscosity, which at the time was thought to be the dominant regulator of the speed of shortening against different loads. Later experiments by Fenn (1923, 1924) and Hill himself (1938) led to the rejection of the viscosity hypothesis (for reviews, see Hill, 1965; Zatsiorsky, 1997).

[4] The present explanation is that changes in muscle temperature affect the rate of chemical reactions associated with cross-bridge dynamics (Woledge et al., 1985).

[5] A good drawing of this device can be found in Gasser and Hill, 1924.

[6] Otto Fritz Meyerhof shared the 1922 Nobel Prize in physiology or medicine with Hill (see "Introduction"). Meyerhof was born in Hanover, Germany, on April 12, 1884. He studied medicine and graduated in 1909. He became interested in psychology and philosophy and, later on, physiology and physical chemistry. He was head of the Department of Physiology in the Institute for Medical Research in Heidelberg from 1929 to 1938. He worked at the Institut de Biologie Physico-Chimique in Paris (1938-1940) and then at the University of Pennsylvania in the United States. Professor Meyerhof died on October 6, 1951 (Nobel Lectures, 1999).

[7] Or 343 N.

[8] Or 19 mm.

[9] 1 kilogram-meter = 9.81 J.

[10] It appears that the upper arm could slide away from the flywheel and thus contribute to unrealistically large values of work obtained in these experiments (see endnote 13).

[11] It is unlikely that other muscles crossing the elbow joints were not involved in the elbow flexion task (see, for example, Flanders and Soechting, 1990).

[12] Or 78.5 J.

[13] Or 314 J. This amount of work exceeds approximately four times the theoretical maximum work that 1 kg of vertebrate skeletal muscles can do. This theoretical maximum work can be estimated (see, for example, Alexander, 1992) from known maximum muscle stress ($3 \cdot 10^5$ N m^{-2}), maximum muscle shortening (25%), and muscle density (1060 kg m^{-3}):

$$3 \cdot 10^5 \cdot 0.25 / 1060 = 71 \text{ J kg}^{-1}.$$

This discrepancy might have been caused by underestimation of muscle mass involved in the tested task (see also endnote 10).

[14] This time period yields power of $314/2.5 = 126$ W kg^{-1}. This power is within the range of power output obtained from skeletal muscles using the work loop technique (Josephson, 1993) and using in vivo measurements of muscle force and fiber length changes during flight in pigeons (Biewener et al., 1998a) and during steady-speed hopping in the tammar wallaby (Biewener et al., 1998b).

[15] Or 9.3 mJ.

[16] Or 19.6 mJ. This amount of work done by a muscle weighing 0.33 g yields a mass-specific work of 59 J kg^{-1}, which is consistent with the estimated maximum value (see endnote 13).

[17] In 1965 (p. 93), commenting on his 1922 paper and several others that followed, Hill wrote, "The results were rather exact, but their interpretation in terms of muscle 'viscosity' was realized by 1938 to be unsatisfactory." See also endnote 3.

[18] Or 116 J.

[19] Or 4415 N. This value appears to be largely overestimated. Given that the upper limit of the cross-sectional area of major elbow flexors (biceps brachii [two heads], brachialis, and brachioradialis) is $17 \cdot 10^{-4} m^2$ (estimated from Yamaguchi et al., 1990), the corresponding muscle stress is $4414/ (17 \cdot 10^{-4}) = 26 \cdot 10^5$ N m^{-2}, or approximately 8.5 times larger than the value typically assumed for vertebrate skeletal muscles (see endnote 13).

[20] C.G.S. stands for centimeter-gram-second system.

[21] The K.E. of a uniformly rotating arm of mass M, the end of which is moving with velocity v, is $1/6Mv^2$. (This is Hill's footnote.)

[22] This fact was confirmed later (Dickinson, 1928; Fenn and Marsh, 1935; Hill, 1938 and others) and now is known as the force-velocity relation.

[23] Today it can be considered proven that stronger voluntary efforts of heterogeneous muscles involve a relatively larger number of fast-twitch motor units than weaker efforts (size principle; Henneman et al., 1965). Since muscles consisting of primarily fast-twitch motor units are less efficient than those consisting of slow-twitch units (Barclay, 1994), stronger efforts may actually be less efficient.

[24] The issue of determining efficiency in human movements, and specifically the baseline subtraction, is not completely resolved at present (for a recent review and discussion, see van Ingen Schenau et al., 1997).

References

Aleshinsky, S. Yu. (1986) An energy 'sources' and 'fractions' approach to the mechanical energy expenditure problem.—I-V. *J. Biomech.* 19: 287-315.

Alexander, R. McN. (1992) The work that muscles can do. *Nature* 357: 360-361.

Barclay, C.J. (1994) Efficiency of fast- and slow-twitch muscles of the mouse performing cycling contractions. *J. Exp. Biol.* 193: 65-78.

Biewener, A.A., Corning, W.R. and Tobalske, B.W. (1998a) In vivo pectoralis muscle force-length behavior during level flight in pigeons. *J. Exp. Biol.* 201: 3293-3307.

Biewener, A.A., Konieczynski, D.D. and Baudinette, R.V. (1998b) In vivo muscle force-length behavior during steady-speed hopping in tammar wallabies. *J. Exp. Biol.* 201: 1681-1694.

Blix, M. (1894) Die laenge und die spannung des musckels. *Skand. Arch. Physiol.* 5: 149-206.

Dickinson, S. (1928) The dynamics of bicycle pedalling. *Proc. Roy. Soc. B.* 103: 225-233.

Fenn, W.O. (1923) A quantitative comparison between the energy liberated and the work performed by the isolated sartorius of the frog. *J. Physiol. (London)* 58: 175-203.

Fenn, W.O. (1924) The relation between the work performed and the energy liberated in muscular contraction. *J. Physiol. (London)* 58: 373-395.

Fenn, W.O. and Marsh, B.S. (1935) Muscular force at different speeds of shortening. *J. Physiol. (London)* 85: 277-297.

Flanders M. and Soechting J.F. (1990) Arm muscle activation for static forces in three-dimensional space. *J. Neurophysiol.* 64: 1818-1837.

Gasser, H.S. and Hill, A.V. (1924) The dynamics of muscular contraction. *Proc. Roy. Soc. B.* 96: 398-437.

Hatze, H. (1977) A myocybernetic control model of skeletal muscle. *Biol. Cybernetics* 25: 103-119.

Henneman, E., Somjen, G. and Carpenter, D.O. (1965) Functional significance of cell size in spinal motoneurons. *J. Neurophysiol.* 28: 560-580.

Hill, A.V. (1910) The possible effects of the aggregation of the molecules of haemoglobin on its dissociation curve. *J. Physiol. (London)* 40: iv-vii.

Hill, A.V. (1911) The position occupied by the production of heat in the chain of processes constituting a muscular contraction. *J. Physiol. (London)* 42: 1-43.

Hill, A.V. (1913) The absolute mechanical efficiency of the contraction of an isolated muscle. *J. Physiol. (London)* 46: 435-469.

Hill, A.V. (1927) *Muscular Movement in Man: The Factors Governing Speed and Recovery from Fatigue.* New York: McGraw-Hill.

Hill, A.V. (1928) The air-resistance to a runner. *Proc. Roy. Soc. B.* 102: 380-385.

Hill, A.V. (1938) The heat of shortening and the dynamic constants of muscle. *Proc. Roy. Soc. B.* 126: 136-195.

Hill, A.V. (1949) The abrupt transition from rest to activity in muscle. *Proc. Roy. Soc. B.* 136: 399-420.

Hill, A.V. (1950) The dimensions of animals and their muscular dynamics. *Science Progress* 38: 209-230.

Hill, A.V. (1960) *The Ethical Dilemma of Science and Other Writings.* New York: Rockefeller Institute Press.

Hill, A.V. (1965) *Trails and Trials in Physiology.* London: Arnold.

Hill, A.V. (1970) *First and Last Experiments in Muscle Mechanics.* Cambridge: University Printing House.

Hill, A.V., Long, C.N.H. and Lupton, H. (1924a) The effect of fatigue on the relation between work and speed in the contraction of human arm muscles. *J. Physiol. (London)* 58: 334-337.

Hill, A.V., Long, C.N.H. and Lupton, H. (1924b) Muscular exercise, lactic acid and the supply and utilization of oxygen. *Proc. Roy. Soc. B.* 96: 438-475; 97: 84-138.

Hill, A.V. and Lupton, H. (1922) The oxygen consumption during running. *J. Physiol. (London)* 56: xxxii-xxxiii.

Johansson, J.E. (1922) Presentation speech. In *Nobel Prize in Physiology or Medicine: 1922.* **http://www.nobel.se/laureates/medicine-1922-1-bio.html.**

Josephson, R.K. (1993) Contraction dynamics and power output of skeletal muscle. *Ann. Rev. Physiol.* 55: 527-546.

Katch, F.I. (1997) *History Makers. A. V. Hill.* **http://www.sportsci.org/news/history/hill/hill.html.**

Lupton, H. (1922) The relation between the external work produced and the time occupied in a single muscular contraction in man. *J. Physiol. (London)* 56: 68-75.

Lupton, H. (1923) An analysis of the effects of speed on the mechanical efficiency of human muscular movement. *J. Physiol. (London)* 57: 337-353.

Nobel Lectures (1999) *Nobel Prize in Physiology or Medicine: 1922.* **http://www.nobel.se/ laureates/medicine-1922-1-bio.html.**

Richman, J.P. (1995) Archibald V. Hill. In E. J. McMurray (ed.), *Notable Twentieth-Century Scientists,* pp. 927-929. New York: Gale Research.

van Ingen Schenau, G.J., Bobbert, M.F. and de Haan, A. (1997) Does elastic energy enhance work and efficiency in the stretch-shortening cycle? *J. Appl. Biomech.* 13: 389-415.

Woledge, R.C., Curtin, N.A. and Homsher, E. (1985) *Energetic Aspects of Muscle Contraction.* London: Academic Press.

Yamaguchi, G.T., Sawa, A.G.U., Moran, D.W., Fessler, M.J. and Winters, J.M. (1990). A survey of human musculotendon actuator parameters. In J. Winters & L.-Y. Woo (eds.), *Multiple Muscle Systems: Biomechanics and Movement Organization,* pp. 718-773. Berlin: Springer-Verlag.

Zajac, F.E. (1989) Muscle and tendon: Properties, models, scaling, and application to biomechanics and motor control. In Boume J.R. (ed.), *CRC Critical Reviews in Biomedical Engineering,* pp. 359-411. Boca Raton, FL: CRC Press.

Zatsiorsky, V.M. (1997) On muscle and joint viscosity. *Motor Control* 1: 299-309.

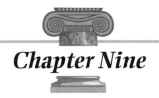

Chapter Nine

First Studies of the Organization of the Human Motor Cortex

John C. Rothwell

MRC Human Movement and Balance Unit, Institute of Neurology, London, UK

Revisiting the work of John Hughlings Jackson

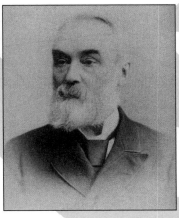

John Hughlings Jackson
From Critchley and Critchley 1998.

John Hughlings Jackson was one of the greatest neurologists of the 19th century and is now best known for his work in epilepsy and aphasia. The former, particularly its relationship to the organization of the motor system, is a subject of the paper in this chapter.

Jackson's Life and Work

John Hughlings Jackson was born of a Yorkshire father (Samuel Jackson) and a Welsh mother (Sarah Hughlings) in Yorkshire in 1835. He left school at 15 and was apprenticed to a general practitioner in York, where his usual tasks would have involved pill rolling, ointment preparation, lotion preparation, and helping at childbirth. Young apprentices were also known to have to serve as drivers of their master's horse-drawn carriage. In 1852, Jackson studied at the York Medical School (which is no longer in existence) in a class of only 12 students. After three years he spent 12 months at St Bartholomew's Hospital in London and qualified in medicine in 1856. He then returned to York and served as a resident medical officer at the York General Hospital, after three years submitting an MD thesis in 1860 to the University of St Andrews in Scotland. In his will, Jackson instructed his executors to destroy all of his personal papers, and consequently there are virtually no records of his performance or even his interests during his adult life.

In 1859, Jackson went to work in London, where he spent several years building up a clinical practice. Through the influence of a friend, Jackson obtained work as a part-time medical journalist at the *Medical Times and Gazette*. This gave him an opportunity to attend interesting medical demonstrations in London and to talk to many senior physicians. At the time, Hughlings Jackson's interests were broad, ranging from ophthalmology and psychology to anatomy and neurology. One of the senior men he met was Dr. Brown-Sequard, whose syndrome of spinal cord injury is now well known; and it may be this connection that sparked Jackson's interest in neurology. In 1860, Dr. Brown-Sequard together with Dr. J.Z. Ramskill founded the National Hospital for the Paralysed and Epileptic (now known as the National Hospital for Neurology and Neurosurgery) in Queen Square London, and in 1862 Brown-Sequard told Hughlings Jackson to apply for the post of assistant physician. Jackson obtained the post and was eventually, in 1867, appointed a full physician at the National Hospital. Before that he had obtained appointments also at the Moorfields Eye Hospital in 1862 and at the London Hospital in 1863. In 1867 he was elected as one of the youngest fellows of the Royal College of Physicians, and in 1878 at the age of 53 he was elected a Fellow of the Royal Society.

Especially to today's readers, John Hughlings Jackson's writings are difficult. They are lengthy and full of qualifications, and have abundant footnotes. This is so, of course, because the style at the time was much more discursive than it is today. However, the difficulty is also a result of Jackson's obsessive desire to be correct: This led him to make so many qualifications to his statements that it is often difficult to remember the original idea. Readers also need to bear in mind that his concepts were often very novel at the time and that Jackson consequently had to resort to new terminology for describing his ideas. Dr. Charles Mercier, one of many neurologists who wrote an appreciation of Jackson's life in the years after his death, commented:

> His writings had the reputation of obscurity, but they were not in the least obscure to those who were familiar with his modes of thought and the subjects of his thought. They had, however, a lack of literary skill and a certain crudity of expression that was in striking contrast with the elaboration and clearness of his thought. Of this lack of skill he was himself conscious. He said that writing on his subjects was like driving 6 horses abreast, each of which needed continuous attention. I know that he wrote one paper 13 times, and was still unsatisfied. (1926, pp. 40-41)

Jackson also did not hesitate to change his mind, and to do so in print. Although laudable, this characteristic makes its difficult for modern readers of any of Jackson's papers to assess the importance of the ideas or even their stage of development.

The extraordinary importance of Jackson's work in the field of epilepsy, particularly in relation to the motor system, can be appreciated only when we realize how little the field was understood in the first half of the 19th century. Neurophysiological recordings did not exist, and the pioneering experiments of Fritz and Hitzig and David Ferrier on electrical stimulation of the exposed cerebral cortex had yet to be performed. There was no idea of the somatotopic organization within specialized areas of the brain devoted to movement control. The cortex was thought to be solely the seat of consciousness and to have no direct motor or sensory functions. It was proposed that epilepsy itself arose in the medulla and that loss of consciousness was a result of cerebral ischemia caused by arterial spasms, the latter provoked by the medullary discharge. Genuine epilepsy was always generalized and always led to loss of consciousness. Focal epilepsies were not considered to be truly epileptic and had received very little attention indeed. The only exception was motor seizures in which the motor manifestations came first and were followed by loss of consciousness. These were sometimes referred to as "epileptiform seizures." John Hughlings Jackson began his work in the neglected area of focal convulsions. This led him over a period of 10 years or so in the 1860s to three main conclusions.

1. Even in his earliest writings it is clear that Jackson did not consider that epilepsy would necessarily have to arise in the medulla. In a short note published in 1864 he described the case of a man (presumably right hemisphere dominant for speech) who had suffered a stroke

that left him with a Broca's aphasia and paralysis of the left arm and leg. Five months later the patient suffered a convulsive seizure of the paralyzed side. This began in the left tongue; movements in the arm and the leg followed, and then the patient became insensible. The patient had four such seizures over the next few months. Jackson also noted that the patient had a valvular disease of the heart. Noting that disease of the middle cerebral artery was probably responsible for both the aphasia and hemiplegia, he then suggested that further irritation of the vessels—perhaps related to the man's heart disease—could have led to excessive discharge of structures in the same area that produced the motor seizures. In other words, the cortex might have been responsible for the seizures rather than the medulla.

2. Careful observation of the order of muscle activity in motor seizures gave Jackson clues as to the way muscles were represented in the brain. Together with data from postmortem studies of patients whom he had observed, this led him to conclude that a center for movement control could exist within the cerebral cortex itself. This work is illustrated by the extracts from one of his papers that are included in this chapter.

3. Jackson's final conclusion was that epilepsy as such was not a condition of the brain, but was simply a symptom of excessive discharge in a particular area of the brain. The quality and the severity of seizures depended only on the location and the amount of nervous tissue involved. As Jackson says in the opening sentence of his study of convulsions, "A convulsion is but a symptom, and implies only that there is an occasional, and excessive, and disorderly discharge of nerve tissue on muscles. This discharge occurs in all degrees; it occurs with all sorts of conditions of ill health, at all ages, and under innumerable circumstances" (1870, p. 162).

When describing these phenomena, Jackson adopted what might now be termed an evolutionary approach to neurology. First, he had noted a parallelism between the organization of motor seizures and hemiplegia. The same muscles that were first and most severely affected in hemiplegia were those most likely to be first affected in motor seizures. From this he concluded that if tissue was destroyed, the muscle would be paralyzed; if damaged, the same tissue might become unstable and activate muscles in a disorderly fashion. "Palsy depends on destruction of fibres, and convulsion on instability of the grey matter" (1870, p. 163). The connection between convulsions and hemiplegia was also evident from the postictal paralysis that Todd had described in the mid-19th century.

The second strand of Jackson's approach to neurology was a strong influence of the then-novel concepts of Darwinism, especially those promulgated by Stanley Spencer, the man who invented the term "survival of the fittest." From this, Hughlings Jackson developed his idea that there were three levels of nervous control of movement from the most automatic to the least automatic. In stroke and in epilepsy, the least automatic movements were affected first. Later in his life Jackson divided epilepsy according to the levels of neural functioning: highest-level fits, middle-level fits, and lowest-level fits. Highest-level fits were due to discharges in the frontal, prefrontal, and occipital lobes, and he proposed that these should be equated with epilepsy proper and loss of consciousness. Discharges beginning in the middle levels, which included the sensory and motor regions of cortex, could be equated with "epileptiform seizures." Spread of the discharge from these middle levels to the higher levels might then produce loss of consciousness and true epilepsy. Jackson also proposed the existence of lower-level fits that originated from the spinal cord and brainstem. These included laryngeal spasm, spasm of asthma, and rigors. Clearly today the three forms of lower-level fits would not be acceptable, and they are perhaps an example of how Jackson wanted to stretch his ideas sometimes beyond their natural limits.

The paper that follows was published in 1875, which was several years after many of the ideas expressed had been confirmed by Fritz and Hitzig and David Ferrier. However, as is the case with many of Jackson's works, this particular paper is simply a reworking of many previous papers, particularly the short reports of individual cases that he had published in the 1860s before the exploration of the cerebral cortex with electrical stimulation. Indeed, the original corpus of this work had been a prime source of inspiration for David Ferrier, who wrote as follows in his description of electrical stimulation of the monkey brain:

> The objects I had in view in undertaking the present research were two-fold: first to put to experimental proof the views entertained by Dr Hughlings Jackson on the pathology of epilepsy, chorea and hemiplegia by imitating artificially the destroying and discharging lesions of disease which his writings have defined and differentiated; and secondly to follow up the path which the researches of Fritz and Hitzig (who have shown the brain to be susceptible to galvanic stimulation) indicated to me as likely to lead to results of great value in elucidation of the function of the cerebral hemispheres, and the more exact localisation and diagnosis of cerebral disease. (1870, p. 130)

At the conclusion of his article, Ferrier writes of the results, "I regard them as an experimental confirmation of the views expressed by Dr Hughlings Jackson. They are, as it were, an artificial reproduction of the clinical experiments performed by disease, and the clinical conclusions which Dr Jackson has arrived at from his observations of disease are in all essential particulars confirmed by the above experiments."

Henry Head, another early 20th-century British neurologist, wrote: "Jackson, who never performed an experiment in his life, and who based his ideas solely on careful clinical observation, influenced neurophysiological science in a remarkable way. Each patient was to him an example of some disturbed process and helped elucidate the laws of normal and morbid function" (1911, pp. 952-953). Strangely enough, Jackson never published a textbook, not even a collected version of his papers. When asked to do so in 1901, he replied, "Many of my papers, all the old ones, are very old-fashioned and are not worthy of reprint (I have been working on neurological subjects for 36 years). As to more recent papers there is much in them too antiquated for republication. As to some others which I do think contain something of little value, there is recapitulation from one to the other—the same thing in various papers" (Mercier, 1926, p. 25).

Hughlings Jackson became deaf in later life and was seen less and less frequently in the hospital at Queen Square or at the meetings of the London Medical Societies. He died of pneumonia at number 3 Manchester Square, London, on October 7, 1911.

The following are two extracts from a long paper, "On the Anatomical and Physiological Localisation of Movements in the Brain," which was published as a pamphlet by J and A Churchill in 1875. Much of the substance of the paper had appeared in earlier papers in the 1860s. The full version of the text is available in *The Selected Writings of John Hughlings Jackson*, which was originally edited by James Taylor, Gordon Holmes, and F.M.R. Walshe in 1931 and published by Hodder and Stoughton. A reprint version of this text, published by Arts and Boeve, Nijmegen, The Netherlands, is available.

The original text begins with a long preface that occupies more space than the main text. In it Jackson tries to fit his observations into the new work of the time, including that of David Ferrier. The body of the paper continues with a series of numbered points introduced by the initial paragraph reproduced here. I have selected points 1 and 2 and 6-12 as illustrative of Jackson's approach.

On the Anatomical and Physiological Localisation of Movements in the Brain

John Huhlings Jackson

[Introduction]

(1) Paralysis and Convulsion are not only "Symptoms of Disease", but supply Evidence bearing on the Localisation of Movements and Impressions in the Brain

For some years I have studied cases of disease of the brain, not only for directly clinical, but for anatomical and physiological purposes. Cases of paralysis and convulsion may be looked upon as the results of experiments made by disease on particular parts of the nervous system of man. The study of palsies and convulsions from this point of view is the study of the effects of "destroying lesions" and of the effects of "discharging lesions." And for an exact knowledge of the particular movements most represented in particular centres, we must observe and compare the effects of each kind of lesion. It is just what the physiologist does in experimenting on animals; to ascertain the exact distribution of a nerve, he destroys it, and also stimulates it. Indeed, this double kind of study is essential in the investigation of cases of nervous disease for physiological purposes. For limited *destroying lesions* of *some* parts of the cerebral hemisphere produce no obvious symptoms; whilst *discharging lesions* of those parts produce very striking symptoms. By this double method we shall, I think, not only discover the particular parts of the nervous system where certain groups of movements are most represented (anatomical localisation), but, what is of equal importance, we shall also learn the order of action (physiological localisation) in which those movements are therein represented.

I. Movements Lost From "Destroying Lesions"

(2) The Order of Loss of Movements, Faculties etc., is from the Special or Voluntary to the General or Automatic; Illustrated by Hemiplegia

I begin by speaking of destroying lesions, and take the simplest case— hemiplegia of the common form from lesion of the corpus striatum. A blood clot which has destroyed part of the corpus striatum has made an experiment, which reveals to us that movements of the face, tongue, arm, and leg are represented in that centre. This is the localisation of the movements anatomically stated. Physiologically we say that the patient whose face, tongue, arm, and leg are paralysed has lost the most voluntary movements of one side of his body, and it is equally important to keep in mind that he has not lost the more automatic movements. The study of cases of hemiplegia shows that from disease of the corpus striatum those external parts suffer most which, psychologically speaking, are most under the command of the will, and which, physiologically speaking, have the greater number of different movements at the greater number of different[1] intervals. That parts suffer more as they serve in voluntary, and less as they serve in automatic operations, is, I believe, the law of destroying lesions of the cerebral nervous centres. It may be illustrated in the hemiplegic region itself: that limb which has the more voluntary uses – the arm – suffers more. I have illustrated by a case of hemiplegia of limited range from a lesion of moderate gravity. But from lesions of different degrees of gravity we have hemiplegia of very different ranges, varying gradually from palsy of the face, tongue, arm, and leg of one side, to universal powerlessness.[2] Or, physiologically speaking, there are all degrees, from paralysis limited to the most voluntary parts of one side of the body to paralysis of the most automatic parts of the whole body. The movements of the heart and respiration are less frequent, and the temperature is abased (soon after the seizure, of course, is meant). The patient, to put it in the shortest way, *is reduced to a more or less automatic condition*, according to the gravity of the lesion.

It must be added, that degrees of hemiplegia are not simple degrees; that is to say, they are not either degrees of more or less loss of power only, nor degrees of more or less range only, but of both. They are Compound Degrees. For example, if there be paralysis not only of the *most* voluntary parts of the body—face, tongue, arm, and leg—but also of those next[3] most voluntary, *vis.* loss of certain movements of the eyes and head and side of the chest, we find that the most voluntary parts (face, arm, and leg) *are very much paralysed*. In other words, the graver the lesion not only the more are the most voluntary parts paralysed, but the further spread to automatic parts is the paralysis.

From these facts, supplied by cases of destroying lesions of the centre producing *loss* of movements, we may conclude that the physiological order of representation of movements in the corpus striatum is such that action in health spreads from the automatic to the voluntary; or rather (the unit of action of the nervous system being a double unit – a molecule of two atoms) that there is *first* action spreading from the automatic to the voluntary, and then action spreading in the reverse order.[4] The spreading of healthy movements is best illustrated by degrees of "effort," as in lifting weights. There is first fixation of the more automatic parts of the arm, side of chest (and still further in automaticity according to the preconceived degree of heaviness of the object), before the most voluntary part, the hand, grasps the weight and then lifts it. The heavier the weight, not only the more strongly are the most voluntary parts used, but the further does the movement spread to the more automatic parts. This compound spreading of healthy movement corresponds to the compound degrees of hemiplegia. [Here I have omitted points 3, 4 and 5.]

II. Movements Developed By "Discharging Lesions" of Convolutions

I pass now to speak of symptoms resulting from "discharging lesions" of the brain. The movements in chorea as well as those in convulsion, are the result of abnormal discharges; but I shall speak in this paper only of convulsions ordinarily so called. Here, again, it may be objected that I consider still another topic; but I think it will be seen that the facts to be pointed out illustrate the same principle as do the symptoms already spoken of as resulting from "destroying lesions."

(6) The Nature of the Morbid Discharge in Convulsion

The nervous discharge in a convulsion differs from the discharge which occurs in a healthy movement in that it is sudden, excessive, and of short duration. The discharge being of the grey matter of processes for *movements*, there is caused by it a development of movements in the related and connected external regions. But the development of the movements is so abrupt, and the number of movements developed at once is so great, that the visible result is apparently a mere heedless struggle of muscles, in which at first glance it seems unlikely that we shall trace any kind of order. If we take for first investigation cases of *general* convulsions (such as are sometimes called "idiopathic epilepsy"), we shall, I believe, make little out. The paroxysms are too sudden, too quickly universal, and of too short duration for precise investigation. But if we take simple cases we shall, I think, accomplish a great deal. Most unquestionably the simplest cases of convulsion are those in which the spasm begins deliberately on one side of the body and affects that side only, or affects it more than the other. Such fits are often very limited in range, and then the patient is not unconscious, and can describe the seizure. As they begin deliberately, and as they may last many minutes, we are able, if we are present at a paroxysm, to note the place of onset and the order of spreading of the spasm. But even these simple convulsions represent the healthy movements contained in the region discharged only in outline and, so to speak, in caricature. For besides the facts already mentioned (that the discharge is sudden, excessive, and soon over) the discharge is of a *limited part of the brain*—of a part picked out, as it were, somewhat at random, by disease. The presumption is that there are no more isolated discharges of parts of the brain—an *excessive* discharge of a small part—*in health* than there are movements of single muscles in health. (Movements of single muscles, except perhaps in the face, are, Duchenne insists, only producible artificially—that is, by galvanism.)

(7) Convulsion beginning Unilaterally, the Mobile Counterpart of Hemiplegia

These seizures I used to call unilateral convulsions, but since the spasm (although it affects one side first and most) may *become* universal, it is more correct to call them "convulsions beginning unilaterally." Indeed, as is well known to careful clinical observers, they occur in all degrees, from twitching of a finger to universal convulsion. It is important to bear this in mind, especially as the same patient may have fits of several degrees; unless we do, we may erroneously suppose that he has several *varieties* of convulsions. Convulsions beginning unilaterally depend on disease of the same *cerebral* region as does hemiplegia of the common form, but hemiplegia depends on "destroying lesion" of the corpus striatum, the convulsion on a "discharging lesion" of the convolutions near to this body—convolutions in the region of the middle cerebral artery. We have, indeed, not only "corpus striatum paralysis," but a "corpus striatum convulsion." To prove that the convulsion is one of the mobile counterparts of hemiplegia, we find both in the same case. After a severe fit which has begun in the hand, we occasionally find hemiplegia like that which is so often produced by a clot in the corpus striatum, like it in degree and in range, but unlike it in being transitory. When the convulsion is partial, the palsy left by it is partial too. Thus I have recorded the case of a patient who had paralysis limited to the arm after a convulsion of that limb dependent on tumour in the hinder part of the first (superior) frontal convolution.[5] (There was a tumour in each lobe of the cerebellum as well.) There can, in short, be no doubt that these convulsions are the mobile counterparts of hemiplegia.

(8) The Convolutions near the Corpus Striatum re-represent the Movements represented in that Centre

When in such cases we do discover disease of the brain, we do find it in the region of the corpus striatum, but occasionally no local morbid change is found in any part of the brain. Nevertheless, the very fact that the convulsion has been one-sided, or has begun on one side, warrants the inference that there *is* in such cases also a local lesion, although we are unable to detect it. The lesion—when a lesion is discovered—involves more or less of convolutions which are near to, and, I suppose, *discharge through* the corpus striatum. I suppose that these convolutions represent over again, but in new and more complex combinations, the very same movements which are represented in the corpus striatum. They are, I believe, the corpus striatum "raised to a higher power." *Discharge*[6] of the grey matter of these convolutions *develops* the same groups of movements which are *lost* when the corpus striatum is *destroyed*.

(9) The most Voluntary or most Special Movements first and most affected by the Discharge of Convolutions

But there are several varieties of convulsions beginning unilaterally. They may be classified according to the places of onset of the spasm. There is nothing more important than to note where a convulsion begins, for the inference is, that the first motor symptom is the sign of the beginning of the central discharge.

There are three parts where fits of this group mostly begin: (1) in the hand; (2) in the face, or tongue, or both; (3) in the foot. In other words, they usually begin in those parts of one side of the body which have the most voluntary uses. The order of frequency in which parts suffer illustrates the same law. I mean, that fits beginning in the hand are commonest; next in frequency are those which begin in the face or tongue, and rarest are those which begin in the foot. The law is seen in details. When the fit begins in the hand, the index-finger[7] and thumb are usually the digits first seized;

when in the face, the side of the cheek is first in spasm; when in the foot, almost invariably the great toe.

(10) Leading Movements; Compound Order of spreading of Spasm

In each of these varieties there must be some difference in the situation of the grey matter exploded. In one part the movements of the hand have the leading representation, in another part those of the cheek and tongue, and in a third those of the foot. I say *leading* representation because spasm of the hand, etc., is only the *beginning* of the seizure. I had under my care a patient whose fits always *began* in his left thumb. [Case recorded *Medical Times and Gazette,* November 30, 1872.] We found, after death, a tubercle the size of a hazel-nut in the hinder part of his third right frontal convolution. Now in this case the most that one could say was, that in the convolution or region first discharged there lay processes for movements in which the thumb had *the leading part.* For although the spasm *began* in that digit, it went up the arm, and at length probably all over the body.

Besides, since the movements of the thumb and fingers could scarcely be developed for any useful purpose without fixation of the wrist (and of parts further and further in automaticity according to the force required), we should *a priori* be sure that the centre discharged, although it might represent movements in which the thumb had the leading part, must represent also certain other movements of the forearm, upper arm, etc., which serve subordinately. These remarks have partly anticipated the next topic—the march of the spasm.

(11) The Order in which Movements are developed by Discharge of Convolutions. The March of Spasm

After noting the part in which the fit begins, we have to observe how the spasm spreads (the "march of the fit"), and this for two purposes. We have not only to learn *how much* of the body is ultimately involved by the spasm, but also to note the *order* in which the several parts involved are affected. For example, we have not only to report of a case that the spasm "affected the whole of one side of the body," but also that "the spasm began in the hand, spread *up* the arm, next took the face, and then passed *down* the leg." We have to note not only the range of a fit, but the *order* of development of movements one after another in that range. Or, speaking now of the nerve centres, we have to study convulsion not only to learn what particular movements are represented in a nervous centre (anatomical localisation), but also to learn the particular order in which those movements are therein represented (physiological localisation).

As already remarked, the movements first developed in a fit probably represent those which take the lead; those next developed are, we may suppose, the subordinately associated movements. Let me illustrate by a healthy movement. When we grasp strongly, although the flexors take the lead the extensors must be in subordinate, and yet in associated action, or the grasp would not be vigorous; and the more strongly the hand is used, the farther up the arm does the movement spread. The observation therefore of the order of development of spasm will enable us, it is reasonable to hope, to determine the association of leading with subordinate movements. For example, if a fit begins in the thumb and index-finger, there will probably[8] be developed as the spasm spreads that series of movements which in health serves subordinately when the thumb and index-finger are used. Of course we can only make very rough observations, as in a convulsion a great number of movements are developed all at once.

It is to be observed that, just as degrees of hemiplegia are compound degrees, so the order of development of spasm is a compound order. For example, when the fit begins in the hand, the spasm does not leave the hand when it involves the rest of the arm. Two things occur: the spasm of the hand becomes more powerful, and the spasm spreads up the arm. This compound order—as are degrees of hemiplegia (*ante*, No. 2)—is roughly in accordance with the order of development of movements in increasing strains, as in lifting things of different weight (in what is technically called "effort"). It is important to note this compound order, especially when we consider that it implies that increasing discharge of a centre has not only the effect of intensifying movement, but also the effect of increasing the range of movement. It has an important bearing on the method of mental operations. For brevity and clearness, we shall, however, in what follows, speak of the spreading of spasm as if it were simple.

(12) The Same Muscles represented in Different Order in Several Places

To show, further, the importance of noting sequence as well as range, I would mention that there are two varieties of fits, in each of which, so far as I can learn, the same muscles are involved, but in each they are involved in a different order. The range is the same; the sequence is different. Thus one man's fits begin in his hand, go up his arm and down his leg; another man's begin in his foot, go up his leg and down his arm. But, though the same muscles are in action in each of the two fits, the fact that parts of both limbs are involved in different order, and probably in very different degrees, renders the inference irresistible that the two fits depend on discharge of two different centres. For the nervous centres do not represent muscles, but very complex movements in each of which many muscles serve. In each of the two centres discharged the *very same muscles* are represented in two different orders of movements. In one there are represented movements in which the arm leads and the leg is subordinate; in the other, movements in which the leg leads and the arm is subordinate. The very same notes are made up into two different tunes; in chemical metaphor, the fits are isomeric.[9]

My impression is, that the face is differently affected according as the spasm *begins* there and then goes to the arm, or comes there after the arm has been first seized. In the former case the spasm, I believe, begins in the mouth (both sides of the lips, or in the cheek near the angle of the mouth), and spreads all over the face. When the spasm begins in the hand, I believe the orbicularis palpebrarum is the part of the face first in spasm. If the order be as I suppose, the muscles of the face will be represented in movements of different orders, and therefore in several parts of the nervous system.

Thus, then, the three fits may be looked upon as experimental stimulations, each of some different part in the region of the corpus striatum, and as showing us (1) what movements have the leading representation in each part; (2) the movements which are sequent and subordinate to those having the leading representation. It is freely granted that no definite results have as yet been obtained on the second point. Very few cases have been carefully observed, very few autopsies indeed have been obtained on cases which *have been* observed carefully; and, lastly, as I shall point out very prominently later on, there are complications which impede our attempt to draw exact conclusions. It is for the very reason that so little has been done that I urge the careful investigation of these seizures.

[Endnotes]

[1] I shall use (and, after the physiological definition, without any psychological implication) the words "voluntary" and "automatic." It is not to be implied that there are abrupt demarcations betwixt the two classes of movements; on the contrary, there are gradations from the most voluntary to the most automatic.

[2] Of course, the term "hemiplegia" becomes a misnomer when there is universal powerlessness. I shall have more to say of the universal powerlessness which occurs from disease of but one side of the brain when I consider convulsive seizures.

[3] Or, in equivalent terms, of those next least automatic.

[4] That the unit of action of the nervous system is double the unit of composition is inferable from the fact that the whole nervous system is double. This conclusion runs physiologically parallel with the psychological law that all mental operations consist, fundamentally regarded, in the double process of tracing relations of likeness and unlikeness. The lower parts of the nervous system are plainly double in function, and it would be marvellous if the higher parts were not so too. The most automatic of the visible movements of the body "practically" constitute a single series, although we see that they are in duplicate. The two sides of the chest act so nearly together in time and so nearly equally in range that there is "practically" but one movement. But the very highest movements—those for words—are *apparently* in single order too, but for the very opposite reason. It is because we only consider the *end* of word processes (speech), and neglect altogether the prior automatic reproduction of words. In the double action, of which the second part is speech, there is first, I suggest, the automatic and unconscious reproduction of words. Later in this paper will be given facts which tend to show – (1) that the unit of action of the nervous system is double the unit of composition; (2) that the higher the nervous processes are the more unlike become the two components of the unit of action; (3) that the unlikeness is first in time, one acting before the other; and second in range, one being in stronger action than the other.

[5] See *Medical Mirror*, September 1869.

[6] It is supposed that in the part which is occasionally discharged the grey matter is highly

unstable. This, indeed, seems to me to be a truism; the difficulty is to discover the *patho-logical process* by which that instability results. In the cases I shall mention later on it has been *associated with* tumour; the tumour does not discharge, but in some way it leads to changes involving instability of grey matter. My speculation is that, speaking in chemical language, the highly unstable grey matter of disease remains of the same Constitution as the comparatively stable grey matter of health, but that it is of a different Composition; and a further speculation is that the phosphorus ingredient is replaced by its congener nitrogen—that the nervous matter is more nitrogenised, and therefore more explosive. If this be so, we see that although the nutrition of grey matter is carried on abnormally, in cases of convulsion, chorea, etc., we cannot say without much qualification that its nutrition is *defective*. The supposed therapeutical value in nervous affections of the other member of the group of triads (arsenic) is significant.

7 Perhaps it may be well here to mention again that the word "voluntary" is used for a part like the hand, which has the greater number of different movements and the greater number of different intervals of movements, and that the word "automatic" is used for a part like the chest, which has the greater number of nearly similar movements and the greater number of nearly equal intervals. The hand is a more "voluntary" part than either the cheek (or articulatory organs altogether) or the leg. Indeed, the hand is the most important part of the body from any point of view. Hence the significance of the fact that in disease of the highest centres it usually suffers first and most.

8 In the case mentioned we had no opportunity of noting the march of the spasm.

9 I have recently had two patients under my care whose fits begin in the foot. When the spasm does get to the arm in these cases, it begins in the fingers and goes up the limb; but even in these cases the centre discharged must be a different one from that discharged when the fit begins first of all in the hand.

Summary

1. One of the confusing aspects of Hughlings Jackson's writings on motor epilepsy is his ambiguity about the relative role of the corpus striatum and the overlying cortex in producing seizures. Before about 1875, the cortical origin of the pyramidal tract was not generally accepted, and the majority opinion was that the pyramidal tract arose within the corpus striatum, and thus lesions of that body were supposed to be involved in producing hemiplegia. In the extract, Jackson seems to stick with the prevailing view that damage to the striatum produces hemiplegia, but also cites evidence from cases in which convulsions appeared to have arisen from verified postmortem damage to the overlying cerebral cortex. In this case he seemed to believe that the discharge arose within the cerebral cortex and was conducted through the corpus striatum and then to the muscles.

2. Up until the time that this particular paper was published, Jackson seems to have been of the impression that he was the first to describe the details of a motor seizure. However, at about the time this paper was published, he became aware from writings of a French neurologist, Charcot, that a French author named Bravais had written a thesis in 1824 describing such attacks. In writings after 1876, Jackson always conscientiously inserted in parentheses the words "they were first described by Bravais in 1824" whenever he referred to epilepti-

form seizures. Indeed, in 1887 Charcot wrote that he had often spoken of this type of disorder as Jacksonian epilepsy and that many others since had done the same. "Such was just. I do not regret it. I have done Bravais a little injustice but in fact the work of Monsieur Jackson is so important that truly his name deserves to be attached to that discovery. If one could link Bravais and Jackson, the Frenchman and the Englishman, and speak of the Bravais-Jacksonian epilepsy that would be more correct; it is true that this would be a little lengthy."

3. By a tragic twist of fate, Jackson had ample opportunity in his own life to observe the consequences of his eponymous epileptic fits. In 1865 he married his cousin, a writer of children's tales. The marriage is said to have been very happy but lasted only 11 years. Mrs. Jackson contracted what was described as cerebral thrombophlebitis and developed focal motor seizures, later to be known as Jacksonian epilepsy.

References

Charcot, J.M. (1887). *Leçons du mardi à la Salpêtrière*. Paris: Bureau du Progrès Médical.

Head, H. (1911). *Obituary*. British Medical Journal, II, 952-953.

Hill, A.V. (1922). "The maximum work and mechanical efficiency of human muscles, and their most economical speed." Journal of Physiology (London), 56, 19-41.

Jackson, J.H. (1864). Medical Times and Gazette, vol. ii, 166.

Jackson, J.H. (1870). *A study of convulsions*. Transactions St. Andrews Medical Graduates Association, vol iii, 162.

Ferrier, D. (1873). West Riding Asylum Reports, vol iii, 130.

Mercier, C. (1926). *Neurological Fragments*. Ed. J. Taylor. Oxford University Press.

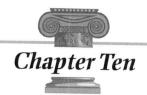
The Action of Two-Joint Muscles: The Legacy of W.P. Lombard

Arthur D. Kuo
University of Michigan

Revisiting the work of W.P. Lombard

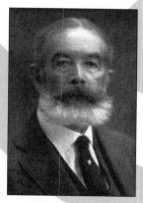

W.P. Lombard
Reprinted from Fenn 1968.

In a five-page missive, W.P. Lombard (1903a) helped lay the foundation for a new and rational approach to understanding how muscles are coordinated. Although investigators dating back to Borelli (1685) had described the relationship among muscle, joint, and limb in a logical, intuitive, and physically meaningful manner, Lombard made an astonishing, counterintuitive claim. He asserted that muscles with apparently opposing actions, termed pseudo-antagonists, can be used together in a productive way (see also Lombard, 1903b; Lombard and Abbott, 1907). This concept came from a remarkable intuition—one that we have been challenged to state more quantitatively and objectively for nearly 100 years. Though Lombard expressed his ideas qualitatively, the definitive nature of his statements implied that they could be translated into precise mathematical descriptions. The enduring influence of his work stems perhaps from its tantalizing character, a mix of biological description and bold prediction. We might classify Lombard's theory of the pseudo-antagonist as a conjecture—a theorem waiting for definitive proof. In our attempts to find the proof, we have adopted the principles of mechanics, carving out a new field of biomechanics. A review of Lombard's influence will suggest that much of our as-yet-incomplete understanding of muscular function has been fed from and driven by this remarkable source.

As with any developing field, advances in biomechanics have come on a variety of fronts. Motor tasks have been differentiated in terms of upper and lower extremity, unconstrained and constrained, isometric and otherwise. In taking stock of Lombard's impact on biomechanics, it is expedient to use a single mathematical notation to assess and compare the many contributions made by different researchers studying different motor tasks. Mathematics is a precise and unambiguous language, but it is also somewhat inaccessible. Fortunately, there is a geometric interpretation that will be both accessible and mathematical. We will use Lombard's main thesis as a vehicle for introducing the mathematics and geometry, after which contributions by others will motivate appropriate extensions but all within a single framework.

Historical Perspective

The existence of two-joint muscles was remarked upon long before the time of Lombard. For example, Ingen Schenau (1990) cites Galen's (131-201 A.D.) *De Usu Partium* (translated by May, 1968) as an early description of the effect of the rectus femoris in flexing the hip and extending the knee. Borelli (1685, cited by Fick, 1879) described the dependence of knee joint torque on the hip angle, and some think that his mechanistic arguments pioneered the field of biomechanics. Prior to (Hunter, 1797) and more contemporary with Lombard, several authors (Cleland, 1867; Fick, 1879; Langer, 1879) remarked on how two-joint muscles could link movement of joints, and how this would enable transfer of energy to the periphery from other muscles closer to the trunk. Of particular interest was the fact that by extending one joint and flexing another, a two-joint muscle is able to maintain a constant length and thereby stay within a length range for which significant force can be produced (Hüter, 1863, 1869; Fick, 1879).

Up to the early 20th century, however, muscle coordination was mostly discussed in terms of combinations of muscles all located at different joints. Few considered how the joint coupling provided by a two-joint muscle could be harnessed by another muscle crossing the opposite side of one of the same joints. One early exception was Duchenne (1885), who described the ability of hamstrings to work with rectus femoris to extend the knee, a concern identical to Lombard's. Although earlier in this century Duchenne was cited more extensively in the literature than Lombard was, he is presently given little credit for his earlier observation. (This unfortunate fact is not due to any inferiority in Duchenne's contribution; the primacy of English as a scientific language is a likely reason.) In his time, Duchenne was well known for his treatises on muscle function (1867, 1885), in which he also described the ability of one- and two-joint muscles to stabilize a joint—a relevant concern to this day (e.g., Markee et al., 1955; Baratta et al., 1988). Another early contributor was Hering (1897), who predated Lombard in the use of the term pseudo-antagonist and made observations very similar to those of Lombard.

Lombard's Conjecture

Lombard stated that opposing two-joint muscles can reinforce each other; he also stated, "A muscle can cause the extension of a joint which it can flex." He gave the following necessary conditions for such behavior:

a. [The muscle] must have the better leverage at the end by which it acts as extensor.

b. There must be a two-joint muscle that flexes the joint which the muscle in question extends, and extends the joint which it flexes.

c. [The muscle] must have sufficient leverage and strength to make use of the passive tendon action of the other muscle. (1903a)

Lombard further asserted:

When all the two-joint muscles are contracting at the same time . . . the energy is transmitted by the muscles, as by an endless chain, having the form of a figure 8. . . . Thus each muscle helps all the rest to produce the extension of hip, knee and ankle, and all the two-joint muscles act as a unit. . . . (1903a)

Lombard gives no specific definition for condition (c) regarding passive tendon action. The statement appears to refer to a muscle that is activated isometrically, in a manner similar to Cleland's (1867) "ligamentous action" and to the work of others (Hüter, 1869; Fick, 1879; Duchenne, 1885; Hering, 1897; Strasser, 1917; Baeyer, 1921, 1922). We will see that an isometric interpretation of passive tendon action is merely a simplifying assumption and not critical to the understanding of muscle coordination.

We will first apply the concept of passive tendon action to studying the ability of a muscle to couple joints kinematically, using a simple two-joint system as an example (see figure 10.1). Kinematic behavior serves as an ideal introduction to musculoskeletal function, but for many motor tasks, intersegmental dynamics are also relevant. We will therefore consider the role of dynamics of both unconstrained and constrained two-joint systems in the coordination of muscles. As alluded to by Lombard, there are also energetic concerns in coordination, leading us to study the production and absorption of power, and relation to efficiency. Finally, we will examine the actions of muscles of all types and arrive at a more general interpretation, based on the summation of vector contributions, of muscle function in any type of motor task.

Kinematic Coupling of Joints

The first concern in studying a multijoint system is the set of kinematic constraints that connect the links. Joints and muscles both constrain movement. A ball-and-socket joint, for example, constrains the relative positions of the ends of two limbs. A muscle viewed kinematically—that is, with an

Two-joint, six-muscle system

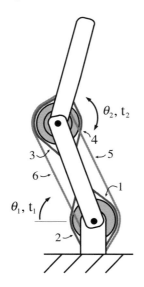

Figure 10.1
Example system illustrates muscle actions. Two-joint, six-muscle system illustrates many principles of muscle function. Four of the muscles cross a single joint, each with a moment arm that is independent of configuration (moment arms in diagram are for schematic purposes and are not to drawn to scale). Muscles 5 and 6 are two-joint muscles and illustrate Lombard's (1903a) concept of pseudo-antagonists. Muscle 5 has a larger extension moment arm about joint 1 than its flexion moment arm about joint 2, and muscle 6 has a larger flexion moment arm about joint 2 than its extension moment arm about joint 1. Joint torques t_1 and t_2 and joint angles θ_1 and θ_2 are defined to be positive in the direction corresponding to joint extension.

output in terms of length rather than force—also constrains movement. This is the case regardless of the rate of shortening or lengthening, although the concept is conceptually easier to understand when the length is fixed. Physiologically, there is some significance to isometric action, because a muscle can stay near optimum length and thereby generate large forces. More generally, the force-velocity relationship limits muscle's ability to generate force when the rate of shortening is high. This implies that there is some advantage to be gained from the ability of a two-joint muscle to act nearly isometrically during a motion in which two joints are simultaneously extended or flexed (Cleland, 1867; Duchenne, 1867; Fick, 1879; Fischer, 1902a, 1902b; Fenn, 1932, 1938).

In interpreting kinematic coupling, we must first establish a few definitions. First, instead of leverage, it is preferable to discuss a muscle's moment arm about each joint. Supposing that there are m muscles and n joints, we define the moment arm r_{ij} as the moment arm of muscle j (numbered from 1 to m) about joint i (numbered from 1 to n). It will also be convenient to place the list of all n moment arms for a muscle j into a vector, denoted

$$\mathbf{r}^{(j)} \equiv \begin{bmatrix} r_{1j} & r_{2j} & \cdots & r_{nj} \end{bmatrix}^T.$$

In each muscle's moment arm vector, the moment arm will be zero for each joint the muscle does not cross. There will be only one non-zero moment arm for one-joint muscles, and two for two-joint muscles (see figure 10.1).

The moment arms determine the shortening speed of a muscle-tendon unit as a function of the joint angular velocities. (For convenience, we will use "muscle" informally to refer to the muscle-tendon unit.) Defining the shortening speed to be positive when the muscle is contracting,

$$v_j \equiv \left\{ \mathbf{r}^{(j)} \right\}^T \dot{\boldsymbol{\theta}}$$

where

$$\dot{\boldsymbol{\theta}} \equiv \begin{bmatrix} \dot{\theta}_1 & \dot{\theta}_2 & \cdots & \dot{\theta}_n \end{bmatrix}^T$$

is the vector of joint angular velocities. Of particular interest, primarily for simplicity, is the case when the muscle is held isometric,

$$v_j = 0, \tag{1}$$

which specifies the relationship between joint angular velocities necessary for the muscle to be kept at constant length. This isometric case is what was studied by Cleland (1867) and his contemporaries and later used as a requirement for Lombard's conjecture.

Graphical methods are particularly well suited to describing these kine-matic constraints. Enklaar (1954) used graphical methods to show that, in the space of joint positions or velocities, equation (1) can be expressed as a straight-line constraint (for a two-joint system). More generally, $\mathbf{r}^{(j)}$ may be regarded as a vector normal to an isometric constraint surface passing through the origin in the coordinate system of joint angular velocities. When the joints move such that the joint velocities lie on the constraint surface, muscle j is held at constant length (see figure 10.2a). It is obvious that the constraint surface for a one-joint muscle requires that one joint be held stationary. For a two-joint muscle, however, the corresponding constraint requires that the two joints move in a fixed proportion. As noted by Landsmeer (1961), constant, non-zero muscle speeds appear as additional constraints parallel to the isometric constraint surface.

Enklaar (1954) examined the case of two muscles, both crossing two joints on the same side but with different moment arms (see figure 10.2b). Not only are there motions in which both muscles must shorten or lengthen; there are also motions in which one muscle must lengthen while the other

a. Muscle moment arm vectors and isometric constraints

b. Muscle shortening/lengthening sectors in joint velocity space

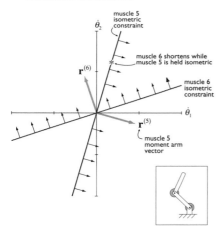
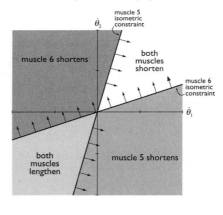

Figure 10.2
Isometric constraints for two-joint muscles. *(a)* Each muscle's moment arm vector defines a constraint surface (a line in this example) in joint velocity space. The constraint divides joint velocity space into motions for which the muscle shortens (denoted by arrows) or lengthens. Motions that lie on the constraint are achieved with the corresponding muscle held isomet-ric. Only constraints for muscles 5 and 6 are shown. *(b)* Isometric constraints in combination divide joint velocity space into sectors. Depending on the direction of motion, any combina-tion of lengthening or shortening of the two muscles is possible. The constraints show that a muscle with an extension moment arm about joint 1, such as muscle 5, can still shorten while joint 1 flexes.

shortens, even though these muscles might naively be labeled agonists. We can see that this phenomenon takes place whenever two muscles have differing moment arms, and that the more the moment arms differ, the larger the set of such lengthening/shortening motions.

This same example also applies directly to Lombard's conjecture. Here we will use muscle 6 as the primary muscle, which produces flexion torque about joint 1 (i.e., $r_{16} < 0$) and extension torque about joint 2 (i.e., $r_{26} > 0$), satisfying condition (a). The pseudo-antagonist, muscle 5, satisfies condition (b) and, when held isometric, constrains joint 1 to extend when muscle 6 shortens (see figure 10.2a). Stated mathematically, the isometric constraint from equation (1) is

$$v_5 = \left\{ \mathbf{r}^{(5)} \right\}^T \dot{\theta} = r_{15}\dot{\theta}_1 + r_{25}\dot{\theta}_2 = 0 \qquad (2)$$

and if muscle 6 is shortening,

$$v_6 = \left\{ \mathbf{r}^{(6)} \right\}^T \dot{\theta} = r_{16}\dot{\theta}_1 + r_{26}\dot{\theta}_2 > 0. \qquad (3)$$

Together, these equations imply that joint 1 will extend, that is, $\dot{\theta}_1 > 0$ if

$$r_{16} - r_{26} \frac{r_{15}}{r_{25}} > 0. \qquad (4)$$

Condition (b) guarantees that $r_{15}/r_{25} < 0$; the requirement that muscle 6 be an extensor of joint 2 implies that $-r_{26}r_{15}/r_{25}$ is positive, and must outweigh r_{16}, which is negative. We can therefore see that Lombard was very nearly correct in his conjecture. With condition (a) he stated the equivalent of $r_{26} > |r_{16}|$, which is helpful but not actually necessary for inequality (4) to be true.

We therefore conclude that a more precise version of Lombard's claim is that the two-joint muscle can extend a joint for which it has a flexor moment arm, if inequality (4) is true. Geometrically, this is equivalent to stating that the other two-joint muscle, the pseudo-antagonist, must have an isometric constraint line that both passes through the quadrant in joint velocity space for which both joints extend (the first quadrant in figure 10.2a) and does so on the shortening side of the primary muscle's isometric constraint.

Stated in this way, Lombard's claim is neither mysterious nor paradoxical. What might make it seem paradoxical is the potential misconception that the direction of torque produced by a muscle is equivalent to the direction of the resulting motion. Any two-joint muscle with such a flexor moment arm is capable of a range of motions that include extension of that same joint (see figure 10.2b). This property is moreover not exclusive to pairs of two-joint pseudo-antagonists. A two-joint muscle, held isometric, can act as a pseudo-antagonist to a single-joint muscle so that the latter can extend a joint that it does not even cross. Again, the joint velocities are constrained to the pseudo-antagonist's isometric surface, and joint extension lies on the shortening side of the primary (single-joint) muscle's isometric constraint.

Joint Torques Due to Muscle

Although Lombard did not explicitly consider joint torques in his paper, his secondary claim regarding transfer of energy hinted at the importance of kinetic variables. In fact, many later developments regarding two-joint muscles have involved joint torques. We will first review the relationship between torques and the isometric constraint lines already discussed, and then apply this relationship to the coordination of multiple muscles in order to gain additional insight about the action of single- and two-joint muscles.

Landsmeer (1961) was the first to observe that the same moment arm relationship that determines the joint motions for which a muscle is isometric applies to joint torques as well. Plotted in joint torque space, the individual torque vectors for each muscle are perpendicular to the isometric constraint lines (see figure 10.2a), and the joint torque vector associated with the activation of muscle j is

$$\mathbf{t}^{(j)} = \mathbf{r}^{(j)} \cdot f_j^{\max} \cdot f_j \tag{5}$$

where $f_j^{\max}$ is the maximum isometric (tensile) muscle force, and f_j is the normalized force or activation level allowed to vary between 0 and 1 (Kuo, 1994). The net torque due to muscle, $\mathbf{t}^M$, is the sum of the individual muscle torques, which can alternatively be interpreted as a weighted sum of maximal torque vectors $\mathbf{t}_{\max}^{(j)}$,

$$\mathbf{t}^M = \sum_{j=1}^{m} \mathbf{r}^{(j)} \cdot f_j^{\max} \cdot f_j = \sum_{j=1}^{m} \left(\mathbf{r}^{(j)} \cdot f_j^{\max} \right) \cdot f_j = \sum_{j=1}^{m} \mathbf{t}_{\max}^{(j)} \cdot f_j \tag{6}$$

where

$$\mathbf{t}_{\max}^{(j)} \equiv \mathbf{r}^{(j)} \cdot f_j^{\max}.$$

Landsmeer (1961) noted that the net torque due to muscle is simply the vector sum of individual muscle torque vectors. Static equilibrium can therefore be achieved if the torques due to gravity and other external forces balance those produced by the muscles.

A geometric interpretation of this vector summation demonstrates that each muscle's torque vector has a unique direction in torque space, determined by the relative moment arms (An et al., 1981; Kuo, 1994). The maximal torque vectors $t_{max}^{(j)}$, are equal to the moment arm vectors scaled by the maximal muscle force, and so must also be perpendicular to the isometric constraint lines (see figure 10.3a). The vector lengths depend on both the absolute moment arms and the maximal force that can be generated by each muscle. The central nervous system (CNS) must weight each of the possible torque vectors in such a way as to achieve a desired task (see figure 10.3b).

Elftman (1939a, 1939b, 1966) also understood the summation properties of joint torques, although without using a geometric interpretation. He calculated the joint torques associated with human locomotion and noted that a single muscle crossing the ankle, knee, and hip with appropriate moment arms could potentially replace the actions of the existing muscles and with greater efficiency. The torques associated with such a muscle would require the minimum summed absolute torque as opposed to any group of less specialized muscles with the same resultant torque. This point was also illustrated by Herzog and Binding (1994).

We can use the vector summation approach to gain a greater understanding of Elftman's observation. Any two vectors that are not collinear will

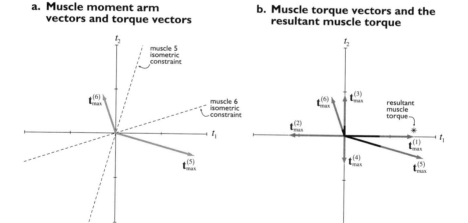

a. Muscle moment arm vectors and torque vectors

b. Muscle torque vectors and the resultant muscle torque

Figure 10.3

Muscle joint torque vectors. *(a)* Each maximal torque vector $t_{max}^{(j)}$ is proportional to that muscle's moment arm vector and perpendicular to the isometric constraint line. *(b)* Maximal torque vectors for all six muscles, of which a weighted sum is formed to produce a net muscle torque t^M. Shown in black are normalized activation levels f_j for each muscle such that a net joint torque (denoted by asterisk) of almost pure extension about joint 1 is formed. There is no unique solution, but this example distributes forces between muscles so as to minimize the sum of squared activation levels. Both single- and two-joint muscles will typically be activated to minimize this objective.

have components both normal and tangent to their resultant. The normal components cancel out; and because there is a metabolic cost to producing force or torque whether or not work is performed, this cancellation is costly. Any net muscle torque produced by a group of muscles could therefore be replaced by a single more efficient but more specialized muscle, with moment arms chosen so as to produce the same torque without cancellation. Elftman recognized that even single-joint muscles that cross different joints will act together such that there is a normal component to the resultant, an inefficiency that can be eliminated by substituting an appropriately located muscle in their stead.

It is therefore advantageous, in terms of the efficiency of vector summations, to have a large variety of muscles pointing in many directions in joint torque space (Kuo, 1994). These advantages are of course weighed against possible difficulties in routing a physical muscle to achieve some torque combinations, as well as the probable fact that efficiency is a concern in only a subset of all motor tasks. Nevertheless, the significance of different muscle types is partially to provide a repertoire of directions in torque space that are both achievable and efficient when used with other muscles. This basis of this observation, properly attributed to Elftman (1939a), has never been adequately recognized—perhaps because it was overshadowed by the many other contributions from that same paper, not least of which was Elftman's original use of dynamics to study human movement.

Dynamic Coupling at Joints

Most studies of two-joint muscles have concerned the flexion or extension of joints without consideration of the role of dynamics. A flexion or extension torque is therefore implicitly assumed to equate to flexion or extension motion. However, intersegmental forces can couple joint motion such that a pure flexion torque about a single joint will generally be expected not only to cause that joint to accelerate in flexion but also to cause other joints to move. We can distinguish between joint torques and joint accelerations by regarding them as separate sets of outputs and examining the action of muscles in each case. This examination is made simpler by the fact that the dynamical equations of motion map torque space to acceleration space.

The control implications of dynamical coupling were not appreciated until relatively recently. Dynamical equations of motion were first employed by Elftman (1939a) and later applied by many others to perform inverse dynamics and other calculations. Interest in motor control led Hollerbach and Flash (1982) to examine the problem of compensating for intersegmental forces. Zajac and Gordon (1990) offered an accessible tutorial on dynamical coupling based on a simple two-segment system, showing how muscles can accelerate joints they do not cross. This concept can be illustrated by examination of the dynamical equations of motion,

$$\ddot{\theta} = \mathbf{M}(\theta)^{-1} \cdot \left(\mathbf{t}^{M} + v\left(\theta, \dot{\theta}\right) + \mathbf{g}(\theta) \right). \tag{7}$$

where $\mathbf{M}(\theta)$ is the mass matrix, $\mathbf{g}(\theta)$ is a vector of gravitational terms, and $v\left(\theta, \dot{\theta}\right)$ is a vector of Coriolis and centripetal terms (see appendix for details). Neglecting the latter two terms for now, combining equations (5)-(7) with the following definition for maximal acceleration vectors for each muscle j,

$$\ddot{\theta}^{(j)}_{max} \equiv \mathbf{M}(\theta)^{-1} \cdot \mathbf{r}^{(j)} \cdot f_j^{max}$$

yields

$$\ddot{\theta} = \mathbf{M}(\theta)^{-1} \cdot \mathbf{t}^{M} + \cdots = \mathbf{M}(\theta)^{-1} \cdot \sum_{j=1}^{m} \mathbf{t}^{(j)}_{max} \cdot f_j + \cdots =$$

$$\sum_{j=1}^{m} \left(\mathbf{M}(\theta)^{-1} \cdot \mathbf{r}^{(j)} \cdot f_j^{max} \right) \cdot f_j + \cdots = \sum_{j=1}^{m} \ddot{\theta}^{(j)}_{max} \cdot f_j + \cdots \tag{8}$$

This equation demonstrates that the mass matrix transforms $\mathbf{t}^{(j)}_{max}$ from joint torque space to $\ddot{\theta}^{(j)}_{max}$ in joint acceleration space (Hogan, 1985; Kuo, 1994), and that each muscle induces an acceleration that contributes to the net acceleration vector.

In the output space of joint accelerations, the inverse of the mass matrix $\mathbf{M}(\theta)$ transforms the effect of each muscle. Figure 10.4a shows the muscle-induced joint angular acceleration vectors for our two-segment example, demonstrating that none of the muscles accelerate the joints in the same direction that they do in joint torque space nor in the same relative amounts. For example, muscle 1, which produces a pure extension torque about joint 1, accelerates both joints in nearly equal proportions. Muscle 6 produces a flexion torque about joint 1 and an extension torque about joint 2 but actually accelerates both joints into extension. Muscle 3 produces significantly less torque than muscle 1, yet it accelerates the joints by nearly twice as much for the configuration shown. The torques produced by a muscle can therefore not be assumed to indicate the direction or amount of accelerations that actually occur. It is also interesting to note that even the extension of a single joint requires coordination of many muscles, including some that do not even cross that joint (Fujiwara and Basmajian, 1975).

Despite the effect of these transformations, however, the fundamental role of the CNS is still to form (at each instance in time) an appropriate weighted sum of vectors. In acceleration space, it is typical that the mass matrix $\mathbf{M}(\theta)$ will exhibit significant dependence on the configuration of the limbs, more so than the moment arms. Added to the muscle-induced accelerations are those due to gravity, Coriolis, and centripetal terms.

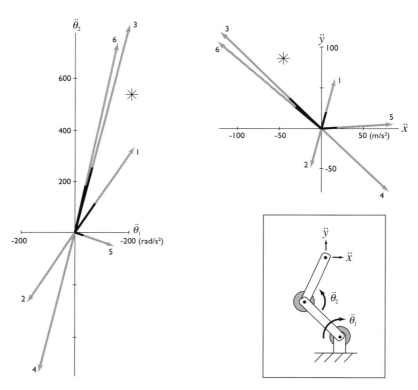

a. Muscle-induced accelerations in joint acceleration space

b. Muscle-induced accelerations in cartesian endpoint space

Figure 10.4

Muscle-induced acceleration vectors. *(a)* Each maximal joint angular acceleration vector $\ddot{\theta}^{\varphi}_{max}$ points in a direction in acceleration space that generally differs in direction from $\mathbf{t}^{\varphi}_{max}$. As in torque space, a weighted sum of muscle-induced acceleration vectors (plus Coriolis, centripetal, and gravity terms, if any) produces the net joint angular acceleration $\ddot{\theta}$. Shown in black are normalized activation levels necessary to produce the net acceleration denoted by an asterisk. This acceleration vector is the result of the net torque produced in figure 10.3. *(b)* An alternative output space can be defined in terms of accelerations of the endpoint in the Cartesian plane. Maximal acceleration vectors are shown, along with normalized activation levels necessary to form the net acceleration, which is upward and to the left (denoted by asterisk). Inset diagram shows configuration of links. See appendix for details.

The choice of output space is somewhat arbitrary. Joint torques, joint angles, and other coordinates are quantities that are derived, measured, and analyzed for the convenience of the observer and are not necessarily relevant to the CNS. An alternative to joint angular acceleration output space for our two-joint system is the accelerations of the endpoint or body center-of-mass in the plane (see figure 10.4b), which is of interest in cases such as reaching (Sergio and Ostry, 1994; Gielen et al., 1990), leg extension or sit-to-stand tasks (Soest et al., 1993; Ingen Schenau et al., 1995; Jacobs and Ingen Schenau, 1992), and posture (Kuo and Zajac, 1993). The vector summation properties apply here as well; and as in most output spaces, it is difficult (and not necessarily helpful) to distinguish between single- and two-joint muscles. Again, there is an advantage to be gained from the availability of muscles distributed in a variety of directions in the output space of interest.

Contact and Force Tasks

When a motor task involves contact with the environment, the consequences of muscle activation are different than for unconstrained tasks. This is so because external constraints limit the kinematically admissible motions. A number of investigators (Fischer, 1927; Donskoi, 1961; Molbech, 1966; Carlsöö and Molbech, 1966; Ingen Schenau, 1989a-c; Ingen Schenau et al., 1990; Gielen et al., 1990; Jacobs and Ingen Schenau, 1992; Doorenbosch et al., 1994, 1995; Prilutsky and Gregor, 1997) reported various kinematic constraint analyses demonstrating cases in which a two-joint muscle can exhibit behaviors similar to those reported by Lombard, and some (Ingen Schenau, 1990) thought that these behaviors were due to the presence of constraints. Closer analysis, however, reveals that these behaviors are fundamentally no different from those for unconstrained tasks and that they can be understood using the same mathematics as considered previously. We will begin by adopting the kinematic analysis of Enklaar (1954) and then consider the role of dynamics and reaction forces in contact tasks.

When the limbs form a closed kinematic chain with the environment, the joints are kinematically constrained. If this constraint is expressed as

$$\gamma(\theta) = 0 \qquad (9)$$

the corresponding constraint on joint velocities is

$$\frac{d\gamma(\theta)}{dt} = \frac{\partial \gamma}{\partial \theta} \cdot \dot{\theta} = \mathbf{J} \cdot \dot{\theta} = 0 \qquad (10)$$

where $\mathbf{J}$ is referred to as the Jacobian matrix (see appendix for details). This constraint is similar in form to that of isometric constraints such as equations (2) and (3), and can therefore be interpreted as a surface in joint velocity space.

As an example, let us consider the previous two-joint system except with the endpoint constrained to move in a slot (see figure 10.5). For the particular configuration shown, the corresponding constraint in joint velocity space is nearly aligned with the isometric constraint of equation (2). (In fact, an appropriately designed slot could have an identical constraint surface in joint velocity space.) Just as in the isometric case, the slot constrains motion so that joint 1 must extend when muscle 6 is shortening, even though that muscle produces a flexion torque about that joint.

These kinematic observations must in any case be discarded when dynamic coupling is significant. In contact tasks, the external constraints produce reaction forces that are a function of the joint torques and velocities similar in nature to the equations of motion (7). These reaction forces could be thought of as producing virtual accelerations that add to the unconstrained accelerations to produce motion along the constraint. Mathematically, the constrained accelerations must satisfy the constraint

$$\mathbf{J} \cdot \ddot{\theta} + \dot{\mathbf{J}} \cdot \dot{\theta} = 0 \tag{11}$$

which is simply the time-derivative of equation (10). The fact that the reaction force equations are similar in form to the equations of motion allows for a remarkably simple interpretation of constrained motion.

External kinematic constraint

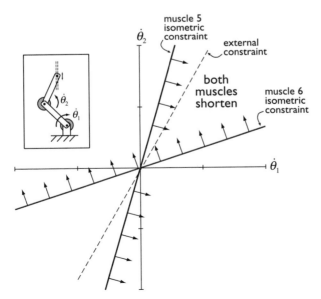

Figure 10.5
External kinematic constraints limit possible joint motions. A slot constrains motion of the endpoint as shown, limiting joint motions to the dashed line. Upward motion of the endpoint corresponds to shortening of both muscles 5 and 6. Muscle 6, which produces a flexion torque about joint 1, actually causes kinematic extension of that joint while shortening with the constraint in place. Inset diagram shows configuration of links and slot constraint.

We illustrate the dynamical effects of a constraint with our two-joint example with the endpoint moving in a slot (see figure 10.6a). To each muscle's unconstrained acceleration vector is added the virtual acceleration imposed by the constraint reaction force. The effect is such that muscle 1, which produces no torque about joint 2 but accelerates that joint into extension in the unconstrained case, will actually reverse the direction of that acceleration in the presence of the slot. In fact, with the exception of

a. Muscle-induced accelerations in joint acceleration space, with constraints

b. Muscle-induced accelerations in constraint/reaction force space

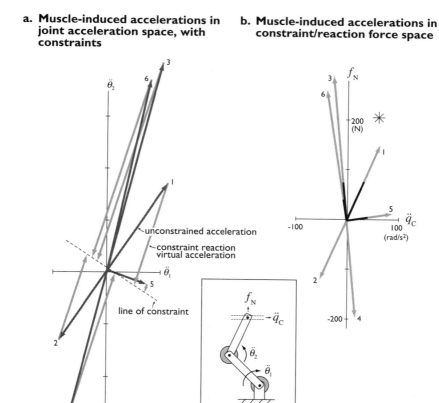

Figure 10.6
Muscle-induced acceleration vectors for constrained system, in two output spaces. In joint angular acceleration space (a), slot constraint adds virtual accelerations in reaction to the accelerations of the unconstrained system, so that each muscle induces an acceleration that must satisfy constraint (11). Constraint/reaction force space (b) defines the horizontal axis for accelerations along constraint (11) and the vertical axis for the normal force exerted against the slot. Also shown in both (a) and (b) are normalized activation levels necessary to produce a net output of 60 m/s² endpoint acceleration to the right and 200 N normal force, with an instantaneous endpoint velocity of 1 m/s to the right. Inset diagram shows configuration of links and slot constraint.

muscle 5, every muscle exhibits a change in direction of acceleration about one joint or another. As tempting as it may be to attribute these changes to the properties of two-joint muscles, they are changes merely in degree rather than in type. The fundamental significance is that constraints generally produce quantitative changes in the muscle-induced acceleration vectors.

Even though the constraint reduces the number of degrees of freedom of acceleration, there remain other degrees of freedom that are of interest. For contact tasks, most significant of these is typically the actual reaction force against the constraint, such as the pedal force (Gregor et al., 1985). Andrews (1985, 1987) advocated using alternative outputs such as motion along a constraint. Because there is acceleration but no reaction force *along* the constraint (11), and reaction force but no acceleration normal to the constraint, we will combine acceleration along and reaction force normal to the constraint as outputs of interest. For our example system we denote these two quantities $\ddot{q}_C$ and f_N, respectively. The corresponding output equations are

$$
\begin{bmatrix} \ddot{q}_C \\ f_N \end{bmatrix} = \begin{bmatrix} K_1 & K_2 \\ S_1 & S_2 \end{bmatrix} \cdot \mathbf{t}^M + \begin{bmatrix} K_0 \\ S_0 \end{bmatrix}
\tag{12}
$$

where the quantities K_0, K_1, K_2, S_0, S_1, and S_2 are defined in the appendix.

Combining equations (6) and (12), it is apparent whether viewing accelerations, reaction forces, or some combination thereof, that at each instance in time each muscle produces a vectorial contribution to these outputs. As shown in figure 10.6b, the directions of each muscle-induced acceleration vector in this output space are again different from those of the torque vectors of figure 10.3. Each muscle produces components of both acceleration and reaction force. For the configuration shown, muscle 1, with an extension moment arm about joint 1 only, produces a substantial reaction force in addition to its acceleration. It is evident that even a motor task calling for no reaction force will require that the muscles be coordinated carefully so that the weighted sum of the output vectors produces no resultant reaction force.

It is therefore clear that even though contact tasks produce different motions of the limbs, they do so in a manner no different from isometric or other constraints. In fact, so-called unconstrained tasks are subject to the action of joint constraints that are fundamentally no different from the external constraints considered here. Again, we must be careful not to assume that the direction of torque produced by a muscle is equivalent to the direction of the resulting motion. It is advantageous to rely on the mathematics to determine how the joints will move, whether we are considering kinematics alone or dynamics and reaction forces.

Positive and Negative Muscle Power

Although Lombard's conjecture describes the isometric behavior of a two-joint muscle, it is clear that Lombard was also concerned with the production and transfer of energy. Quantitative estimates of the net power produced at each joint were first made by Elftman (1939a), who was studying human gait. A number of methods have been proposed to quantify the transfer of energy between body segments (e.g., Aleshinsky, 1986; Ingen Schenau and Cavanagh, 1990; Bobbert et al., 1986a, 1986b; Bobbert et al., 1987; Prilutsky and Zatsiorsky, 1994), although not without controversy (Wells, 1988; Ingen Schenau, 1998). The controversy arises because there is no objective means to attribute energy transferred from one body segment to another to a particular muscle when there are multiple joints and muscles. Fortunately, for the purpose of understanding two-joint muscles, it is sufficient merely to determine whether a muscle is producing or absorbing power rather than where the power goes. From this information it can be demonstrated that a wide selection of muscles, with a variety of directions in torque space, allows many tasks to be performed efficiently.

One of the most-studied tasks in which power is a concern is cycling, which has typically been regarded as an example of Lombard's conjecture. The quadriceps must lengthen during the propulsive phase and might be thought of as antagonists to the hamstrings. However, Gregor et al. (1985) showed that when pedal forces are considered along with crank motion, the muscles contribute to the overall output in a consistent manner—especially in the second half of the propulsive phase, during which knee flexor moments were reported. Andrews (1987) also found more agreement when considering crank rather than knee motion. Ingen Schenau (1990) demonstrated that for some motor tasks, two-joint muscles make it possible to perform tasks more efficiently, in metabolic terms, than would be possible using single-joint muscles alone. In the absence of two-joint muscles during a positive work task such as cycling, it would be necessary for some single-joint muscles to actively lengthen and therefore absorb power even as others produce power. With two-joint muscles, this inefficiency can be avoided.

These phenomena can be understood by applying our mathematical approach. The net power produced or absorbed at a joint is given by the equation

$$p_i^M = t_i^M \cdot \dot{\theta}_i \tag{13}$$

where p_i^M is the total muscle power produced or absorbed at joint i and t_i^M is the i'th component of $\mathbf{t}^M$. An individual muscle produces power when it actively shortens and absorbs power when it actively shortens. The power produced by muscle j is

$$p^{(j)} = f_j \cdot v_j . \tag{14}$$

An equivalent relation is found using joint torque space, where the power is equal to the inner (dot) product of the muscle torque and angular velocity vectors (Kuo, 1994),

$$p^{(j)} = \left\{ \mathbf{t}^{(j)} \right\}^T \dot{\theta} .$$ (15)

The net power generated by all muscles is

$$p^{\mathrm{M}} = \sum_{j=1}^{m} p^{(j)} = \sum_{j=1}^{m} \left\{ \mathbf{t}^{(j)} \right\}^T \dot{\theta} = \left\{ \mathbf{t}^{\mathrm{M}} \right\}^T \dot{\theta} .$$ (16)

The inner product equation allows us to ascertain whether a muscle is producing or absorbing power by plotting the angular velocity and muscle torque vectors and measuring the angle between the two. If the included angle is less than 90°, the muscle is producing power; if greater, it is absorbing power.

These equations can be applied to the case of a positive work task performed first using single-joint muscles alone, and then with the addition of two-joint muscles. Even though the net torque vector has an acute angle with the angular velocity vector $\dot{\theta}$, as is required of positive work tasks, this need not be true for each individual muscle's torque vector (see figure 10.7a). When two-joint muscles are included (see figure 10.7b), they may make it possible to perform the same task but with all muscles producing positive work. There is therefore no need for one muscle to dissipate the power produced by another.

Ingen Schenau et al. (1987, 1988) claimed that this efficiency advantage is a unique property of two-joint muscles during contact and force tasks, but in fact the advantage can apply to other situations. First, any task can be described in terms of joint angles and angular velocities (which comprise the state of the system) and individual muscle torques (which may be thought of as the control input). The same power relationships demonstrated by Ingen Schenau, which are mathematically described in terms of torque and angular velocity vectors here, can occur in noncontact tasks. In fact, the example of figure 10.7 can apply to both contact and noncontact tasks because the presence of a constraint has not been specified and is not necessary. Second, because the efficiency advantage simply depends on the availability of a muscle whose torque vector is more closely aligned to the angular velocity vector than the torque vector of another muscle, a single-joint muscle can also function in this capacity.

We may therefore augment our previous conclusion regarding the distribution of torque vectors. A selection of torque vectors provides the potential to produce certain net torques with increased efficiency. Poor efficiency is not only a case of muscles producing torques that cancel each

a. Positive work task performed
with single-joint muscles

b.   Positive work task
performed with single- and two-

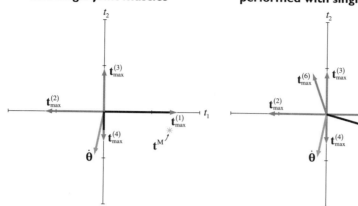

Figure 10.7

Example of a positive work task that is more efficient with a wider variety of muscles. *(a)* The task involves exerting an extensor torque about joint 1 and a flexor torque about joint 2, at a point in time when the joint angular velocities are such that both joints are flexing. This is a positive work task because the inner product of the net muscle torque vector $\mathbf{t}^M$ and angular velocity $\dot{\theta}$ is positive. In a system with few muscles—in this case single-joint muscles only—it is necessary for muscle to perform negative work, thereby absorbing power produced by muscle 4. *(b)* When the variety of muscles is increased—in this case with two-joint muscles— the same task can be performed with only one muscle. Here, muscle 5 performs positive work only. In other tasks, the roles of the single- and two-joint muscles may be reversed.

other; it may also involve some muscles absorbing the power produced by others. A wider variety of muscles increases the potential for the CNS to avoid both torque and power cancellation.

Are Two-Joint Muscles Really Unique?

We have reviewed a substantial body of literature addressing the role of two-joint muscles in a variety of tasks. The analyses we have considered are by and large correct. However, the majority of them have been used to argue that two-joint muscles have unique properties not shared by single-joint muscles—a conclusion that appears to be too narrow. It may seem contradictory, given the body of evidence, that we could arrive at such a conviction; but the preferable conclusion is that uniqueness is not exclusive to two-joint muscles. All muscles, by nature of unique origins, insertions, and moment arms, have unique actions. The differences between muscles are a matter of degree rather than of type, and to emphasize a classification based on the number of joints crossed is to disregard more important issues. Moreover, we conclude that different types of motions, such as contact or reaching tasks, alter the quantitative effect of each muscle but that they can all be explored using the same fundamental mathematics, for which all relevant distinctions are also a matter of degree rather than of type.

The mathematical approach reveals the fundamental principles of muscle coordination. Whether viewed in an output space of joint torques, joint angular accelerations, contact or reaction forces, or any combination of these outputs, each muscle contributes a vector component to a net output. These vectors point in different directions in output space, and there is an advantage, in terms of efficiency of force, torque, or power production, to having a variety of vector directions to choose from. Differences in vector directions are quantitative rather than qualitative in nature; and in most output spaces such as joint acceleration, there are no distinguishing features between single- and two-joint muscles.

Torque space is one output space in which single- and two-joint muscles might superficially appear to be distinct because single-joint muscles have output vectors aligned to the coordinate axes, and two-joint muscles do not. The choice of joint torque space is, however, somewhat arbitrary and subjective. The concept of joint torque is an abstraction made for our convenience of analysis rather than a quantity that is measurable or known to the CNS. In an alternative and equally sensible output space of segment torques, the distinction between single- and two-joint muscles is lost. Moreover, the classification of single joints is subjective because common "single joints" such as the ankle or shoulder are actually composed of multiple joints. Mathematically, an accurate and complete dynamical representation of a biomechanical system must in any case be given in terms of degrees of freedom (DOFs) rather than number of joints. Even when one considers the knee, there are varus/valgus moments that are relevant to joint and ligament loading. Lombard himself was careful, in his first paragraph, to qualify his claims by recognizing that he was neglecting DOFs such as abduction/adduction and inward/outward rotation. In nature, single-DOF or single-joint muscles are quite rare. In the human, the numerous muscles of the spine cross many DOFs, and in the lamprey there may not be any single-DOF muscles to be found; they may very well be a relatively recent evolutionary improvement upon multi-DOF muscles. There are significant concerns of objectivity and relevance for a classification scheme based on the number of joints crossed.

The legacy of Lombard's findings should therefore be that in explaining the function of two-joint muscles, he was exposing two common misconceptions. The first is the assumption that antagonism occurs only when two muscles cross opposite sides of a joint, and the second is that the moment arms or directions of torque production associated with a single muscle are sufficient to determine the direction of motion that occurs as the muscle shortens. Lombard's example disproves both of these assumptions. The analyses of Elftman (1939a), Enklaar (1954), and Landsmeer (1961) have further shown that in a multijoint system, the consequences of muscle activation occur about joints that are not even directly actuated.

These misconceptions arise because what is true of a single-joint system does not apply to multijoint systems. In a single-joint system, antagonism can occur only when two muscles are on opposite sides of the joint, and shortening of a muscle implies movement of the joint in the shortening direction. However, when we consider a multijoint system, no joint can be viewed in isolation. Vectors are useful for representing muscle function because they summarize how a muscle affects motion about all joints simultaneously. Using the vector approach, it is evident that there is an antagonistic component when practically any pair of muscles is activated. Even two single-joint muscles, crossing two different joints but on the same side, produce components of torque that cancel each other. Isometric constraint lines (figure 10.2) show that shortening of a muscle only restricts movements to a region of angular velocity space, admitting, as Lombard states, "extension of a joint which [the muscle] can flex" (Lombard 1903a, p. 143).

One advantage to the mathematical approach is that understanding of muscle coordination is made simpler. Instead of examining each muscle individually to decide if it should be activated as part of a motor task, it is more comprehensive simply to consider whether a muscle produces moments that contribute to the desired net action (Capozzo et al., 1976; Wells and Evans, 1987; Wells, 1988). In fact, a number of researchers have employed optimization to successfully predict muscle activation patterns without special classifications of two-joint muscles at all (Crowninshield and Brand, 1981; Dul et al., 1984; Pedersen et al., 1987; Patriarco et al., 1981; Herzog and Binding, 1992; Prilutsky et al., 1997; Pedotti et al., 1978). The large number of muscles and the large number of motor tasks make it unwieldy to classify and qualitatively describe how these muscles are used, in comparison to an approach that requires no special classification and can make quantitative predictions.

This approach is not meant to suggest that two-joint muscles are not interesting. The rectus femoris, hamstrings, and gastrocnemius muscles, for example, surely contribute to human gait in a unique manner (Elftman, 1939b; Prilutsky et al., 1998). However, for other motor tasks, there are other muscles crossing one or more joints that will act efficiently, allow transfer of energy, or exhibit other phenomena that have sometimes been attributed to two-joint muscles alone. Each muscle is unique and each provides a unique contribution to certain motor tasks. In turn, many motor tasks are likely to be coordinated so as to harness the action of these muscles. It is this important realization that has emerged from the pioneering studies of Duchenne, Lombard, and their contemporaries.

Acknowledgments

This work was supported in part by a grant from the Whitaker Foundation, NSF Grant IBN-9511814, and NIH Grant R29DC02312-01.

References

Aleshinsky, S.Y. (1986) An energy 'sources' and 'fractions' approach to the mechanical energy expenditure problem I-V. *J. Biomechanics* 19: 287-315.

An, K.N., Hui, F.C., Morrey, B.F., Linscheid, R.L., and Chao, E.Y. (1981) Muscles across the elbow joint: A biomechanical analysis. *J. Biomech.* 14: 659-69.

Andrews, J.G. (1985) A general method for determining the functional role of a muscle. *J. Biomech. Eng.* 107: 348-353.

Andrews, J.G. (1987) The functional roles of the hamstrings and quadriceps during cycling. Lombard's paradox revisited. *J. Biomech.* 20: 565-575.

Baeyer, H. von (1921) Zur Frage der mehrgclenkicen Muskeln. *Anat. Anz.* 54: 289-301.

Baeyer, H. von (1922) Modell zur Demonstration der Wirkung mehrgelenkiger Muskeln. *Z. fur Anat. und Entw.* 64: 276-278.

Baratta, R., Solomonov, M., Zhou, B.H., Leson, D., Chuinard, R., and Ambrosia, R.D. (1988) Muscular coactivation: The role of the antagonist musculature in maintaining knee stability. *Am. J. Sports Med.* 16: 113-122.

Bobbert, M.F., Hoek, E., and Ingen Schenau, G.J. van (1987) A model to demonstrate the power transporting role of bi-articular muscles. *J. Physiol.* 387: 24P.

Bobbert, M.F., Huijing, P.A., and Ingen Schenau, G.J. van (1986a) A model of human triceps surae muscle-tendon complex applied to jumping. *J. Biomech.* 11: 887-898.

Bobbert, M.F., Huijing, P.A., and Ingen Schenau, G.J. van (1986b) An estimation of power output and work done by human triceps surae muscle-tendon complex in jumping. *J. Biomech.* 11: 899-906.

Borelli, J.A. (1685) *De motu animalium. Pars prima* (cited by Fick, 1879).

Capozzo, A., Figura, F., Marchetti, M., and Pedotti, A. (1976) The interplay of muscular and external forces in human ambulation. *J. Biomech.* 9: 35-43.

Carlsöö, S., and Molbech, S. (1966) The functions of certain two-joint muscles in a closed muscular chain. *Acta Morphol. Neerl.-Scand.* 6: 377-386.

Cleland, J. (1867) On the actions of muscles passing over more than one joint. *J. Anat. and Physiol.* 1: 85-93.

Crowninshield, R.D., and Brand, R.A. (1981). A physiologically based criterion of muscle force prediction in locomotion. *J. Biomech.* 14: 793-801.

Donskoi, D.D. (1961*) Biomechanik der Körperübungen.* Berlin: Sportverlag.

Doorenbosch, C.A.M., Harlaar, J., Roebroeck, M.E., and Lankhorst, G.J. (1994) Two strategies of transferring from sit-to-stand; the activation of monoarticular and biarticular muscles. *J. Biomech.* 27: 1299-1307.

Doorenbosch, C.A.M., and Ingen Schenau, G.J. van (1995) The role of mono- and bi-articular muscles during contact control tasks in man. *Hum. Movement Sci.* 14: 279-300.

Duchenne, G.B. (1867) *Physiologie des mouvements.* Paris: J.B. Baillière. Translated by E.B. Kaplan (1949). Philadelphia: W.B. Saunders & Co.

Duchenne, G.B. (1885) *Physiologie tind Bewegungen.* Th. Fischer u. Cassel.

Dul, J., Townsend, M.A., Shiavi, R., and Johnson, G.E. (1984) Muscular synergism—1. On criteria for load sharing between synergistic muscles. *J. Biomech.* 17: 663-673.

Elftman, H. (1939a) Forces and energy changes in the leg during walking. *Am. J. Physiol.* 125: 339-356.

Elftman, H. (1939b) The function of muscles in locomotion. *Am. J. Physiol.* 125: 357-366.

Elftman, H. (1966) Biomechanics of muscle. *J. Bone Joint Surg.* 48A: 363-377.

Enklaar, M.J.E. (1954) Antagonisme entre demi-tendineux et demi-membraneux chez l'homme, 6ième Congrès de la Société Internationale de Chirurgie orthopédique et de Traumatologie, 558-572. Bruxelles: Impr. Des Sciences.

Fenn, W.O. (1932) Zur Mechanik des Radfahrens in Vergleich zu der des Laufens. *Pflügers Arch. ges. Physiol.* 229: 354.

Fenn, W.O. (1938) The mechanics of muscular contraction in man. *J. Appl. Physics* 9: 165-177.

Fick, A.E. (1879) Über zweigelenkige Muskeln. *Archiv. Anat. u. Entw. Gesch.* 3: 201-239.

Fischer, K. (1927) Zur geführten Wirkung der mehrgelenkigen Muskeln. *Zeittschr. F. Anat. u. Entw. gesch. Anat. I. Abt.* 83: 752-770.

Fischer, O. (1902a) Kritik der gebrauchlichen Methoden die Wirkung eines Muskelns zu bestimmen. *Abhandlungen der Königlich sächsischen Gesellschaft der Wissenschaften. Mathematische-Physische Klass* 22: 483-590.

Fischer, O. (1902b) Das statische und kinetsche Mass für die Wirkung eines Muskels, erläutert an ein- und zweigelenkigen Muskeln des Obserschenkels. *Abhandlungen der Königlich sächsischen Gesellschaft der Wissenschaften. Mathematische-Physische Klasse* 27.

Fujiwara, M., and Basmajian, J. (1975) Electromyographic study of two-joint muscles. *Am. J. Phys. Med.* 54: 234-242.

Gielen, C.C.A.M., Ingen Schenau, G.J. van, Tax, A.A.M., and Theeuwen, M. (1990) The activation of mono-articular muscles in multi-joint movements. In: J. Winters and S. L. Y. Woo (eds.), *Multiple muscle systems*, pp. 302-311. New York: Springer-Verlag.

Gregor, R.J., Cavanagh, P.R., and Lafortune, M. (1985) Knee flexor moments during propulsion in cycling—A creative solution to Lombard's Paradox. *J. Biomech.* 18: 307-316.

Hering, H.E. (1897) Über die Wirkung zweigelenkiger Muskeln auf drei Gelenke und über die pseudo-antagonistische Synergie. *Archiv. für die gesammte Physiologie* 65: 627-637.

Herzog, W., and Binding, P. (1992) Predictions of antagonistic muscular activity using nonlinear optimization. *Math. Biosci.* 111: 217-229.

Herzog, W., and Binding, P. (1994) Effects of replacing 2-joint muscles with energetically equivalent 1-joint muscles on cost-function values of nonlinear optimization approaches. *Hum. Movement Sci.* 13: 569-586.

Hogan, N. (1985) The mechanics of multi-joint posture and movement control. *Biol. Cybernetics* 52: 315-331.

Hollerbach, J., and Flash, T. (1982) Dynamic interactions between limb segments during planar arm movement. *Biol. Cybernetics* 44: 67-77.

Hunter, J. (1797) Croonian lectures on muscular motion, no. II. In: J.F. Palmer (ed.), *The works of John Hunter.* London: Longman, Rees, Orme, Brown Green and Longman, 1837, pp. 195-273.

Hüter, C. (1863) Anatomische Studien an den Extremitatengelenken Neugeborenen und Erwachsener. *Arch. f. path. Anat. und Physiol. und klinische Medizin* 28: 253-281.

Hüter, C. (1869) Über Längeninsufficienz der bi- und polyarthrodalen Muskeln. Ihre Bedeutung für die Muskelkraft. *Arch. f. path. Anat. und Physiol. und klinische Medizin* 46: 37-40.

Ingen Schenau, G.J. van (1989a) From rotation to translation: Constraints on multi-joint movements and the unique action of bi-articular muscles. *Hum. Movement Sci.* 8: 301-337.

Ingen Schenau, G.J. van (1989b) From rotation to translation: Implications for theories of motor control. *Hum. Movement Sci.* 8: 423-442.

Ingen Schenau, G.J. van (1989c) Dynamical approaches and biomechanics. *Hum. Movement Sci.* 8: 543-546.

Ingen Schenau, G.J. van (1990) On the action of bi-articular muscles, a review. *Netherlands J. Zool.* 40: 521-540.

Ingen Schenau, G.J. van (1998) Positive work and its efficiency are at their dead-end: Comments on a recent discussion. *J. Biomech.* 31: 195-198.

Ingen Schenau, G.J. van, Bobbert, M.F., de Graaf, J.B., and Tettero, W.E. (1988) The action of bi-articular muscles in explosive movements. In: N. Berme and A. Cappozzo (eds.), *Biomechanics of human movement.* Dordrecht: Martinus Nijhoff.

Ingen Schenau, G.J. van, Bobbert, M.F., and Rozendal, R.H. (1987) The unique action of bi-articular muscles in complex movements. *J. Anat.* 155: 1-5.

Ingen Schenau, G.J. van, Bobbert, M.F., and van Soest, A.J. (1990) The unique action of biarticular muscles in leg extensions. In: J. Winters and S. L. Y. Woo (eds.), *Multiple muscle systems*, pp. 639-652. New York: Springer-Verlag.

Ingen Schenau, G.J. van, and Cavanagh, P.R. (1990). Power equations in endurance sports. *J. Biomech.* 23: 865-881.

Ingen Schenau, G.J. van, Dorssers, W.M.M., Welter, T.G., Beelen, A., de Groot, G., and Jacobs, R. (1995) The control of mono-articular muscles in multijoint leg extensions in man. *J. Physiol.* (London) 484: 247-254.

Jacobs, R., and Ingen Schenau, G.J. van (1992) Control of external force in leg extensions in humans. *J. Physiol.* (London) 457: 611-626.

Kuo, A.D. (1994) A mechanical analysis of force distribution between redundant, multiple degree-of-freedom actuators in the human: Implications for the central nervous system. *Hum. Movement Sci.* 13: 635-663.

Kuo, A.D. (1998) A least-squares estimation approach to improving the precision of inverse dynamics computations. *J. Biomech. Eng.* 120: 148-159.

Kuo, A.D., and Zajac, F.E. (1993) Human standing posture: Multijoint movement strategies based on biomechanical constraints. In: J.H.J. Allum, D.J. Allum-Mecklenburg, F.P. Harris, and R. Probst (eds.), *Progress in Brain Research* 9: 349-358. Amsterdam: Elsevier.

Landsmeer, J.M.F. (1961) Studies in the anatomy of articulation H. *Acta Morphol. Neerl.-Scand* 3: 304-321.

Langer, C. (1879) Die Muskulatur der Extremitäten des Orang als Grundlage einer vergleichendmytoiogischen Untersuchung. *Sitztingsberichte der kaiserlichen Akademie der Wissenschaften Math-Naturwissens. Class. Bd.* 79: 177-219.

Lombard, W.P. (1903a) The action of two-joint muscles. *Am. Phys. Educ. Rev* 9: 141-145.

Lombard, W.P. (1903b) The tendon action and leverage of two-joint muscles of the hind leg of the frog, with special reference of the spring movement. In: G. Wahr (ed.), *Contributions to medical research,* pp. 280-301. Ann Arbor, MI: Ann Arbor Science.

Lombard, W.P., and Abbott, F.M. (1907) The mechanical effects produced by contraction of individual muscles of the thigh of the frog. *Am. J. Physiol.* 20: 1-60.

Markee, J.E., Logue, J.T., Williams, M., Stanton, W.B., Wrenn, R.N., and Walker, L.B. (1955) Two-joint muscles of the thigh. *J. Bone Joint Surg.* 37: 125-142.

May, M.T. (1968) *Galen: On the usefulness of the parts of the body.* Ithaca, NY: Cornell University Press.

Molbech, S. (1966) On the paradoxical effect of some two-joint muscles. *Acta Morphol. Neerl.-Scand.* 4: 171-178.

Patriarco, A.B., Mann, R.W., Simon, S.R., and Masour, J.M. (1981) An evaluation of the approaches of optimization models in the prediction of muscle forces during gait. *J. Biomech.* 14: 513-525.

Pedersen, D.R., Brand, R.A., Cheng, C., and Arora, J.S. (1987) Direct comparisons of muscle force predictions using linear and nonlinear programming. *J. Biomech. Eng.* 109: 192-199.

Pedotti, A., Krishnan, V.V., and Stork, L. (1978) Optimization of muscle-force sequencing in human locomotion. *Math. Biosci.* 38: 57-76.

Prilutsky, B.I., and Gregor, R.J. (1997) Strategy of muscle coordination of two- and one-joint leg muscles in controlling an external force. *Motor Control* 1: 92-116.

Prilutsky, B.I., Gregor, R.J., and Ryan, M.M. (1998) Coordination of two-joint rectus femoris and hamstrings during the swing phase of human walking and running. *Exper. Brain Res.* 120: 479-486.

Prilutsky, B.I., Herzog, W., and Allinger, T.L. (1997) Forces of individual cat ankle extensor muscles during locomotion predicted using static optimization. *J. Biomech.* 30: 1025-1033.

Prilutsky, B.I., and Zatsiorsky, V.M. (1994) Tendon action of two-joint muscles: Transfer of mechanical energy between joints during jumping, landing, and running. *J. Biomech.* 27: 25-34.

Sergio, L.E., and Ostry, D.J. (1994) Coordination of mono- and bi-articular muscles in multidegree of freedom elbow movements. *Exper. Brain Res.* 97: 551-555.

Soest, A.J. van, Schwab, A.L., Bobbert, M.F., and Ingen Schenau, G.J. van (1993) The influence of the biarticularity of the gastrocnemius muscle on vertical-jumping achievement. *J. Biomech.* 20: 1-8.

Strasser, H. (1917) *Lehrbuch der Muskel- und Gelenkmechanik. III: Die untere Extremität.* Berlin: Julius Springer.

Wells, R.P. (1988) Mechanical energy costs of human movement: An approach to evaluating the transfer possibilities of two-joint muscles. *J. Biomech.* 11: 955-964.

Wells, R.P., and Evans, N.C. (1987) Functions and recruitment patterns of one- and two-joint muscles under isometric and walking conditions. *Hum. Movement Sci.* 6: 349-372.

Zajac, F.E., and Gordon, M.E. (1990) Determining muscle's force and action in multi-articular movement. In: K. Pandolf (ed.), *Exerc. and Sport Sci. Reviews* 17 (ch. 6): 187-230. Baltimore, MD: Williams & Wilkins.

Appendix

The example system consists of two links that rotate in the plane about two hinge joints. There are six muscles actuating the links, four of which cross a single joint and two of which cross two joints. The mass of each link is $M = 3$ kg, and the length is $L = 0.3$ m. Each link is also of uniform density with the inertial properties of a thin rod. The equations of motion are described in equation (7), where the following quantities are defined:

$$\mathbf{M}(\theta) \equiv \begin{bmatrix} \frac{5}{3}ML^2 - ML^2\cos\theta_2 & -\frac{1}{3}ML^2 + \frac{1}{2}ML^2\cos\theta_2 \\ -\frac{1}{3}ML^2 + \frac{1}{2}ML^2\cos\theta_2 & \frac{1}{3}ML^2 \end{bmatrix},$$

$$\mathbf{v}(\theta,\dot{\theta}) \equiv \begin{bmatrix} \sin\theta_2\left(-ML^2\dot{\theta}_1\dot{\theta}_2 + \frac{1}{2}ML^2\dot{\theta}_2^2\right) \\ \frac{1}{2}ML^2\dot{\theta}_1^2\sin\theta_2 \end{bmatrix}, \mathbf{g}(\theta) \equiv \begin{bmatrix} 0 \\ 0 \end{bmatrix}.$$

The muscles are specified as follows. The moment arm matrix is

$$R \equiv \begin{bmatrix} 0.03 & -0.03 & 0 & 0 & 0.035 & -0.01 \\ 0 & 0 & 0.03 & -0.03 & -0.01 & 0.03 \end{bmatrix} \text{m}.$$

As an example of the sign convention, muscle 1 has an extension moment arm about joint 1, as does muscle 5 but with the addition of a flexion moment arm about joint 2. The maximum isometric forces are

$$\mathbf{f}^{\max} \equiv \begin{bmatrix} 2500 & 2000 & 1500 & 1000 & 2500 & 1500 \end{bmatrix}^T \text{N}.$$

The transformation from joint angular accelerations to endpoint (or center of mass) accelerations involves a simple matrix multiplication. The endpoint accelerations are

$$\begin{bmatrix} \ddot{x} \\ \ddot{y} \end{bmatrix} = \mathbf{J}(\theta) \cdot \ddot{\theta} + \dot{\mathbf{J}}(\theta) \cdot \dot{\theta}$$

where $\ddot{\theta}$ is found using equation (7) and

$$\mathbf{J}(\theta) \equiv \begin{bmatrix} \left[L\sin\theta_1 - L\sin(\theta_1 - \theta_2) & L\sin(\theta_1 - \theta_2) \right] \\ \left[L\cos\theta_1 - L\cos(\theta_1 - \theta_2) & L\cos(\theta_1 - \theta_2) \right] \end{bmatrix}.$$

Two slot constraints are employed. In the example of figure 10.5, the slot constraint prevents horizontal motion, and the constraint equations (9) and (10) use the quantities

$$\gamma_x(\theta) \equiv -L\cos\theta_1 + L\cos(\theta_1 - \theta_2) - c_x$$

and

$$\mathbf{J}_x(\theta) \equiv \begin{bmatrix} L\sin\theta_1 - L\sin(\theta_1 - \theta_2) & L\sin(\theta_1 - \theta_2) \end{bmatrix}.$$

In the example of figure 10.6, the slot constrains vertical motion, and the corresponding quantities are

$$\gamma_y(\theta) \equiv L\sin\theta_1 - L\sin(\theta_1 - \theta_2) - c_y,$$
$$\mathbf{J}_y(\theta) \equiv \begin{bmatrix} L\cos\theta_1 - L\cos(\theta_1 - \theta_2) & L\cos(\theta_1 - \theta_2) \end{bmatrix}.$$

For the constrained system of figure 10.6, the equations of motion (7) are combined with the constraint (11), yielding the constrained accelerations (figure 10.6a)

$$\begin{bmatrix} \ddot{\theta}_1 \\ \ddot{\theta}_2 \end{bmatrix} = \begin{bmatrix} C_{11} & C_{12} \\ C_{12} & C_{22} \end{bmatrix} \cdot \mathbf{t}^M + \begin{bmatrix} C_{10} \\ C_{20} \end{bmatrix}$$

where

$$C_{11} \equiv \frac{12}{ML^2 d}\cos^2(\theta_1 - \theta_2),\ C_{12} \equiv \frac{12}{ML^2 d}\left(\cos\theta_1 \cos(\theta_1 - \theta_2) - \cos^2(\theta_1 - \theta_2)\right),$$

$$C_{22} \equiv \frac{24}{ML^2 d}\left(\cos\theta_1 - \cos(\theta_1 - \theta_2)\right)\sin\left(\theta_1 - \frac{\theta_2}{2}\right)\sin\frac{\theta_2}{2},$$

$$C_{10} \equiv \frac{1}{d}\begin{pmatrix} \left(-\sin 2\theta_1 + \sin(2\theta_1 - \theta_2) + 5\sin\theta_2 - 3\sin 2\theta_2\right)\dot{\theta}_1^2 + \\ \left(\sin(2\theta_1 - \theta_2) + 5\sin\theta_2\right)\left(2\dot{\theta}_1\dot{\theta}_2 - \dot{\theta}_2^2\right) \end{pmatrix},$$

$$C_{20} \equiv \frac{1}{d}\begin{pmatrix} \left(\sin 2\theta_1 + 5\sin 2(\theta_1 - \theta_2) - 6\sin(2\theta_1 - \theta_2) - 16\sin\theta_2 + 6\sin 2\theta_2\right)\dot{\theta}_1^2 + \\ \left(-5\sin 2(\theta_1 - \theta_2) + \sin(2\theta_1 - \theta_2) + 5\sin\theta_2 - 3\sin 2\theta_2\right)\left(2\dot{\theta}_1\dot{\theta}_2 - \dot{\theta}_2^2\right) \end{pmatrix},$$

$$d \equiv -7 + \cos 2\theta_1 - 5\cos(2\theta_1 - 2\theta_2) + 3\cos 2\theta_2.$$

In terms of the output space of motion along the constraint (11) and the normal force against the constraint, the quantities in equation (12) are

$$K_1 = \frac{-12}{MLd} \cos(\theta_1 - \theta_2)\sin\theta_2, \quad K_2 = \frac{12}{MLd}\left(\cos\theta_1 \sin\theta_2 - \cos(\theta_1 - \theta_2)\sin\theta_2\right),$$

$$K_0 = \frac{L}{d}\left[\begin{array}{l} 4\left(\cos\theta_1 + 5\cos(\theta_1 - \theta_2)\sin\left(\frac{\theta_2}{2}\right)^2\right)\dot{\theta}_1^2 + \\ \left(-9\cos(\theta_1 - \theta_2) + \cos(\theta_1 + \theta_2)\right)\left(2\dot{\theta}_1\dot{\theta}_2 - \dot{\theta}_2^2\right) \end{array}\right],$$

$$S_1 = \cos\theta_1 - 3\cos(\theta_1 - 2\theta_2), \quad S_2 = \cos\theta_1 - 3\cos(\theta_1 - 2\theta_2)$$
$$+13\cos(\theta_1 - \theta_2) - 3\cos(\theta_1 + \theta_2),$$

$$S_0 = \frac{ML}{6d}\left[\begin{array}{l} \left(\sin\theta_1 - 15\sin(\theta_1 - 2\theta_2) + 17\sin(\theta_1 - \theta_2) - 3\sin(\theta_1 + \theta_2)\right)\dot{\theta}_1^2 + \\ 2\left(-17\sin(\theta_1 - \theta_2) + 3\sin(\theta_1 + \theta_2)\right)\left(2\dot{\theta}_1\dot{\theta}_z - \dot{\theta}_2^2\right) \end{array}\right].$$

The constraint forces are derived using application of Newton's law and are described in more detail by, for example, Kuo (1998).

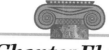

Chapter Eleven

Sir Charles S. Sherrington: Humanist, Mentor, and Movement Neuroscientist

Douglas G. Stuart, Patricia A. Pierce, Robert J. Callister, Alan M. Brichta, and Jennifer C. McDonagh

Department of Physiology, University of Arizona, USA (D.G.S., P.A.P.); Discipline of Anatomy, University of Newcastle, Australia (R.J.C., A.M.B.); and Arizona School of Health Sciences, USA (J.C.M.)

Revisiting the work of Sir Charles S. Sherrington

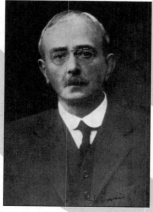

Sir Charles S. Sherrington
Reprinted from Sherrington 1953.

Dedication

This article is dedicated to Emeritus Professor Anders Lundberg, Department of Physiology, University of Göteborg, Sweden, for his research and mentoring contributions to movement neuroscience, and for his development of the concepts of segmental interneuronal convergence and alternative spinal reflex pathways.

Introduction

Standard textbooks on the neural control of movement emphasize the continual interplay between excitation and inhibition within the central nervous system (CNS), from the neurons of the most rostral portions of the forebrain to the brainstem and spinal motoneurons whose output creates movement. Furthermore, much is made of the fact that the cerebellar cortex, a key central structure in the planning and modulation of movement, has an output to deep cerebellar nuclei and brainstem neurons that is exclusively inhibitory (Ito and Yoshida, 1966; Ito, 1970; Llinas, 1997). It is important for students of movement science to appreciate, however, that in the late 19th century it was a daunting challenge to prove that CNS inhibition is indeed an active process rather than simply an abatement (or withdrawal) of excitation. The demonstration of active inhibition led to the awarding of two Nobel Prizes in the 20th century, one (albeit indirectly) in 1932 to Sir Charles Sherrington (1857-1952), and one in 1963 to his former trainee, Sir John Eccles, for work that included the electrophysiological proof of this critically important phenomenon.

In this chapter, we present Sherrington's Nobel Lecture on his study of CNS inhibition. From the outset, we have stressed his admirable humanistic and mentoring capabilities, which are still having a beneficial effect as the 21st century begins.

Three excellent accounts have been written about Sherrington and his contributions by four of his former trainees. These include a biographical memoir for the Royal Society by Eric Liddell (1952) and books by Ragnar Granit (1966) and Eccles and Gibson (1979). In addition, a valuable perspective has been provided by the medical historian, Judith Swazey (1969). These four publications cite innumerable other accounts of Sherrington's contributions to humanism, neuroscience, and philosophy. Also, they are written with such élan and verve that they should be experienced firsthand by a dedicated student of movement neuroscience. In this paper we have focused on selected features of Sherrington's research and mentoring contributions.

Sherrington: The Man and Scientist

After initial medical training at St. Thomas's Hospital Medical School (London, U.K.), Sherrington graduated from Cambridge University with first-class honors in natural science (including botany, human physiology and anatomy, and zoology) in 1883, and with a medical degree in 1885. Although relatively slight of build, he was, from an early age, an enthusiastic and accomplished athlete (soccer, rugby football, rowing, and later, alpine sports). Most remarkably, he was also a lifelong and well-respected classicist, humanist, and poet. His postdoctoral training in neurohistology and pathology included stints at the Universities of Strasbourg (about nine months in 1884-1885; then part of Germany) and Berlin (several months in 1986-1987). This overseas training was undertaken more or less in parallel with valuable and adventurous clinical and fine-arts trips to Spain (summer of 1885) and Italy (summer of 1886). His academic (including teaching) postings were, in order, at St. Thomas's Hospital Medical School (University of London) as an anatomy demonstrator (1883-1984) and later as a lecturer in physiology (1887-1895); in parallel positions as physician-superintendent at the Brown Institution of Preventative Medicine (University of London; 1891-1895) and at Cambridge University as a fellow and tutor (1887-1895); at the University of Liverpool as the professor of physiology (1895-1912); and at the University of Oxford as the professor of physiology (1913-1936). He retired in 1936 at the age of almost 79 years. Sherrington's first scientific paper was published in 1884 when he was 27 years of age; his last in 1953, one year after his death at the age of 95 years. In this 69-year span, he had over 320 scientific publications. Eccles and Gibson (1979) have emphasized that from the age of 68 in 1925 until 75 in 1932, Sherrington was regarded internationally as ". . . the great integrator of knowledge of the central nervous system . . ." (p. ix). Thereafter, until 1936, he returned to neurohistological research. Subsequent to his retirement (1936) and until his death in 1952, he published on the interface between neuroscience and humanistic/philosophical discourse on humankind and its nature. In these later years of his life, he never lost contact with the advances and rigor of neuroscience research. This is exemplified in the precision and fervor of his 1948 BBC radio lecture on the then-current status of neuroscience, which he delivered at the remarkable age of 91 years (Sherrington, 1948).

Scientific Achievements

It has been claimed that Sherrington ". . . achieved for the nervous system what William Harvey achieved for the circulation" (Liddell, 1952; p. 259). In support of this strong statement, table 11.1 lists Sherrington's major contributions to neuroscience in general and to movement science in particular. For his substantial contributions to other areas of biomedical science (including academic clinical medicine, public health, and educational issues), the reader is referred to Liddell (1952) and Eccles and Gibson (1979).

Table 11.1   A Selected List of Sherrington's Major Contributions to Overall Neuroscience and to Movement Neuroscience

	Delineation	Concept(s)	Current state-of-the-play
Overall neuroscience			
with Foster (1897); with Schäfer (1900); (1906a)		Importance of synapse in reflexes and behavior	Kandel et al. (2000)
(1925a, 1932, 1934)		Active inhibition as a coordinative CNS mechanism	Strauss et al. (1992); Strausfeld et al. (1998); Mizunami et al. (1998a-b); Rothwell (1994)
(1893 to 1909[1]); (1925a)	Reciprocal innervation	Active inhibition	Davidoff (1997); Jonas et al. (1998)
Suprasegmental motor control			
(1889)	Cortex-pyramidal degenerations	Function of the corticomotoneuronal system	Fetz et al. (1989); Wiesendanger (1997a, b)
with Mott (1895)	Arm movements following limb deafferentation	Segmental convergence of descending command and sensory feedback signals	Jankowska and Lundberg (1981); Georgopoulos (1996a)
with Grunbaum[2] (1901, 1917)	Functional organization of sensorimotor cortex		Wise (1997); Georgopoulos (1996b, 1997)
Segmental motor control			
A			
(1894, 1924)	Sensory nature of muscle spindles and Golgi tendon organs	Muscles as sense as well as force organs	Matthews (1972); Taylor and Prochazka (1981); Hasan and Stuart (1988); Gandevia and Burke (1992); Taylor et al. (1995); Prochazka (1996, 1999); Proske et al. (2000)
(1918)	Sensory role of extraocular muscles		
(1892a, 1910a)	Functional anatomy of spinal cord-muscle connectivity		Lundberg (1969b); Baldissera et al. (1981); Burke (1985); McCrea (1992); Jankowska (1992); Jordan (1998);

	Delineation	Concept(s)	Current state-of-the-play
(1892a, 1910a) (continued)			Matsuyama and Mori (1998); Fetz et al. (1999); Katz and Pierrot-Deseilligny (1999); Schieppati and Nardone (1999)
(1904, 1906b, 1910a, 1925a, 1931[2]) with Liddell (1924, 1925b) with Eccles (1931) with Creed et al. (1932)	Reflex play of one muscle's (and/or dermatome's) sensory input upon another muscle and/or movement	Central excitatory vs. inhibitory state; disynaptic pathway; final common path; integrative reflex action; spatiotemporal summation	
(1898)	Decerebrate rigidity		
B			
with Liddell (1925b); (1929a, 1931)		Motor unit (i.e., motoneuron and its muscle unit)	Burke (1981); Henneman and Mendell (1981); Binder and Mendell (1990); Binder et al. (1996); Cope and Sokoloff (1999)
with Creed et al. (1932)		Discharge zone and subliminal fringe	
C			
(1906b, 1910b-c)	Scratch reflex, spinal stepping, and reflex standing	Sensory feedback modulation of movement	Stein et al. (1997); Kiehn et al. (1998)

Note: This table divides a selection of Sherrington's movement neuroscience contributions into three themes (neuroscience in general; suprasegmental motor control; segmental motor control), and one of these, segmental motor control, into three areas of the modern-day definition of the segmental motor system (A, properties and central action of muscle and other limb receptors; B, motoneurons, motor units, and the size principle; and C, spinal pattern generation). For each, two categories of contribution are considered: *delineation,* i.e., those in which experiments were undertaken to advance general understanding of the functional organization of the CNS and the peripheral neuromuscular system; and *concept,* those in which the goal was somewhat more theoretical (almost teleological) in order to arrive at a far-reaching concept. Each finding and/or concept is considered to have modern-day follow-ups, the most recent of which is/are cited. For further details, see the text.

Footnotes: [1]Sherrington devoted 13 articles specifically to reciprocal inhibition, including that of antagonistic eye muscles. A 14th article addressed double reciprocal innervation. [2]After his early 1880s training (table 11.2), Sherrington published several articles on corticospinal connections (1901 to 1917, the experimental work for the most definitive of which [1917: with Leyton nee Grunbaum] was completed over a decade earlier [see Swazey, 1969; p. 18]).

Contributions to Neuroscience

Sherrington made three lasting conceptual contributions to neuroscience: incorporation of the synapse into reflexology and behavioral science; active inhibition as a *coordinative* mechanism within the CNS; and the closely allied concept that inhibition is an *active* rather than passive process.

Incorporation of the Synapse Into Reflexology and Behavioral Science. Even though Santiago Ramón Y Cajal (1852-1934; Madrid University, Spain) shared a Nobel Prize in 1906 with Camillo Golgi (1843-1926; Pavia University, Italy) for their work on the structure of the nervous system, they differed profoundly on their concept of brain organization. Until his demise, Golgi favored the concept of a reticular syncytium of neurons, whereas Cajal promulgated the "neuron doctrine" involving an organization of essentially separate neurons. The latter took hold quite early on. This was due in part to the work of Augustus Waller (1816-1870), who had shown (1850) that degeneration in the peripheral portion of a cut nerve (Wallerian degeneration) generally stopped short of the next neuron (for additional references, see Langley and Sherrington, 1891; p. 284). Other early important contributors to the neuron doctrine were Hans Held and Leopold Auerbach II (Granit, 1966; ch. 2). Of particular importance were Sherrington's published viewpoints that emphasized the functional significance of the neuron doctrine. Presumably, he was convinced that his own results on the physiology of spinal reflexes (see later) were best explained by Cajal's essentially morphological (albeit remarkably intuitive) concepts. Sherrington and Sir Michael Foster (1836-1907) together coined the term "synapsis" (Greek origin; a "clasp," "connection," or "junction") and used it in Foster's 1897 textbook (p. 929) with the anatomical findings and theories of Cajal well in mind. Synapsis later became "synaptic knob" for the morphological structure of a unitary presynaptic-postsynaptic complex. Shortly thereafter, Sherrington introduced the term "synapse" (Greek verb for "to join"; later employed for function and/or general usage) in Sir Edward Schäfer's (1900) widely read textbook of physiology: "The synapses are fewest; in some, perhaps there intervenes but one synapse . . ." (p. 834). In his renowned 1906 text, *Integrative Action of the Nervous System*, which was the published version of his 1904 Silliman Lectures at Yale University, Sherrington stated with even more impact that "in the neurone-chains of the grey-centred system of vertebrates, histology on the whole furnishes evidence that a surface of separation does exist between neurone and neurone [later called the "synaptic cleft"; about 20-40 nm in width]. . . . The characters distinguishing reflex-arc conduction from nerve-trunk conduction may therefore be largely due to intercellular barriers. . . . It is convenient to have a term for it. The term introduced has been synapse [i.e., citing his chapter in Foster (1897)]" (p. 17).

Thus, the functional jump-start that Sherrington (and others) provided to Cajal's neuron doctrine had a resounding worldwide effect on neuroscience research. It is still thought-provoking to review Cajal's 1933 final summing (English translation in 1954), one year before his death, and to consider that some still argue that ". . . the definitive disproof of the reticular doctrine and confirmation of the neuron doctrine had to await the electron microscope [i.e., demonstration of the existence of the synaptic cleft by Palade and Palay in 1954]. . ." (Gross, 1997; p. 1). Irrespective of this argument, to provide the modern-day follow-up to Sherrington's contributions on the synapse, the authors have simply cited in table 11.1 two current, widely used textbooks of neuroscience. Virtually all aspects of these textbooks (Kandel et al., 2000; Zigmond et al., 1999) cover material requiring consideration of synaptic mechanisms, the key device employed by nature to create and process information, including the ideation, planning, elaboration, and ongoing control of movement.

Active Inhibition As a Coordinative Central Nervous System Mechanism. Sherrington entitled his 1932 Nobel Lecture "Inhibition as a Coordinative Factor." By this he meant that within the CNS, inhibition is (1) as important as excitation in the control of CNS mechanisms that initiate and control movement and (2) continually interacting (coordinating) with excitation to achieve a smooth control of movement. For example, in the cyclical elaboration of a locomotor step cycle, it is necessary for the CNS to provide a cyclical excitation of motoneurons supplying extensor muscles that is coordinated with a similarly cyclical inhibition of motoneurons to flexor muscles (and vice versa). Without such coordination of excitation and inhibition to the relevant motoneurons, the step cycle could not ensue in a smooth and efficient manner.

In his lecture, Sherrington went well beyond his own results, which were largely restricted to the spinal cord, to expound the concept that "In the working of the central nervous machinery inhibition seems as ubiquitous and as frequent as is excitation itself. The whole quantitative grading of the operations of the spinal cord and brain appears to rest upon mutual interaction between the two central processes «excitation» and «inhibition», the one no less important than the other" (1932; p. 288). For Western neuroscience in 1932, this was an original and bold concept—while for Russian neuroscience, influenced as it was by Ivan Sechenov (1829-1905; Brazier, 1959) and the 1904 Nobel laureate, Ivan Pavlov (1849-1936; Schultz and Schultz, 1992), Sherrington's approach to inhibition was a critically challenging, albeit important and fresh (i.e., with its *synaptic* emphasis) complement to their neuroscientists' collective work on central inhibition (Jeannerod, 1985; see also endnote 8). As emphasized by Granit (1966), "Whatever other mechanisms could be forced [meaning found] to explain central excitation and inhibition, as the balance of evidence stood when Sherrington, after forty years of experimentation, laid down his tools, it must be concluded that he had definitely established *synaptic* excitation and *synaptic* inhibition as the mirror images of two genuine and opposite processes. These had been endowed with properties which in a decisive manner guided experimentation in this field in the future" (p. 83).

The coordinative nature of inhibition has subsequently been borne out time and again. For example, for modern-day follow-ups, the movement neuroscience reader is referred to the higher centers in insect brains in which the central body complex (Strauss et al., 1992) may play crucial roles in orchestrating limb movements with another center, the mushroom bodies, having a cardinal position in context-dependent sensory selection, motor reafferent integration, and place memory (Strausfeld et al., 1998; Mizunami et al., 1998a-b). The reader is also referred to chapters on the mammalian motor cortex, basal ganglia, and cerebellum in Rothwell (1994). In all these cases, including interactions between key structures in both the invertebrate and vertebrate brain, there are numerous examples of the interplay between excitatory and inhibitory processes, as demonstrated with techniques far more advanced than were available in Sherrington's day.

Inhibition As an Active Rather Than Passive Process. Sherrington emphasized in his Nobel Lecture that he was not the first to propose that within the CNS, inhibition was an active process. His results on this issue were far more convincing, however, than those of previous workers or of Sherrington's contemporaries. His most clear-cut demonstration of active inhibition was based on results described in 13 reports between 1893 and 1908 on the reciprocal innervation (term first used in his 1897 report) of antagonistic, largely hindlimb (but also eye) muscles of the decerebrate cat. A 14th note in 1909 addressed double reciprocal innervation.

Early on, Sherrington realized that reflex inhibition was the key to understanding reciprocal innervation and that by its action, reflex muscle activation could be *graded* (i.e., the origin of his focus on inhibition as a coordinative mechanism, as previously discussed). Interestingly, Sherrington was ever willing to concede that reciprocal innervation had originally been described by the Bell brothers (Charles and John) in 1822. These earlier observations had been long forgotten, however, before their resurrection by Sherrington himself.

The modern-day follow-up to active CNS inhibition spans more than a century of technological developments to allow, for example, paired patch-clamp recordings from synaptically connected neurons to advance understanding of inhibitory postsynaptic currents across selected ion channels (for review, Davidoff, 1997; for the current state-of-the-play, Jonas et al., 1998).

Contributions on Suprasegmental Motor Control

To evaluate Sherrington's contributions to movement science, we should first consider his work on the cerebellum and suprasegmental release phenomena, as well as the cerebral sensorimotor cortex and its connections with the spinal cord in a variety of nonhuman primates. For the cerebellum, the reader is referred to Granit (1966; pp. 89, 94-95) for some of Sherrington's contributions to cerebellospinal connectivity and function. This work, while valuable, lacked the historical significance of his work on the sensorimotor cortex and corticospinal connectivity and function. He is best known for three studies: (1) his 1889 report showing the diffuse pattern of pyramidal tract degeneration following selective lesions of the precentral gyrus; (2) his 1895 report with Frederick (later Sir Frederick) Mott showing in the monkey that the voluntary movement of a forelimb was more impaired by section of that limb's dorsal roots than by a cortical ablation, the inference being then drawn that a coactivation of sensory input was required for the spinal cord's effective utilization of descending corticospinal command signals; and, most importantly, (3) his 1901-1903 and 1917 work with Arnold Leyton (nee Grunbaum), in which motor responses were carefully noted when the anesthetized nonhuman primate's sensorimotor cortex was subjected to punctate electrical stimulation. The findings from these latter studies have recently been reviewed in depth by Porter and Lemon (1993), who emphasized that this work set "... the scene for the histological descriptions of identifiable and separable structural zones within the cerebral cortex of both apes and man ... on which foundations the electrical stimulation experiments in human subjects performed [subsequently] by Penfield, Foerster [Otfrid], and others were to be interpreted" (p. 4). Similarly, Granit (1966) proposed that it had not been "... necessary to alter in any fundamental way the picture Leyton and Sherrington gave of the functional organization of the motor cortex even though the number of sites in the cortex from which motor effects can be elicited has increased" (p. 90). Still thought-provoking today is the statement of Leyton and Sherrington (1917), "The acquirement of skilled movements, though certainly a process involving far wider areas ... of the cortex than the excitable zone itself, may be presumed to find in the cortex an organ whose synthetic properties are part of the physiological basis that renders that acquirement possible" (p. 165).

The modern-day follow-ups to the work just mentioned comprise the continuing delineation of corticospinal projections (Wiesendanger, 1997a), including those obtained with spike-triggered averaging (Fetz et al., 1989); the concept of interneuronal convergence whereby it is largely segmental neurons that integrate the input to the spinal cord of descending command and sensory feedback signals (Jankowska and Lundberg, 1981); and the functional organization of the motor cortex (Georgopoulos, 1996a-b; Wise, 1997).

Ironically, according to Liddell (1952; pp. 249-250), Sherrington himself was not particularly enamored of his motor cortex results, particularly because U.K. law dictated that his preparations had to be anesthetized. Despite his well-deserved prominence in the history of work on corticospinal function, as emphasized so strongly by Porter and Lemon (1993), it did not give Sherrington the prominent position that he now holds in movement neuroscience. Rather, it is to the spinal cord that we must now turn. For his research in this area ". . . he was able to avail himself of every parallel advance in the histology of the spinal cord, being a good enough histologist to be able to sift the wheat from the chaff" (Granit, 1966; pp. 29-30).

Segmental Motor Control

Regarding this area, it is useful for the reader to keep in mind the modern-day phrase, "segmental motor system." This terminology refers to the properties and segmental actions of muscle and other somatic (cutaneous, joint) sensory receptors; the properties of motoneurons, motor units, and the size principle (the latter a rubric for studies on the mechanisms underlying orderly motor unit recruitment); and spinal pattern generation (i.e., the mechanisms whereby spinal cord [and brainstem] interneuronal circuitry can produce rhythmic outputs without rhythmic command and/or sensory feedback signals). Sherrington's contributions to each of these areas, which he summarized in his Hughlings Jackson Lecture (1931) and in chapter VII of Creed et al. (1932), are evaluated in the following sections, along with consideration of their modern-day follow-ups.

Properties and Central Actions of Muscle and Other Limb Receptors

Sherrington published only one experimental paper on muscle receptors (1894). He used Wallerian degeneration to prove that the mammalian muscle spindle (first shown to have both neural and muscular components by Kölliker [1862a-b; frog] and Kühne [1863a-b; mammal]) was a sense organ, and to show that Golgi tendon organs (identified by Golgi in 1880) were supplied by sensory afferents. Sherrington also showed that about one third of the axons in a muscle nerve are sensory, with a relatively large representation of spindle and tendon organ afferents. These were important discoveries, and Sherrington continued to have an impact on the significance of skeletal muscles' sensory signals for both spinal reflexes and kinesthesis by virtue of his early textbook (1897, 1900) and monograph (1906a) writings; a 1918 article on the kinesthetic significance of sensory input from extraocular muscles; and especially his 1924 Linacre Lecture. In the latter, he implicated spindles as length detectors, albeit activated by muscle contraction, and tendon organs as force transducers. The authors would urge the interested reader to read Matthews' (1972, 1977) detailed and well-considered views on Sherrington's impact on all these areas.

In his 1924 Linacre Lecture, Sherrington argued that ". . . through their own nervous arcs the muscles have a voice in their own management and coordination . . . they are, moreover, not motor machines only but sense organs as well. Only by the fuller study of them in these aspects can we know how best to use them" (p. 932). Ironically, in otherwise prescient work that Sherrington undertook with Eccles a few years later (Eccles and Sherrington, 1930), these talented investigators failed to attribute the innervation of fusimotor fibers in muscle spindles to the population of motor axons of clear-cut smaller diameter in cat hindlimb muscle nerves. This key finding was left to Leksell in 1945 (see Matthews, 1972 for earlier tentative observations; pp. 12-15). Just how their incorrect interpretation came about is told with admirable candor by Eccles (Eccles and Gibson, 1979; pp. 49-52), an example of his ever-evident willingness to acknowledge his own misinterpretations and to give credit where credit was due.

Table 11.1 documents the intensive, largely post-World War II responses to Sherrington's 1924 Linacre gauntlet. These developments have included Matthews' remarkable capturing of the science and spirit of this field of inquiry up to 1972 and the advances made throughout the 1970s (Taylor and Prochazka, 1981) and subsequently (Taylor et al., 1995; Proske et al., 2000). This has comprised work on both freely moving animals (Prochazka, 1996) and, for more limited movements, humans (Gandevia and Burke, 1992; Proske et al., 2000). On the basis of "outside-to-inside" and comparative considerations, it has also been argued that proprioceptors play far more roles in the control of movement than had hitherto been considered. Further advances seem now to require a collective, interdisciplinary attack by neurophysiologists and investigators of biomechanics and robotics (Hasan and Stuart, 1988).

Functional Anatomy of Spinal Cord-Muscle Connectivity. Between 1892 and 1894 mainly, Sherrington reported on the relationship among the cat lumbosacral portion of the spinal cord, the ventral root arrangement in the lumbosacral plexus, and the motor nerves to hip and hindlimb muscles. For this effort, he used very precise and exacting surgery combined with electrical stimulation of ventral roots and their subcomponents in the spinal canal. From this work came such fundamental information as which muscles were physiological (vs. anatomical) flexors and which were extensors and their overlapping function in double-joint muscles. For example, one widely held belief at that time was that a single muscle's nerve supply came from but one ventral root. Sherrington showed that a single ventral root supplied parts of many muscles, some of which were antagonists to each other. He further delineated the nature of pre (headward-located motoneuron efferent axons)- and post (hindward-located efferents)-fixed lumbosacral plexuses, a tricky technical issue for even today's experimentalists. Between 1893 and 1897, he provided data on the sensory input to the companion dorsal roots and the segmental projection pattern of dorsal root input. These advances were made by again using visual observation to note reflex muscle responses to electrical stimulation of the skin and de-efferented muscle nerves. "In later life, Sherrington was known to say that this early work on spinal roots and the innervation of muscles was dull and boring but he had to do it because anatomical knowledge of the time was so inaccurate and useless" (Liddell, 1952; p. 247). Indeed, generations of subsequent spinal cord neurophysiologists, extending well past World

War II (and including the present authors), used this information to advance the understanding of segmental motor mechanisms. In retrospect, Sherrington felt that this effort had required ". . . an undue amount of time refuting . . . 'laws' [e.g., Pfluger's laws on spinal reflexes; see Liddell, 1960] . . . which had obtained doctrinal importance and were as erroneous as they were widely accepted" (Liddell, 1952; p. 250).

Reflex Play of One Muscle Upon Another. This rubric is appropriate for considering Sherrington's ad seriatim 1891-1932 experimental and theoretical contributions about the tendon-jerk reflex (i.e., the monosynaptic component of the stretch reflex; the latter term introduced by Liddell and Sherrington in 1924 and 1925); the extensor thrust reflex (1899; still understudied by mammalian segmental motor workers; Hasan and Stuart, 1988); muscle tone and the "full" stretch reflex (i.e., including its oligosynaptic [few-synapse] component); the mechanistic implications of "decerebrate rigidity" (i.e., the clasp-knife reflex via autogenetic inhibition; see endnote 20); the "lengthening reaction" (see Liddell, 1952; pp. 251-252); the flexor reflex (both its relatively low-threshold and high-threshold nociceptive components); integrative reflex actions (i.e., the interaction of one spinal reflex with that of another of different type); spatiotemporal summation of sensory input (e.g., the scratch reflex; see later); and the concept of the "common final path" (introduced in a 1904 report). This body of work emphasized that "Reflex action of short latency, the long [meaning long duration] recruitment of motoneurones through [presumed] multiple synapses, afterdischarge and well-timed inhibition all worked together to ensure speed, smoothness and adequate endurance of muscular acts" (Liddell, 1952; p. 254). It should also be noted that in his studies on reciprocal innervation (see further on), Sherrington addressed the issue of the extent to which it could be modulated by descending command and sensory feedback signals. These findings, together with the emphasis on reciprocal innervation as an active CNS mechanism, were probably his greatest personal achievements in the laboratory. Sherrington himself apparently favored reciprocal innervation as his single best contribution (Granit, 1966; p. 50-51).

As an example of the long-range significance of Sherrington's early-20th-century experiments, consider the following one. In his 1906b report, Sherrington described the use of two pairs of stimulating electrodes, each at a different site in the scratch receptive field of a decerebrate (sometimes also spinalized) cat—that is, one pair in one dermatome and the second pair in another dermatome. He stimulated each pair alone with a subthreshold stimulus for the scratch. When the two subthreshold stimuli were combined within 1.6 s of each other, however, a full-blown scratch was elaborated, thereby demonstrating spatiotemporal summation in the CNS!

To further emphasize the vast sweep of this work, two simple anecdotes suffice. First, the authors would emphasize to modern-day motor control trainees that those who work on the in vivo cat spinal cord must read

Sherrington's 1910b report time and time again to glean its vast amount of detailed technical information, the mastery of which is so critical to the successful execution of an experiment. Second, the authors would urge such trainees to read about Eccles' ". . . vivid remembrances of the heroic experimental procedures required in those days [i.e., 1928; work undertaken in collaboration with Granit and Sherrington] to carry out some simple tests" (Eccles and Gibson, 1979; pp. 55-56). The group was attempting to measure the time course of the central excitatory state (c.e.s.) for various reflex-initiated muscle responses. In their parlance at that time, the c.e.s. referred to the rise and fall of motoneuronal excitatory response to a then-presumed postsynaptic action. Despite a major initial disappointment whose resolution required taking up electromyographic (EMG) recording, Eccles and Sherrington were indeed later able to measure the c.e.s. for the flexor reflex in response to a single afferent shock (for background, see Eccles and Sherrington, 1931; Figures 5 and 6 in the first of their six reports). It had a time course of about 15 ms: that is, within the 10 to 20 ms range (for the c.e.s. and the c.i.s.; the latter the inverse of the former; i.e., the excitatory postsynaptic potential [EPSP] and the inhibitory postsynaptic potential [IPSP], respectively) of that measured precisely more than two decades later in Eccles' Dunedin (New Zealand) laboratory by use of intracellular recording. Interestingly, Sherrington had presented this time frame speculatively in his now-renowned 1925 paper (1925a), criticized at the time for being too teleological (Eccles and Gibson, 1979; pp. 61-62)! This multifaceted story not only exemplifies the intuition, tenacity, and experimental skill of Sherrington, even in ideas and experiments developed when he was in his 70s; it also shows how his work continually set the stage for more precise measurements when technological advances provided the requisite instrumentation.

In table 11.1, the two areas just mentioned are grouped in terms of selected post-Sherringtonian advances. These include Lundberg's (1969b) extension of Sherrington's 1906a introduction of the term "disynaptic" pathway to consideration of oligosynaptic (few-synapse) pathways and the critical role of segmental interneurons as the primary sites of integration (convergence) of descending command signals and sensory feedback—and, as a major conceptual leap forward, the concept of alternative reflex pathways (i.e., the pathway chosen by the CNS depending on the phase and intent of a movement); the further progressive elaboration of essentially Lundberg's ideas and experimental strategies for unraveling spinal cord circuitry (Baldissera et al., 1981; Burke, 1985; McCrea, 1992); the significant progress on the identification and functional morphology of segmental interneurons (Jankowska, 1992; Jordan, 1998; Matsuyama and Mori, 1998; Fetz et al., 1999; McDonagh et al., 1999); the application of the ideas just mentioned to human segmental motor control (e.g., Katz and Pierrot-Deseilligny, 1999; Schieppati and Nardone, 1999); and, finally, the call for the application of modern engineering control theory as a means for future advances (Prochazka, 1996, 1999).

Motoneurons, Motor Units, and the Size Principle

Sherrington and Liddell coined the term "motor unit." While they were probably not the first to consider the concept and its functional signifi-cance for the graded development of muscle force (see endnote 14), Sherrington's group brought power to the term by considering the rela-tionship between the firing pattern of motoneurons and force development. Consider also the significance of Liddell's (1952) comments: "Experiments interpreted on the basis of motor units excited or inhibited revealed much information about the convergence of nerve impulses on a group of spinal motor units with a single function—'spinal centre' as they were vaguely called before, but now 'motoneuron pool' [i.e., motoneurons supplying a single muscle and its close synergists]. Into that pool streamed streams of excitation or of [actually "and"] inhibition from various axones of distant origin" (p. 253). Furthermore, after the 1924 introduction of the term "mo-tor unit," the Sherrington group emphasized a quantitative interpretation of the interaction between reflexes in terms of the activation of motor units (for several examples, see Creed et al., 1932). Finally, the 1930 report of Sherrington's trainees, Sybil Cooper and Eccles, on the isometric forces of cat hindlimb muscles, helped set the stage for post-World War II advances on the properties of different "types" of motor units and their association with the properties of the motoneurons that innervate them (Burke, 1981). This was still a fruitful line of inquiry as of the late 1990s (Binder et al., 1996).

Orderly Motor Unit Recruitment and the Size Principle. Granit (1966) has explained that ". . . the concept of recruitment is a development of Sherrington's fundamental principle of reflex action, which maintains that excitability is graded among the individual motoneurones of a pool. Sherrington himself did not call this fact a principle—a term he reserved for reciprocal innervation—but everything that has happened since in the study of the central nervous system justifies the elevation of the discovery of such liminal grades of excitation to the rank of a principle" (p. 72).

Fixed motor unit recruitment refers to an invariant order of unit recruit-ment during voluntary and reflex contractions. Apparently, it was first observed in the 1930s by several groups, and it may possibly have been known to the Sherrington group (see later); but it was not mentioned by Denny-Brown in a major report (1929), nor was it mentioned by the group as a whole in their summing-up text (Creed et al., 1932). Furthermore, in his masterful 1949 review on the EMG, Denny-Brown cited only two pre-cedents (Smith, 1934; Lindsley, 1935) to his and Pennybacker's (1938) brief discussion of fixed recruitment. Denny-Brown also mentioned that "oth-ers" had observed fixed recruitment, presumably in the early 1930s. (Note further that Denny-Brown and Pennybacker [1938] cited Liddell and Sherrington [1923] and Sherrington [1929a] for their work on fixed recruitment. This was an error. Neither paper mentioned fixed recruitment order!)

Denny-Brown and Pennybacker (1938) went on to report an *orderly* (small before large) motor unit recruitment pattern, there being no further such reports in the 1930s (see Seyffarth, 1940). It is important to note, however, that Denny-Brown focused solely on fixed recruitment in his 1949 review. This may suggest that he was less certain by then about the validity of the orderly recruitment he had reported in his 1938 paper with Pennybacker (Stuart, 1999). Such uncertainty would surely have been appropriate because of the brief and equivocal nature of Denny-Brown and Pennybacker's (1938) results on orderly recruitment, as well as technical limitations in EMG interpretation at that time (Stuart, 1999). Clearly, it remained for Henneman (1915-1996; Young, 1997) to firmly establish orderly recruitment (1957) using a far less equivocal method than was available to Denny-Brown and Pennybacker (1938) and, far more importantly, to add to it his size principle as an explanation of the underlying mechanisms.

From what has been said, it is clear that Sherrington's work up to the Creed et al. (1932) textbook had no direct effect on subsequent developments on orderly motor unit recruitment and the size principle (Henneman and Mendell, 1981; Binder and Mendell, 1990). Nonetheless, all post-1960s workers in this field would agree that the emphasis in Creed et al. (1932) on the c.e.s., recruitment, the discharge zone of a pool of motoneurons, and the "subliminal fringe" (defined in endnotes 18-19) all had a major impact on post-1957 work and interest in Henneman's size principle. It would certainly delight both Sherrington and Henneman that this interest is still to the forefront. Orderly recruitment is now thought to result from a still-undetermined combination of neural membrane and synaptic-input properties, the most relevant of which are correlated with motoneuron size (for review: Stuart and Enoka, 1983, 1990; Enoka and Stuart, 1984; Gustafsson and Pinter, 1985; Cope and Clark, 1991; Binder et al., 1996; Cope and Sokoloff, 1999).

Spinal Pattern Generation

To introduce this topic, it is necessary to present an overview of the current state-of-the-play on spinal pattern generation. A quote from the preface to a recent volume (Stein et al., 1997), which followed a 1995 symposium (Stein et al., 1995), provides such an overview. According to Stein et al.,

> . . . understanding the control of movement requires a multilevel approach . . . [emphasizing] the importance of synthesis and analysis. Reductionist analysis reveals properties of components of the system: specific motor patterns generated by networks, neurons, and neuromolecules (channels, receptors, transmitters, and modulators). Synthesis uses a systems approach regarding the levels of networks and behavior: motor patterns

generate movements that are modulated by movement-related sensory feedback. Such a multilevel approach has been reported elsewhere: Bunge (1989) stressed the importance of multilevel approaches in neuroscience; Stein (1995) applied Bunge's perspectives to the neural control of movement; and Getting (1989) emphasized the utilization of reductionist results in the construction of synthetic mathematical models of neuronal networks that generate motor patterns. . . . Prior to the 1975 conference [Valley Forge, PA], researchers of vertebrate systems tended to view only vertebrate research as relevant, whereas researchers of invertebrate systems tended to focus only on invertebrate research. The 1975 symposium and its accompanying 1976 volume [i.e., Herman et al., 1976] revealed common neuron, network, and behavior organizational principles for both vertebrates and invertebrates. That discovery led to a change in the way many investigators and university training programs approached the neural control of movement. The 1985 conference (Stockholm, Sweden) and its 1986 volume (Grillner et al., 1986) offered further support for the view that the nervous system of lower vertebrates share important common features with the nervous system of mammals. Incorporating these previous insights, the 1995 conference (Tucson, AZ) and this volume [Stein et al., 1997] add the emerging concept of the current decade: the modulatory abilities of the neurons that make up a neuronal network confer abilities onto the modulated network that allow it to generate an array of motor patterns responsible for a set of motor behaviors. (paragraphs 3-5 of preface)

Viewed from this perspective, the one enigma about Sherrington's experimental and theoretical contributions to segmental motor control is his ambivalent and somewhat confusing attitude toward the results of his former trainee and close collaborator, Thomas Graham Brown. His statements to this effect are provided in endnotes 28-30 because this ambivalence is also evident in his Nobel Lecture. Here it is sufficient to point out that from the early 1960s onward, an overwhelming body of evidence has shown, for a wide variety of species including the human (Gurfinkel et al., 1998), that interneuronal networks in the brainstem and spinal cord (and their analogues in invertebrates) have the intrinsic capacity (i.e., do not depend on descending command and sensory feedback signals) to generate rhythmical activation of motoneurons such as to produce rhythmical movements like chewing, licking, scratching, and locomotion (Stein et al., 1997; Kiehn et al., 1998). While Sherrington's trainee at the University of Liverpool (1910-1913) and shortly thereafter at the University of Manchester (i.e., up to 1916), Graham Brown undertook highly original experiments in support of this essentially segmental control system and was its primary pre- and post-World War II supporter among mammalian workers. His 1911-1915 reports and summary 1916 review on stepping are evaluated in depth in Wetzel and Stuart (1976).

As discussed in detail in endnotes 28-30, Graham Brown was clearly ahead of his time. It is fair to think that if Sherrington had thrown his considerable weight behind the need for parallel advances in the quantitative unitary and interactive reflex approach he personally favored focusing on and the more novel, holistic approach of Graham Brown, there could have been a far more rapid advance in the study of spinal pattern generation than occurred prior to the 1960s. Furthermore, if Sherrington had accommodated Graham Brown's theories on a central segmental rather than sensory feedback primary genesis for rhythmical locomotor movements, then Sherrington's own work on the scratch reflex (see later), spinal stepping (Wetzel and Stuart; pp. 42-60; Sherrington's contributions on pp. 43-44), and so-called reflex standing (Liddell, 1952; pp. 252-253) would be held in much higher regard today. As it is, the careful work that Sherrington did in these three areas has been marginalized over the years. Admittedly, it was reviewed in depth by Liddell (1952) and Granit (1966) but again, unfortunately, without a spinal pattern generation orientation. This is a pity, because in the history of segmental motor control, this body of work included many important observations. For example, consider Liddell's assessment of Sherrington's 1906b paper on the scratch reflex in the spinal dog: "Sherrington seldom displayed his powers better than in this paper. 'Electric tickling,' as he was to call it in after years, from the artificial flea on a tiny point on the skin, brought into vigorous action nineteen muscles beating rhythmically five times a second, and kept seventeen muscles in steady postural action. The main characteristic of reflex action due to interneuronal synapses could all be depicted inspiringly on the grand canvas of the scratch reflex: summation of stimuli, facilitation, long latent period, long refractory phase, after-discharge, irritability, the 'law' of forward direction, postinhibitory rebound" (p. 250). All of this true and valuable, and such a demonstration is extremely impressive even today; but as with the full 1906 article and Liddell's comments quoted earlier, it lacks the conceptualization of the activation of a spinal pattern generator (e.g., Stein et al., 1997).

Because of the problem just discussed, the sense of Sherrington's contribution to modern-day spinal pattern generation is limited to the widely held perception that he offered important examples of how sensory input from the proprioceptors (defined in endnotes 23-24) could enhance the quality of rhythmical movements but failed to grasp the overall gestalt, even though from time to time he conceded in passing that Graham Brown's position on spinal pattern generation would eventually have to be accommodated into the overall scheme of locomotor control.

Despite their presumably philosophical differences concerning the best strategy to advance segmental motor research, it would seem that Sherrington and Graham Brown remained close friends and effective collaborators. They published together seven times between 1911 and 1913, with one report on the pilomotor system, one on segmental reflexes, and five on the motor cortex (references in Liddell, 1952). Many years later, Graham Brown was an active and successful promulgator of the case for Sherrington's being awarded a Nobel Prize (Eccles and Gibson 1979; p. 70; see also Graham Brown (1947) and parts of his touching letter in Granit, 1966; p. 96). Furthermore, Sherrington did include important comments on Graham Brown's work on spinal pattern generation in his 1931 Hughlings Jackson Lecture (p. 25) and the influential Creed et al. (1932) text (p. 146), and he did mention Graham Brown in his Nobel Lecture (see endnotes 28-30).

The key to the enigma may lie in the attitude of the coauthors of the Creed et al. (1932) text. At least Eccles and Denny-Brown held Graham Brown in low regard as judged by their perception of the cavalier nature and strategy of his experiments (personal communication from Eccles in a spirited, strong-minded conversation with D.G.S. in 1973 while they were watching the Graham Brown movie; see later). This attitude may have affected the extent to which Sherrington was prepared to emphasize the potential significance of Graham Brown's 1911-1922 findings on spinal pattern generation. Sherrington was, after all, an essentially shy and self-effacing person, with ". . . a friendly unassuming manner. . ." (Liddell, 1952; p. 255). At the age of 75 years, he may simply have lacked the energy to support Graham Brown in the face of well-meant (albeit misguided) criticisms offered by his aggressive collaborators from the antipodes! Also exacerbating the problem was Graham Brown's early "retirement" from active research. Perhaps as a result of the general lack of enthusiasm and support for his ideas and results, and/or personal eccentricities, he published little after his 1922 review. He did return to rhythmical movements, however: ". . . in 1935 he began to use a moving platform to induce walking movements in the decerebrate cat, and a few years later he studied the wing beat of the decerebrate pigeon moved through the air at different speeds. He had made some excellent films to illustrate these experiments and they were shown to the Physiological Society, but he could never be induced to publish an account of what he had found" (Adrian, 1966; p. 28). Thirty-two years later, Lundberg and Phillips (1973) set the record straight by providing an insightful description and interpretation of the contents and thrust of this valuable film (see also Wetzel and Stuart, 1976), viewing and discussion of which should be considered an essential component of training in movement neuroscience.

Use of Relatively Unsophisticated Techniques

Much of Sherrington's pre-1920s work was undertaken with quite simple electrical stimulation apparatus combined with visual observations of muscle contractions: He used ". . . careful surgery . . . meticulous care . . . and a mind which pondered" (Liddell, 1952, p. 253). He was one of the first to quantitate reflex outputs in terms of muscle-length changes of antagonistic muscles (see figure 11.1 in the endnotes); and, taking the lead from

Sir David Ferrier (1875), he was also one of the first to use repetitive (then called "faradic") stimulation of peripheral nerves rather than the previously used sustained (then called "galvanic") stimulation. Sherrington did not use an accurate length-measuring device, however, until arriving at Oxford in 1914. This was a spring-loaded isotonic myograph, with muscle-twitch recordings made on a stationary smoked drum (Sherrington and Sowton, 1915). By 1918, he was working with his own newly developed isometric torsion-wire optical myograph (Sherrington, 1921; see figure 11.2 in the endnotes), which he did not combine with the EMG (with Eccles) until the late 1920s—"Together we learnt the technique of electrical recording from muscle, one of us near the end of his experimental life, the other near the beginning" (Eccles and Gibson, 1979; p. 56). The EMG was first applied to spinal reflexology by Cooper and Sherrington's co-1932 Nobel laureate, Lord Edgar Adrian (1924), at Cambridge University. In Sherrington's group, it was first combined with force measurements by John Fulton and Liddell (1926).

Work Ethic

For most of his career, Sherrington labored long into the night. The last of his experimental collaborators, Eccles, remembered with admiration that their ". . . experiments were complicated and one hesitated to break off once they were running well. So in this arduous life during the years 1929, 1930, and even into 1931 our experiments went all day with no lunch break. Then usually at about 4 p.m. we went downtown for an enormous afternoon tea before returning for a final session. Lady Sherrie was rightly concerned about this strenuous existence—often with two such experiments a week, and early in 1931 the last physiological experiments were done, Sir Charles then being in his seventy-fourth year" (Eccles and Gibson, p. 56). Of such stuff many of his trainees were also made (see further on), to the lasting benefit of movement neuroscience!

Summary and Reflection

Sherrington's contributions to neuroscience place him to the forefront of 19th- and 20th-century workers in this field. The synapse was incorporated into the overall workings of the CNS, as was inhibition both as an active process and as an equal partner of excitation in brain function. These were Sherrington's greatest personal scientific achievements. For movement neuroscience, he set the stage for post-World War II advances in both suprasegmental and segmental motor control. He is best known for the latter and is held in the highest regard for advancing understanding of the properties and central actions of muscle and other limb receptors, the spatiotemporal summation of sensory input, and the workings of motoneurons and motor units—thereby indirectly leading others into the study of orderly motor unit recruitment and the size principle. The single, puzzling blemish on his career is for not advancing spinal pattern generation, particularly because one of his own former trainees had made such a promising start in this area. It should be remembered, however, that Sherrington operated within an intellectual community that strongly favored a single-cell (vs. systems) approach to the study of the CNS. This inside-out approach was most successful in setting the stage for post-World War II advances using the intracellular microelectrode. In parallel, Nicolai Bernstein (1896-1966), the Russian clinician/mathematician/biomechanist, was making major conceptual advances using an outside-in approach (Latash, 1998; Stuart, 1998), as was the Swiss 1949 Nobel laureate, Walter Hess (1881-1973; see Stuart, 1998; Wiesendanger, 1997b).

The two approaches did not converge in pre-World War II neuroscience, however. For example, the distinguished and imaginative German neurologist, Richard Jung (1911-1986; Stuart, 1998), commented in an inspirational memoir (1975/92) that while he was most impressed with the scientific rigor of the pre-World War II Oxford and Cambridge neuroscientists, he was pleased with his own personal change from ". . . fact-oriented [i.e., unitary cellular] British physiology to the systems-oriented physiology of W. R. Hess . . . [who] considered single facts [i.e., single-cell results] only in their context with functional systems or in their significance for the organism" (pp. 488-489). Ironically, if Keith Lucas (1879-1916), Adrian's brilliant mentor (Adrian, 1934), had survived a 1916 plane crash (Sherrington, 1927) and gone on with his stellar career, the U.K. pre-World War II outlook may have broadened. For example, even as early as 1909, Lucas was deploring and seeking to change ". . . the lack of interaction between evolutionary concepts and physiological research . . . In advocating a reunion of physiology and evolutionary concepts, Lucas emphasized that 'the primary problem of comparative physiology . . . [is] the question to what extent and along what lines the functional capabilities of animal cells have been changed by evolution'" (Gillespie, 1973; p. 534; citing Lucas, 1909b; p. 325). Since Lucas' last research paper, published posthumously (1917), dealt with the neuromuscular physiology of the crayfish, and since he was so extraordinarily inventive, he might truly have reshaped British mammalian cellular neuroscience toward far closer relations between departments of physiology (usually in medical schools) and zoology (on the main campus) than existed then, and most unfortunately, even today. We will never know, of course, and it hardly seems fair to have expected Sherrington (influenced as he was by the comparative orientation of Walter Gaskell; see later) to have accomplished this convergence on his own.

Mentoring Contributions

In many biographical memoirs, too little is said about the academic lineage of scientists like Sherrington: who trained them, whom in turn they trained and whom they collaborated with, and what the subsequent lineage of these trainees and collaborators was (for several examples in movement neuroscience, see Stuart, 1998). This is unfortunate, because with more emphasis on such lineages and the importance of the mentoring process there would be less focus in present-day academic life on short-range, immediate, transient, and self-serving success and more on long-range, longer-lasting, and more altruistic contributions (for further such dialogue, see Kennedy, 1997).

Sherrington's primary mentors in experimental neuroscience were John Langley (1852-1925), who contributed substantially to late-19th-century neuroscience, particularly on the mammalian autonomic nervous system (Sherrington, 1925c); and Gaskell (1847-1914), a cardiovascular, autonomic nervous system, and comparative neurobiologist (Gillespie, 1972c). About the latter Sherrington once wrote, "My own work began by chance at the wrong end—the cortex-pyramidal degenerations, etc. It was certainly through Gaskell that I very soon felt that . . . the cord offered a better point of attack physiologically . . . he was still always a bulwark to me about inhibition and voluntary muscle . . . In a hundred ways I owe him help and inspiration" (Liddell, 1952; pp. 244-245). Sherrington was also strongly influenced by the writings of Cajal, whom, most strangely, Sherrington met only once (in London, U.K., in 1894), even though his work was critical for the development of Sherrington's own contributions (Sherrington, 1935).

After Sherrington's initial two publications with Langley in 1884 and the pathologist Walter Hadden (1856-1893; Sherrington, 1892b) in 1886, most of his subsequent coauthored publications on subjects pertaining directly to movement science involved coauthors who had a junior role or who, if established investigators, were far younger and had less overall experience. The full list of these coauthors is provided in table 11.2; the legend includes a selected list of coauthors in other areas of clinical science and academic or societal endeavor. If space and the overall theme of this book permitted, much more could be made of the significant contributions of this latter group (see discussion further on).

Table 11.2 emphasizes several points of relevance to modern-day motor control research and training.

Relative Lack of Coauthorship

Among Sherrington's 300-plus publications, fewer than 75 were coauthored. This was the pre-World War II custom. Neuroscience then lacked the post-1950s interdisciplinary techniques and theory that continue to gain ground today. Even when Sherrington was working on his single-authored publications, however, "At no time was he a secluded worker. He had a welcome for nearly every visitor to the laboratory" (Liddell, 1952; p. 256). In retrospect, it would have been fitting for Sherrington to mentor his trainees even further by encouraging their coauthorship of even his more theoretical (and sometimes philosophical) approaches to the nervous system, but this was not the custom of the day.

Table 11.2 Sherrington's Academic Lineage in Movement Neuroscience

Epoch	Coauthors on segmental motor control	Coauthors on suprasegmental motor control	Selected visits (V)/trainees and visiting workers
1884-1887		John Langley (1884, 1891) Walter Hadden (1886-88)	V-*Eduard Pflüger* (1884) V-*Friedrich Goltz* (1884-85)[1] V- *Rudolph Virchow* (1886) V-*Robert Koch* (1886-87)
1887-1895	R.W. Reid (1890) Frederick Mott (1895)		
1895-1913	**Michael Foster** (1895-97) Heinrich Hering (1897-99) **Walter Gaskell** (1897) Edward Schäfer (1900) Alfred Frohlich (1901-02) Ernest Laslett (1902-03) Robert Woodworth (1904) Herbert Roaf (1910) S.C.M. Sowton* (1911-15) Thomas Graham Brown (1912)	Heinrich Hering (1899) Arnold Grunbaum (1901-03)[2] Herbert Roaf (1906) Frederick Mott (1911) Edward Schuster (1911) Thomas Graham Brown (1911-13)	*Harvey Cushing* (1901)[3] *Rudolph Magnus* (1908) *Paul Hoffman* (~1912)
1913-1936	Alexander Forbes (1914) Nicholas Dreyer (1918) K. Sassa* (1921) Eric Liddell (1923-32) Richard Creed (1926-32) Sybil Cooper (1926-40) Derek Denny-Brown (1926-32) John Eccles (1929-32) John Fulton (1930-32)	Alexander Forbes (1914) Arnold Leyton[2] (1917)	*Wilder Penfield* (1915-16, 1919-20) *Grayson McCouch* (1919-20) *Francis Walshe* (1920-23) *Stanley Cobb* (1923-25) *Theodore Ruch* (1929-32) *George Lindor Brown* (1932) *John Young* (1932) *John Magladery* (1935) *David Lloyd* (1935-36)
1936-1952	Sybil Cooper (1940)		

Note: Table shows the years of Sherrington's coauthored publications, with his primary and other mentors in **bold** and his other coauthors in regular type (span of publication years with him in parentheses). For the specific citations, see the references and/or those in Liddell (1952). The epochs are for Sherrington's various academic appointments and/or locales. They include 1884-1887, Cambridge University, St. Thomas's Hospital Medical School, and Europe; 1887-1895, St. Thomas's Hospital Medical School and the Brown Institution of Preventative Medicine; 1895-1913, University of Liverpool; 1913-1936, University of Oxford; 1936-1952, academic retirement years in Ipswich and Eastbourne. His visits (V) to others' laboratories for training, and his own laboratory's visitors and trainees in the field of movement neuroscience, are shown in *italics*. The visitors' and trainees' years of association with him are indicated. Other well-known and often illustrious scientists and humanitarians who collaborated with, and/or were mentored/trained by Sherrington while abroad (1884-87), at St. Thomas's Hospital (1887-1895), and/or at the Universities of

Liverpool (1895-1913) and Oxford (1913-1936) include, in their chronological order: Jacques Loeb (1884-85); Harold Forster (1907-1909, 1910); Henry Bazett (~1913-14); James Olmsted (~1914); Emil Holman (1914-17); Wilburt Davison (1915-19); Harold Carleton (~1916-1927); Henry Viets (1916-17); Walter Russell Brain (1919-20); Howard Florey (1921-24); Marshall Fulton (1920-1923); Hugh Cairns (~1923); Leon Ballif (~1925); John Balsdon (~1925-27); Ian Marcou (~1927); Frank Ingrahan (1929); David Rioch (1929-30); Ebbe Hoff (1930-32); Karl Matthes (1931); Hebbel Hoff (1931-34); J.H. Wolfenden* (~1934); Jose Odoriz (1934-35); Sixto Obrador (1934-35); John Pritchard (1934-35); David Witteridge (1934-35); and William Gibson (1935). Still others** who worked with Sherrington included Gordon Holmes, Geoffrey Jefferson, Lewis Weed, and Charles Wilkinson. Sherrington's coauthors (a few of whom were his trainees) in other areas of clinical and other academic/societal endeavors included, in the chronological order in which Sherrington's efforts were initiated: *cholera pathology,* Charles Roy and John Graham Brown; *scar tissue and other forms of pathlogy and bacteriology,* Charles Ballance, Armand Ruffer, William Herdman, Sidney Hickson, Sir Rupert Boyce, and Ronald Ross; *heart and circulation,* Sydney Copeman, Edward Schäfer, and Stanley Kent; *autonomic nervous system,* Robert Reid, Francis Tozer, Frederick Miller, and Thomas Graham Brown; *health education,* Edward Wallis, E.W. Hope,* and E.A. Brown;* *fatigue,* William MacDougall; *chloroform anesthesia,* Joseph Barr and S.C.M Sowton;* *cancer biology,* Sydney Copeman; *visual neuroscience,* Herbert Roaf; *epilepsy,* F.L.J. Muskens;* and *evolutionary biology,* Francis Mason.

Footnotes: [1]Subsequent brief, intermittent visits in 1885-89; [2]In 1915, name changed by deed from Grunbaum to Leyton; [3]A stay Cushing prolonged from one to eight months.

*First name unknown to authors; **Years with Sherrington unknown to authors.

Relative Lateness of Major Mentoring Efforts and Successes

Sherrington trained few subsequently prominent movement neuroscientists until he was well over the age of 60—that is, in his post-1920 Oxford years and particularly between 1926 and 1932. His international influence had come far earlier, however, with many believing that his work on reciprocal inhibition was deserving of a Nobel Prize in the early 1900s (Eccles and Gibson, 1979; p. 70). Furthermore, while at the University of Liverpool (1895-1912) Sherrington was apparently particularly happy and fulfilled (Granit, 1966; p. 88). He was then (as later at Oxford) exerting a profound influence on academic clinicians, and he must have felt privileged to have such outstanding neuroscience trainees as Robert Woodworth (see later) and distinguished visiting collaborators like Rudolph Magnus (later of righting-reflex fame), Heinrich Hering (later prominent in visual perception), Harvey Cushing (see later), and Paul Hoffman (H-reflex).

Worldwide Impact of Sherrington's Movement-Neuroscience Trainees

Among Sherrington's trainees and collaborators are three Nobel laureates and many who achieved the highest of honors in their native countries for their contributions to neuroscience research and training. Here we highlight, in chronological order of their association with Sherrington, the careers of several of them who contributed to movement neuroscience. Their primary and/or major research/training locales are emphasized.

Robert S. Woodworth (1869-1962; Psychology, Columbia University, United States). Subsequent to his 1902-1903 interactions with Sherrington, Woodworth, a doyen of American experimental psychology, was largely responsible for the golden age of psychology at Columbia University (1920-1940). He promulgated eclectic neuropsychology within a rigorous experimental-statistical orientation (Thorne, 1976). His *Experimental Psychology* (1938; one of his 10 major books) was an internationally favored textbook for several generations of graduate students (Murphy, 1962).

Wilder Penfield (1891-1976; Montreal Neurological Institute, McGill University, Canada). After his 1915-1916 and 1919-1920 interactions with Sherrington at Oxford and neurosurgical training with Harvey Cushing (see later), Penfield, a United States-born Canadian, founded the Montreal Neurological Institute in 1934. Here, along with his United States-born neurophysiological collaborator, Herbert Jasper (1906-1999), he explored the electroencephalogram and behavioral responses to electrical stimulation of the brain of conscious subjects (Penfield, 1972). Together these two researchers made enduring contributions to neuroscience and its motor control component (see Jasper, 1991). Both before and after Penfield's death, Jasper continued the tradition of training and encouraging scores of young fundamental and clinical neuroscientists from North America and elsewhere. For example, with the late Jean-Pierre Cordeau (1922-1971) he founded the Center for Neurological Sciences at the University of Montreal in 1965. For further review, see Penfield's autobiography (1977; see also **http://www.cbhr.ca/pub-awa/can-bchr/1958.htm**). (Jasper's own autobiography is in preparation for publication by his widow, Mary-Lou Jasper.)

John F. Fulton (1899-1960; Physiology, Yale University, United States). Fulton, an American, was associated with Sherrington in 1921-1925 and 1928-1930; he was professor and head of physiology at Yale University from 1929 to 1951. Until his death, Fulton exerted a profound effect on American neurophysiology, including his establishment at Yale in 1931 of the first U.S. laboratory for brain research on nonhuman primates, and, in 1938 with Joannes Dusser de Barenne, the *Journal of Neurophysiology*. He edited this premier journal until his death in 1960. Fulton is best known for his work on functional interrelationships of various brain regions, the effects of experimentally placed brain lesions, and the significance of overlapping somatic and autonomic representation in the sensorimotor cortex (Gillespie, 1972b). He promulgated intense training in neurophysiology for academic neurosurgeons and also made important contributions to aviation medicine and medical history. Above all, he trained and supported scores of young neuroscientists.

Derek Denny-Brown (1901-1981; Neurology, Harvard University School of Medicine, United States). Denny-Brown, a New Zealander, introduced several powerful techniques into Sherrington's laboratory in the late 1920s that are still valuable today (e.g., the antidromic stimulation of motoneurons in in vivo cat spinal cord preparations). Eccles (personal communication to D.G.S. in 1968) has said that he was first taught neurophysiological techniques largely by Denny-Brown when Eccles began experimental work at Oxford in 1927-1928. After leaving Sherrington's laboratory in 1928,

Denny-Brown focused mainly on academic neurology, first in the United Kingdom (1928-1941; World War II military service in 1939-1941) and subsequently in the United States (1941-1972; more World War II military service in 1943-1946). Most remarkably, between 1946 and 1967 at Harvard, he trained over 300 American neurology specialists, more than 20 of whom subsequently became heads of neurology departments or divisions. Another chapter in this book documents his and his trainees' wide and far-reaching contributions to basic and clinical neuroscience (Vilensky and Gilman, chapter 4 of this volume; see also Vilensky et al., 1998; Stuart, 1998).

John C. Eccles (1903-1997; Physiology, Australian National University). Eccles, an Australian, shared his 1963 Nobel Prize with Sir Alan Hodgkin (1914-1998) and Sir Andrew Huxley (1917-present). Eccles' far-reaching contributions to neuroscience, including its motor control component, have recently been documented by Andersen and Lundberg (1997; see also Stuart, 1998; Curtis and Andersen, 2000). For the present purposes, two points suffice. Eccles' first scientific paper (a short technical note with Sherrington, 1929b) was published in 1929 and his last posthumously in 1998 (with Friedrich Beck, a German quantum physicist)—an almost 70-year record of sustained productivity that rivaled that of his mentor. Second, in a posttraining academic career at six institutions in five countries (University of Oxford, United Kingdom; University of Sydney, Australia; Otago University, New Zealand; Australian National University; American Medical Research Institute, United States; State University of New York, Buffalo, United States; retirement, Switzerland; for autobiographical details on this odyssey, see Eccles, 1977), Eccles trained (or cotrained) and collaborated with 120 neuroscientists from 20 countries. Virtually all of these people had successful subsequent research and training records closely related to movement neuroscience. This list includes Argentina, 1; Australia, 14; Canada, 7; Czechoslovakia, 1; France, 2; Germany, 4; Hungary, 1; India, 1; Italy, 5; Japan, 15; Lebanon, 1; New Zealand, 7; Norway, 2; Spain, 2; Sweden, 5; Switzerland, 1; Thailand, 1; The Netherlands, 2; United Kingdom, 18; United States, 31; and the former Soviet Union, 1. For further details, see Stuart (1998). As emphasized by Andersen and Lundberg (1997), "To him can be applied Liddell's words in his obituary on Sherrington: 'He has reached long and found much. His kind come to the world not often in centuries'" (p. 325).

Ragnar Granit (1900-1991; Nobel Institute of Neurophysiology, University of Stockholm, Sweden). A Finn (1900-1940) turned Swede (1940 onward), Granit worked with Sherrington and Eccles in 1928 and to a lesser extent on a return trip to Oxford in 1931-1932 (when he focused largely on visual research). Although sharing a Nobel Prize for his visual research in 1967 (with George Wald and Haldan Hartline), Granit will be remembered largely for work on the properties and central actions of muscle receptors, the repetitive firing properties of motoneurons, and his impressive mentoring of young motor control neuroscientists. After becoming the professor of neurophysiology at his institution in 1946, Granit trained and collaborated with over 30 movement neuroscientists from 7 countries, including Canada, 2; Germany, 1; Italy, 1; Japan, 1; Sweden, 16; United Kingdom, 8; United States, 4. For more details on Granit's movement neuroscience achievements, see Grillner (1995).

John Z. Young (1907-1997; Anatomy, University College, London, United Kingdom). In Sherrington's group in 1931-1932, the Bristol (United Kingdom)-born "Jay Zed" Young collaborated with Eccles and Granit in a study on the giant axons of the earthworm (Eccles et al., 1932). He was another near-70-year scientific author. When awarded the 1973 Francis O. Schmitt Medal and Prize in neuroscience, Young was cited for having ". . . provided generations of students and researchers with both living and conceptual propositions at levels from the single nerve fiber to memory" and for having ". . . introduced the squid giant axon to physiology, pioneered with his coworkers in measuring intracellular potassium concentration, birefringence of axon sheaths . . . the dependence of axon velocity on diameter, and the regeneration of nerves, and in localizing the separate assets of learning and memory within the brain of an advanced vertebrate" (Worden et al., 1992; p. 14). Young trained innumerable invertebrate and vertebrate neuroscientists in several countries who subsequently contributed substantially to comparative movement neuroscience, as well as many other topics in neuroscience (Young, 1992; Messenger, 1997). Of possibly even greater import were his three textbooks (*Life of Vertebrates*, 1950; *Life of Mammals*, 1957; *Introduction to the Study of Man*, 1971), which became, and remain, classic textbooks for generations of students and zoologists.

Jose Bernado Odoriz (1908-1971; Physiology, Buenos Aires National University, Argentina). After his 1934-1935 work with Sherrington and Eccles, Odoriz trained with two similarly distinguished physiologists: in 1936-1937 with the 1944 Nobel laureate Herbert Gasser (Rockefeller Institute, New York), for whom he designed several stimulating and recording devices to study action potentials; and in 1938, with the 1947 Nobel laureate Bernado Houssay (National University, Buenos Aires, Argentina), whom he later succeeded as the chair of human physiology (1953-1956). Odoriz is best known in Latin America for (1) his work as a pioneering neurophysiologist and clinical electroencephalographist—he was the first to make electroencephalogram measurements in Argentina (1937; using a machine Odoriz had constructed in Gasser's laboratory) and neighboring countries; (2) his "Sherrington-like" mentoring of innumerable distinguished medical graduates of his institution; and (3) his introduction of sports medicine as a specialty in medicine (1945) in Argentina. Greatly augmenting his impact on South American neuroscience was his fluency not only in his native tongue,

Spanish, but also in Basque, English, French, German, and Italian, as well as his partial fluency in Portuguese and Russian.

David Lloyd (1911-1985; Rockefeller Institute for Medical Research, United States). The Canadian-born Lloyd completed a BS at McGill University (Canada) in 1932 and, at Oxford, a BA in 1936 (departmental demonstrator in physiology in 1935-1936) and a PhD in 1938 (mentor, Eccles). It is possible that he had substantial interactions with Sherrington, albeit the latter undertook no physiological research after 1931. In 1939, Lloyd began work at the Rockefeller Institute, where up to 1959 he trained some leading movement neuroscientists who have had substantial subsequent impact in Australia, France, New Zealand, the People's Republic of China, and the United States. Lloyd's 1939-1959 work on the spinal cord formed an important extracellular-recording bridge between pre-World War II "Sherringtonian" approaches and the intracellular recording era that began in the late 1940s and flourished in parallel with some of Lloyd's contributions in the 1950s. Lloyd was particularly effective in advancing Sherrington's ideas immediately after World War II. For an interesting account of his career, see Patton (1994).

From this account of Sherrington's mentoring contribution, it should be clear that most modern-day researchers in the field of movement neuroscience have a "familial" connection with Sherrington. Indeed, to at least some extent, he has indirectly mentored virtually all of us!

Impact of Other Collaborators

The legend to table 11.2 documents Sherrington's clinical associations with a wide variety of United Kingdom and North American clinical scientists whose careers spanned many fields. Sherrington inspired them to become leaders in academic medicine, and many helped set the stage for post-World War II advances in all-around biomedical science. Influenced as they were by Sherrington, these physician-investigators presumably had a healthy respect for the role of laboratory experimentation in the physiological instruction of medical and graduate students. For such instruction, Sherrington's physiology laboratory manual is as impressive today as it was when published in 1919.

Special attention should be directed to Sherrington's lifelong intellectual rather than experimental association with the famous U.S. surgeon, Harvey Cushing; his training and mentoring of the Australian Nobel laureate, Lord Howard Florey; and his cotraining (with Eccles) of the Spanish neurosurgeon, Sixto Obrador.

Harvey Cushing (1869-1939; Neurosurgery, Harvard University School of Medicine). Shortly after his 1901 interactions with Sherrington (on the motor cortex of nonhuman primates), Cushing, the father of American academic neurosurgery, set the stage for modern neurosurgery (1904-1910) with his near-unique conceptualization and surgical management of

intracranial pressure (Greenblatt, 1997). A lifelong friend and confidant of
Sherrington (Sherrington, 1939), Cushing, along with William Halsted and
the Swiss Theodor Kocher, is also considered one of the fathers of modern
American surgery in general (Modlin, 1998). "Viewed in the perspective of
thirty years since his death," Gillespie wrote in 1971, "Harvey Cushing
remains the dominant figure in neurosurgery. He set an example in the
application of the scientific method to clinical problems in this developing
field, especially to tumors of the brain; and the influence on succeeding
generations of this broad approach will probably be his greatest contribution to medicine" (p. 518). Two of Cushing's former trainees who made
lasting contributions to the neurosurgical treatment of motor disorders were
Walter Dandy (1886-1946; Johns Hopkins University) and Wilder Penfield
(discussed earlier).

Lord Howard Walter Florey (1898-1968; Pathology, University of Oxford).
After a tour as a ship's surgeon, Florey worked in Sherrington's department in 1921-1924, initially as a Rhodes Scholar and later as a physiology
demonstrator (Gillespie, 1972a). He was encouraged by Sherrington (himself initially a pathologist) to pursue an academic clinical career as a pathologist, biochemist, and microbiologist. For his work on the discovery of
penicillin and its therapeutic applications, Florey shared a 1945 Nobel Prize
with Sir Alexander Fleming (1881-1955) and Sir Ernst Boris Chain (1906-
1979). Apart from that major achievement, Florey is best remembered for
the brilliant international group of experimental pathologists he trained at
Oxford between 1935 and 1962, and for his 1944 report that led to the founding of the Australian National University (Canberra, Australian Common-
wealth Territory) and its John Curtin School of Medical Research, where
Eccles's group subsequently flourished (1953-1966; see earlier).

Sixto Obrador (1911-1978; Neurosurgery, Autonomous University, Spain).
Obrador, the father of Spanish neurosurgery, worked with Sherrington and
Eccles in 1934-1936, after a short (1934) period at the Ramón y Cajal Institute (Madrid, Spain). Between 1941 and 1945 in Mexico City, he founded
the neurological department at the Sanatorio Espanol and the Manicomio
General de la Castaneda, and undertook research at the Instituto de Estudios
Medicos y Biologicos at the National University. After returning to Spain
in 1946 (a time of harsh economic circumstances) he founded, over the next
32 years, five neurological services at different hospitals in Madrid and
trained numerous neurosurgeons who extended the specialty throughout
the country. He was the driving force behind the mid-1970s construction of
the Centro Ramón y Cajal, a hospital and research center in Madrid where
Obrador's ashes were blended into the garden soil surrounding the statue
of Ramón y Cajal. (For further details, see Lassiera, 1979.)

This list of three collaborators of Sherrington is by no means exhaustive.
We could, for example, also highlight the contributions of George Lindor

Brown (U.K. physiology), Hugh Cairns (U.K. neurosurgery), Wilburt Davison (U.S. medical education at Duke University), Emil Holman (U.S. surgery at Stanford University), John Magladery (U.S. neurology at Johns Hopkins University), David Rioch (U.S. psychiatry), Charles Roy (U.K. pathology), Theodore Ruch (U.S. physiology at the University of Washington), and many other premier academic basic scientists and clinicians. In all cases, these people felt that they had a lifelong debt to Sherrington not only for the high quality of their training and/or collaborative experience with him but also for his never-ending support of their careers.

Summary

It is fitting to conclude this section with reference to Liddell's (1952) point that as a mentor, Sherrington wanted to know his trainees' ". . . thoughts and problems and not just live on a pedestal above them" (p. 259). In the modern parlance, Sherrington emphasized ". . . putting students and their needs first . . ." (Kennedy, 1997; p. 287)—as is so urgent in present-day research universities.

Impact of Sherrington's Nobel Lecture and Chapter

Although Sherrington chose to speak and write on coordinative CNS inhibition for his Nobel Lecture, he was actually awarded the prize for his 1920s work on the motor unit. In retrospect, it is puzzling that he was not so rewarded far earlier for his work demonstrating that the reciprocal innervation of antagonistic muscles involved an essentially active synaptic process. Perhaps Sherrington's 1885-onward, outspoken opposition to Prussian militarism (Granit, 1966; Eccles and Gibson, 1979) clouded the judgment of earlier Nobel committees, because there had been much early-1900s international enthusiasm for the bestowal of this prestigious award (Liljestrand, 1962). In any case, he shared the prize in 1932 with his good friend and neuroscience colleague, Adrian (the prize for Adrian was for his work on the unitary discharge of sensory receptors), and it was entirely appropriate for Sherrington to provide a Nobel lecture on a topic of his own choosing.

Historical Significance

For Eccles and Gibson (1979), Sherrington's Nobel Lecture was ". . . a masterly review of the role of inhibition in the central nervous system from the earlier suggestions of Descartes up to our most recent investigations . . . there is a superb discussion of the nature of the central excitatory and inhibitory processes, which so well foreshadows the discoveries by intracellular recording two decades later . . ." (p. 71). For present-day upper-division undergraduate and graduate students, well versed not only in the "inside-out" intracellular approach to describing active inhibition but also in hyperpolarizing ion-channel currents measured with patch-clamp electrodes, the literary style probably seems quaint, as if from a far-distant era. To such students, the authors would ask how they themselves would go about testing for active inhibition in the CNS of any species without intracellular recording electrodes and, for the mammalian CNS, in the face of strongly and widely held misperceptions like Pflüger's "laws on spinal reflexes" (Liddell, 1960). To ponder such issues is the quintessence of the way to approach Sherrington's Nobel Lecture and to gauge its historical significance.

Modern-Day Relevance

The pace of modern cellular neuroscience is so rapid that the mechanisms of CNS inhibition (presynaptic, postsynaptic, lateral, feed-forward, feedback) have moved to the molecular and ion-channel level, as studied by use of patch-clamp microelectrodes (e.g., Jonas et al., 1998; for review, Golowasch and Corey, 1997), an area of probably more potential excitement to Sherrington's co-Nobel laureate, Adrian, than to Sherrington himself. More in Sherrington's cellular-to-systems domain would be the recent identification and modeling of the role of inhibition in the behavior of segmental interneurons implicated in the operation of brainstem and spinal pattern generators for rhythmical movement (references in Stein et al., 1997; Kiehn et al., 1998; Binder, 1999)—even though, ironically, he had slowed (albeit unwittingly) this line of endeavor in the pre-World War II period. Also of immediate interest to Sherrington would be (1) the ongoing refinement of techniques to unravel inhibitory (and excitatory) connections between intercalated interneurons in alternative spinal reflex pathways (McCrea, 1998); (2) advances in the use of cytochemical and physiological markers to locate spinal interneurons that become active during movement in the cat (Jordan, 1998); and (3) the modern-day capability to record (extracellularly) the firing patterns of cervical spinal interneurons in the conscious nonhuman primate during operantly stimulated movement (Fetz et al., 1999). Finally, he would take a particular interest in recent studies on the inhibitory (and excitatory) neuromodulation of the stimulus current-spike frequency relation of spinal motoneurons and interneurons in the cat, and in a recent challenge to doctrinaire thinking on this topic mounted by Brownstone et al. (1992; for review, Stuart, 1999; Hornby, 2000). The reader should note that all of the topics mentioned have evolved from extensions of the work summarized by Sherrington in his Nobel Lecture.

Overall Summary

Sherrington held enormous sway in international neuroscience from the mid-1890s until his death in 1952, the peak of his influence being 1925-

1932. His greatest achievements related to neuroscience in general: that is, the incorporation of the synapse into systems and behavioral neuroscience; the promulgation of inhibition as a ubiquitous feature of CNS control mechanisms; and indirect proof that CNS inhibition is an active rather than passive process. For movement neuroscience, he dispelled many false notions that had accumulated throughout the early 19th century, and he laid the groundwork for several decades of precise and exacting work on the properties and central actions of muscle receptors and on motoneurons, motor units, and the size principle. Enigmatically and unfortunately, his influence on spinal pattern generation, which could have been profoundly positive, was ambivalent and thereby potentially misleading. This was largely due to the overwhelming pre-World War II emphasis in British mammalian physiology on unitary rather than systems neuroscience (Jung, 1975). Perhaps Sherrington's seeming ambivalence about the singular importance of the work of his own trainee, Graham Brown (see endnotes 28-30), would have been resolved if Keith Lucas, Adrian's brilliant cellular-, systems-, and comparatively oriented mentor, had been available to round out post-World War I British neurophysiology, or if Sherrington had spent more time in discussion with two outstanding generalists—the Russian Nicolai Bernstein and the Swiss Nobel laureate Walter Hess—rather than with his immediate British associates, commendable and important as was the unitary, cellular focus of the latter in helping to launch the post-World War II intracellular recording era. Nonetheless, it remained for the trainees of Sherrington's own trainees (particularly Lundberg; e.g., his 1969b treatise; see also Burke, 1985), contributing hand in hand with several groups of invertebrate neuroscientists, to bring about the more seamless integration of motor control neuroscience, from the cellular/molecular to the behavioral level of analysis, that flourishes today (e.g., Stein et al., 1997; Kiehn et al., 1998; Binder, 1999). We all owe Sherrington deep gratitude for the mammalian component of this essentially post-1970s development because it is clear that from the outset of his career his mentoring capabilities were profound, far reaching, and long lasting. It is therefore fitting to conclude this introduction to Sherrington's Nobel Lecture by drawing attention to the end of the preface of Eccles and Gibson (1979), where his former trainees spoke to the quintessence of a principle that should be foremost wherever science and training are undertaken, and particularly at research universities (Kennedy, 1997). In emphasizing the significance of the last chapter in Sherrington's (1951) *Man on His Nature*, Eccles and Gibson posited that "Sherrington very strongly expressed his conviction that in the evolutionary process predacity had gradually given place to man's survival—altruism being exalted above all others. His message is both noble and appealing . . ." (p. x). It is to be hoped that we in movement neuroscience can routinely exhibit the altruism, collegiality, and honor that highlighted Sherrington's own personal life and academic career.

Inhibition As a Coordinative Factor*

Sir Charles S. Sherrington

Note: The footnotes added to the following original text are explained below in the endnotes. These include comments on his reference to the work of others because no citations were provided with the original publication.

That a muscle on irritation of its nerve contracts had already long been familiar to physiology when the 19th century found a nerve which when irritated prevented its muscle from contracting. This observation seemed for a time too strange to be believed. Its truth did not gain acceptance for ten years; but at last in 1848 (*actually 1845*) the Webers[1] accepted the fact at its face value and proclaimed the vagus nerve to be inhibitory of the heart muscle. Two hundred years earlier Descartes[2], in writing the *De Homie,* had assumed that muscle was supplied with nerves which caused muscular relaxation. An analogous suggestion was put forward by Charles Bell[3] in 1819. The inhibition suggested was in each case «peripheral». «Peripheral» inhibition, despite its inherent probability, was however to prove void of the fact for skeletal muscle. As just said, it did in fact prove true for the heart,[4] it was found somewhat later to hold good likewise for visceral muscle,[5] and, somewhat later still, was found for the constrictor muscles of the blood vessels.[6] Peripheral inhibition became thus by the sixties and seventies of the 19th century a recognized fact, save for the one important exception of the skeletal muscles.[7]

The first experimental indication of inhibition as a process working *within* the nervous system itself appeared in 1863. Setschenov (*actually Ivan Sechenov*) then noted in the frog that the local reflexes of the limb are depressed by stimulation of the exposed midbrain.[8] Later (1881), somewhat similarly, stimulation of the foot (dog) was found to restrain movements of the foot excited from the brain (Bubnoff[9] and Heidenhain[10]). Matters had, broadly put, reached and remained at that stage, when in the century's last decade experimental examination of mammalian reflexes detected (1892)[11] examples of inhibition of surprising potency and machine-like regularity, readily obtainable from the mammalian spinal cord in its action on the extensors of the hind limb; the inhibitory relaxation of the extension was linked with concomitant reflex contraction of their antagonistic muscles, the flexors. This «reciprocal innervation» was quickly found to be of wide occurrence in reflex actions operating the skeletal musculature.[12] Its openness to examination in preparations with «tonic» background (decerebrate rigidity) made it a welcome and immediate opportunity for the more precise study of inhibition as a central nervous process.

The seat of this inhibition was soon shown to be central, e.g. for spinal reflexes, in the grey matter of the spinal cord. The resulting relaxation of

*Reprinted from Sherrington 1932. © The Nobel Foundation 1932.

the muscle was found to be both in range and nicety as amenable to grading as is reflex contraction itself. In other words the inhibitory process was found capable of no less delicate quantitative adjustment than is the excitatory process. In «reciprocal innervation» the two effects, excitation and inhibition, ran broadly *pari passu;* a weak stimulus evoked weak inhibitory relaxation along with weak excitatory contraction in the antagonist muscle; a strong stimulus evoked greater and quicker relaxation accompanying greater and speedier contraction of the antagonist. No evidence was forthcoming that the centripetal nervous impulses which on their central arrival give rise to inhibition differ in nature from nerve impulses giving rise centrally to «excitation», or indeed differ from the impulses travelling nerve fibres elsewhere. An «inhibitory» afferent nerve emerged simply as an afferent nerve whose impulses at certain central loci cause, directly or indirectly, inhibition, while at other central loci the same nerve, probably even the same nerve fibre can produce excitation. There was no satisfactory evidence that an afferent nerve fibre whose end-effect is inhibitory ever for its end-effect at that same locus evokes excitation or indeed any other effect than inhibition. That is to say its inhibitory influence never changes to an excitatory influence, or vice versa.[13] Fixity of central effect, inhibitory or excitatory respectively, has to be accepted for the individual afferent fibre acting in a specified direction, i.e. on a specified individual effector unit. That does not of course exclude the contingency that an inhibitory influence on a given unit may under some circumstances be unable to produce effective inhibition there owing to its being too weak to overcome concurrent excitation.

I will not dwell upon the features of reciprocal innervation; they are well known. I would only remark that owing to the wide occurrence of reciprocal innervation it was not unnatural to suppose at first that the entire scope of reflex inhibition lay within the ambit of the taxis of antagonistic muscles and antagonistic movements. Further study of central nervous action, however, finds central inhibition too extensive and ubiquitous to make it likely that it is confined solely to the taxis of antagonistic muscles.

In instance let us take a reflex especially facile and regular to type, the well-known spinal flexion-reflex of the leg, evoked by stimulation of any afferent nerve of the leg itself. Its experimental stimulus may be reduced to a single induction shock evoking a single volley of centripetal impulses in the bared afferent nerve. The reflex effect, observed in an isolated flexor muscle, e.g. of the ankle, is apart from exceptional circumstances, a single contraction wave indicating discharge of a single volley of motor impulses from the spinal centre. This «twitch-reflex», recorded isometrically by the myograph, exhibits a tension proportional to the number of motor units[14] engaged, in other words to the size of the single centrifugal impulse volley. The contraction of each motor unit is on the all-or-nothing principle.[15] The maximal contraction-tension for the reflex twitch will be reached only when all of the motor units composing the muscle are activated. The contraction-tension developed by the reflex being proportional to the number of motor units engaged, an average contraction-tension value for the individual motor unit can be found. The contraction developed by the reflex twitch is less the weaker the induction shock exciting the afferent nerve, in other words the fewer the afferent fibres excited, in short, the smaller the size of the centripetal impulse volley. With a given single-shock stimulus the tension developed by the reflex twitch remains closely constant when sampled at not too frequent intervals. In the case of the spinal flexion-reflex therefore, though with many other reflexes it is not so, a standard reflex twitch of desired size (tension) can be obtained at repeated intervals.

The only index available at present for inhibition is its effect on excitation; thus, a standard twitch-reflex, representing a standard-sized volley of centrifugal discharge, can serve as a quantitative test for reflex inhibition. It serves for this with less ambiguity than does a reflex tetanus. In the tetanus the tension developed will depend within limits on the repetitive-frequency of the contraction waves forming the tetanus. Maximal tetanic contraction is reached only when the frequency reaches a rate which, in many reflex tetani, some of the units do not attain. In reflexes the rate of tetanic discharge can differ from unit to unit in one and the same muscle at one and the same time.[16] The rate will differ too at different stages of the same reflex and according as the reflex is weak or strong. Reflex inhibition acting against a reflex tetanic contraction may diminish the contraction in one or other or all of several different ways. In some units it may suppress the motor discharge altogether, in some it may merely slow the motor discharge thus lessening the wave frequency of the contraction and so the tension. The same aggregate diminution of tension may thus be brought about variously and by various combinations of ways, a result too equivocal for analysis. The same gross result might accrue (a) from total suppression of activity in some units or (b) from mere slackening of discharge in a larger number of units. These difficulties of interpretation are avoided by using as gauge for inhibition a standard reflex twitch.[17] The deficit of contraction-tension then observed shows unequivocally the number of motor units inhibited out of the total activated for the standard. Since the direct maximal motor twitch compared with the standard reflex twitch can reveal the proportion of the whole muscle which the standard reflex twitch activates, we can find further what proportion of the whole muscle is reflexly inhibited. Of course subliminal excitation and subliminal inhibition are not revealed by the test and require other means for detection.

A stable excitatory twitch-reflex as standard allows us to proceed further in our quantitative examination of inhibition. We then find that inhibition can be admixt in our simple-seeming flexion-reflex itself and indeed usually is so. To detect it we have simply to add to the earlier excitation of the reflex a following one at not too long interval; we then find the response to the second stimulus-volley partly cut down by an inhibition latent in the first.

This is usually evident with intervals between 300-1,200 µs. The very shortest interval at which the inhibitory effect occurs is difficult to determine for the reason that the excitatory effect has a subliminal fringe and the second stimulus repeats the subliminal effect of the first, and the two subliminal effects can sum to liminal.[18] The second response is therefore enlarged by summation of subliminal fringe[19] in some of the responsive motor units. This activation by the second stimulus of some motor units facilitated for it by the first though not activated by the first alone tends of course to obscure the inhibitory inactivation; the shrinkage due to the latter is offset by the increment due to the former. The inhibition is traceable only by the net diminution of the second reflex twitch. How quickly the inhibitory element in the stimulus develops centrally is not fully ascertainable, because the sooner the second reflex follows on the first the more the facilitation from it that it gets. This increment will conceal at least in part the decrement due to inhibition. Similarly the beginning of the inhibition may be concealed from observation by concomitant excitatory facilitation. This uncertainty does not attach to the longer intervals between the two stimuli because the central inhibitory process considerably outlasts the central excitatory facilitation.

The reflex therefore, which at first sight seems a purely excitatory reaction, proves on closer examination to be in fact a commingled excitation and inhibition. Usually clearly demonstrable in the simple spinal condition of the reflex, this complexity of character is yet more evident in the decerebrate condition.[20]

We may hesitate to generalize from this example, because a stimulus applied to a bared afferent nerve is of course «artificial» in as much as it is applied to an anatomical collection of nerve fibres not homogeneous in function; and, we may suppose, not usually excited together. If cutaneous, its fibres will belong to such different species of sense as «touch» and «pain» which often provoke movements of opposite direction and are therefore in their effect on a given muscle opposed in effect. That a strong stimulus to such an afferent nerve, exciting most or all of its fibres, should in regard to a given muscle develop inhibition and excitation concurrently is not surprising.

With weak stimuli the case is somewhat different. Such stimuli excite only a few of the constituent fibres of the afferent nerve, and those of similar calibre, presumably an indication of some functional likeness. Nevertheless, as shown above, the reflex result even then exhibits admixed excitatory and inhibitory influence on one and the same given muscle. And this admixture of excitation and inhibition persists when the stimulus is reduced in strength still further so as to be merely liminal.[21] It still is so when the afferent nerve chosen is homogeneous in the sense that it is a purely muscular afferent, e.g. the afferent from one head of the gastrocnemius muscle. But we must remember that the afferent nerve from an extensor muscle has been shown to contain fibres which exert opposite reflex influences upon their own muscle, some exciting and some inhibiting that muscle's contraction.[22] This brings with it the question whether admixture of exciting and inhibiting influence in the reflex effect obtains when instead of stimulation of a bared nerve some more «natural» stimulation is employed.

For this the reflex evoked by passive flexion of the knee in the decerebrate preparation has been taken. The single-joint extensor (vasto-crureus) of each knee is isolated; and nothing but that muscle pair thus retained is still innervated in the whole of the two limbs. The preparation thus obtained is a tonic preparation; one of the two muscles is then stretched by passively flexing a knee. This passive flexion excites in the extensor muscle which it stretches a reflex relaxation, i.e. the lengthening reaction; this relaxation at one knee is accompanied in the opposite fellow vasto-crureus by a reflex contraction enhancing the existing «tonic» contraction. The reflex contraction thus provoked is characteristically deliberate and smooth in performance and passes without overshoot into a maintained extension posture. Let however the manoeuvre be then repeated with the one difference of condition, that the muscle contralateral to that which is passively stretched has been deafferented. In the deafferented muscle contraction is still obtained, and more easily than before, but the deafferented condition of the muscle alters the course of its contraction in two respects. The course is no longer deliberate. The contraction is an abrupt rush, with overshoot of the succeeding postural contraction, and this latter is hardly maintained at all. The severance of the afferent nerve has removed a reflex self-restraint from the contracting muscle. Normally the proprioceptives[23] of the contracting muscle put a brake on the speed of the contracting muscle (autogenous inhibition). The explosive rush and momentum of these deafferented extensor reflexes recall the ataxy of *tabes*. They recall also the abruptness and overshooting of the «willed» movements of a deafferented limb. In both cases a normal self-braking has been lost along with the deprivation of the muscle of its own proprioceptive afferents.[24] These latter mediate both a self-braking and a self-exciting (autogenous excitation) reflex action of the muscle. Thus here again there is admixture of reflex inhibition and excitation, and in this case the admixture obtains in response to a «natural» stimulation. Here therefore the admixture of central inhibition with central excitation is a normal feature of a natural reflex.

This makes it clear that for the study of normal nervous coordinations we require to know how central inhibition and excitation interact. As said above, the centripetal impulses which evoke inhibition do not differ in nature from those which evoke excitation. Inhibition like excitation can be induced in a «resting» centre. The only test we have for the inhibition is excitation. Existence of an excited state is not a prerequisite for the production of inhibition; inhibition can exist apart from excitation no less than, when called forth against an excitation already in progress, it can suppress or moderate it. The centripetal volley which excites a «centre» finds, if preceded by an inhibitory volley, the centre so treated is already irresponsive or partly so.

A first question is, are there degrees of «central inhibitory state»; and are they, like central excitatory state, capable of summation. This can be examined in several ways. Thus: against the central inhibition caused by a given single volley of inhibitory impulses a standard single volley of excitatory impulses can be launched at an appropriate interval.[25] The relatively long duration of the central inhibitory state allows a second inhibitory volley to be interpolated between the original inhibitory volley and the standard excitatory volley. The standard excitation is found to be then diminished (as shown by the twitch-contraction which it evokes) more than it is if subjected to either one inhibitory volley only. This holds even when the second inhibitory volley, launched from the same cathode as the first, is arranged to be clearly smaller than the first. Since the distribution of the effect of the smaller impulse volley (launched from the same cathode as the larger) among the motoneurones of the centre must lie completely included within that of the first, the added inhibition due to the second volley indicates that the combined influence of the two volleys prevents activation of sonic motoneurones which neither inhibitory volley acting alone was able to prevent from being activated. Evidently therefore central inhibition sums; consequently it is capable of subliminal existence. Also, successive subliminal degrees of inhibition can by temporal overlap sum to supraliminal degree. In these ways central inhibition presents analogy with its converse «central excitations»; both exhibit various degrees of intensity in respect to the individual motoneurone.

Summation of inhibition is well exhibited when a given twitch-reflex is evoked at various times during and after a tetanic inhibition. The cutting down of the reflex twitch is progressively greater, as within limits, the inhibitory tetanus proceeds. After cessation of the tetanus the inhibitory state, similarly tested, passes off gradually, more quickly at first than later.

The relatively long persistence of the central inhibitory state induced by a single centripetal impulse volley allows examination of the effect on it of two successive excitation volleys as compared with one of the two alone. An excitatory volley is interpolated between the inhibitory volley and a subsequent standard excitatory volley. The interpolated excitatory volley is found to lessen the inhibitory effect upon the final excitatory volley. The interpolated excitation volley neutralizes some of the inhibition which otherwise would have counteracted the final test excitation. Just as central inhibitory state (c.i.s.) counteracts central excitatory state (c.e.s.) so c.e.s. neutralizes c.i.s. The mutual inactivation is quantitative. There occurs at the individual neurone an algebraic summation of the values of the two opposed influences.[26]

It is still early to venture any definite view of the intimate nature of
«central inhibition». It is commonly held that nerve excitation consists
essentially in the local depolarization of a polarized membrane on the
surface of the neurone. As to «central excitation», it is difficult to suppose
such depolarization of the cell surface can be graded any more than can
that of the fibre. But its antecedent step (facilitation) might be graded, e.g.
subliminal. Local depolarization having occurred the difference of potential
thus arisen gives a current which disrupts the adjacent polarization
membrane, and so the «excitation» travels. As to inhibition the suggestion
is made that it consists in the temporary stabilization of the surface
membrane which excitation would break down. As tested against a standard
excitation the inhibitory stabilization is found to present various degrees
of stability. The inhibitory stabilization of the membrane might be pictured
as a heightening of the «resting» polarization, somewhat on the lines of an
electrotonus. Unlike the excitation-depolarization it would not travel; and,
in fact, the inhibitory state does not travel.[27]

The quantitative character of the interaction between opposed inhibition
and excitation is experimentally demonstrable. Thus: a given inhibitory
tetanus exerted on a certain set of motoneurones fails to prevent their
excitation in response to strong stimulation of a given afferent nerve; but
when the stimulation of the excitatory afferent is weaker the given standard
inhibitory tetanus does prevent the response of the motor neurones to the
excitatory stimulation. With the weaker stimulation of the afferent nerve
there are fewer of its fibres acting, and therefore fewer converge for central
effect on some of the units. On these the standard c.i.s. has therefore less
c.e.s. to counteract.

Many features characteristic of reflex myographic records of various type
become interpretable in light of the stimulus volley from a single afferent
nerve trunk, even small, evoking an admixture of inhibition and excitation,
with consequent central conflict and interaction between them. Features
which find facile explanation in this way are the following. (A) The flexion-
reflex (spinal) commonly has a *d'emblée* opening; that is, a steep initial
contraction passes abruptly into a plateau, giving an approximately
rectangular beginning to the myogram. Here the initial reflex excitation is
closely followed by an ensuing reflex inhibition commingled with and
partially counter-acting the concurrent excitation. (B) Allied to this and of
analogous explanation is the so-called «fountain»-form of flexion-reflex.
After the first uprush of contraction a component of reflex inhibition grows
relatively more potent and the contraction-tension drops low before
continuing-level. Between these extreme forms there are intermediates. The
key to the production of them all is admixture of central excitation with
central inhibition; the excitation is prepotent earlier, and later suffers from
encroaching inhibition. (C) Again, the typical opening of the crossed
extensor reflex (decerebrate) «recruits». A variably long latent period

precedes a contraction which climbs slowly, taking perhaps seconds to reach its plateau. Here, struggling with excitation, inhibition has the upper hand at first. The action currents of the muscle marking the serial stimuli to the afferent nerve are not choked by secondary waves of after-discharge. The concurrent inhibition cuts them out. The inhibition is traceable partly to the proprioceptive reflex mechanism attached to the contracting muscle itself; the progress of the reflex contraction is partly freed from inhibition by deafferenting the muscle, but still not wholly freed. A residuum of inhibition in the reflex is traceable to the crossed afferent nerve employed. This again illustrates the ubiquitous commingling of inhibition and excitation in the spinal and decerebrate reflexes evoked by direct stimulation of afferent nerves.

An instance of combination of excitation and inhibition for coordinative effect is the rhythmic reflex of stepping.[28] In the «spinal» cat and dog there occurs «stepping» of the hind limbs; it starts when the «spinal» hind limbs, lifted from the ground, hang freely, the animal being supported vertically from the shoulders. The extensor phase in one limb occurs with the flexor phase in the other. This «stepping» can also be evoked by a stigmatic electrode carrying a mild tetanic current to a point in the cross-face of the cut spinal cord. The «stepping» then opens with flexion in the ipsilateral hind limb accompanied by extension in the contralateral. To reproduce this stepping movement by appropriately timed repetitions of tetanization of, for instance, a flexion producing afferent of one limb or an extension-producing afferent of the other never succeeds even remotely in exciting the rhythmic stepping. In the true rhythmic movement itself, which has been examined particularly by Graham Brown,[29] the contraction in each phase develops smoothly to a climax and then as smoothly declines, waxing and waning much as does the activity of the diaphragm in normal inspiration. But although this rhythmically intermittent tetanus affecting alternately the flexors and extensors of the limb and giving the reflex step cannot be copied reflexly by employing excitation alone, it can be easily and faithfully reproduced and with perfect alternation of phase and with its characteristic asymmetrical bilaterality, by employing a stimulation in which reflex excitation and reflex inhibition are admixt in approximately balanced intensity. The result is then a rhythmic sea-saw about a neutral point. The effect on the individual motor unit appears then to run its course thus: if we start to trace the cycle with the moment when c.e. and c.i. are so equal as to cancel out, the state of the motoneurone is a zero state, for which the term «rest», although often applied to it, is perhaps better avoided. With supervention of preponderance of c.e. over c.i. the motor neurone's discharge commences and under progressive increase of that preponderance the frequency of discharge increases in the individual motor neurone, and more motor neurones are «recruited» for action until in due course the preponderance of c.e. begins to fail and c.i. in its turn asserts itself more.

The recruitment and frequency of discharge begin to wane, and then reach their lowest, and may cease, and an interval of zero state or quiescense may ensue. The quiescence may be inhibitory or merely lack of excitation. Which of these it were could be directly determined only by testing the threshold of excitation. However brought about, it is synchronous with the excitation-phase in the antagonistic muscle and with the excitation-phase in the symmetrical fellow muscles of the opposite limb. Since reciprocal innervation has been observed to obtain between these muscles, the phase of lapse of excitation is probably one of fuller active inhibition. The rhythm induced by stimulation of the «stepping»-point in the cut face of the lateral column of the cord[30] would seem to act therefore by evoking concurrently excitation and inhibition, and so playing them off one against the other as to induce alternate dominance of each. Intensifying the mild current applied to the point quickens the tempo of the rhythm, i.e. of the alternation.

Another class of events revealing inhibition as a factor wide and decisive in the working of the central nervous system is presented by the «release» phenomenon of Hughlings Jackson.[31] The depression of activity called «shock» supervenes on injury of a distant but related part; conversely there supervenes often an over-action due likewise to injury or destruction of some distant but related part. «Shock» is traceable to loss of excitatory influence, which, though perhaps commonly subliminal in itself, lowers the threshold for other excitation. The over-action conversely is traceable to loss of inhibitory influence, perhaps subliminal in itself and yet helping concurrent influences of like direction to maintain a normal restraint, the normal height of threshold against excitation. Where the relation between one group of muscles and another, e.g. between flexors and extensors, is reciprocal, the effect of removal (by trauma or disease) of some influence exerted by another part of the nervous system is commonly two-fold in direction. There is «shock», i.e. depression of excitability in one field of the double mechanism and «release», i.e. exaltation of excitability, in another. Thus spinal transection, cutting off the hind-limb spinal reflexes from prespinal centres inflicts «shocks» on the extensor half-centre and produces «release» of the flexor half-centre.[32] In this case the direction both of the «shock» and of the «release» runs aborally; but it can run the other way, as in the influence that the hind-limb centres have on the fore-limb. Which way it runs, of course, depends simply on the relative anatomical situation of the influencing and the influenced centres.

The role of inhibition in the working of the central nervous system has proved to be more and more extensive and more and more fundamental as experiment has advanced in examining it. Reflex inhibition can no longer be regarded merely as a factor specially developed for dealing with the antagonism of opponent muscles acting at various hinge-joints. Its role as a coordinative factor comprises that, and goes beyond that.[33] In the working of the central nervous machinery inhibition seems as ubiquitous and as frequent as is excitation itself. The whole quantitative grading of the operations of the spinal cord and brain appears to rest upon mutual interaction between the two central processes «excitation» and «inhibition», the one no less important than the other. For example, no operation can be more important as a basis of coordination for a motor act than adjustment of the quantity of contraction, e.g. of the number of motor units employed and the intensity of their individual tetanic activity. This now appears as the outcome of nice co-adjustment of excitation and inhibition upon each of all the individual units which cooperate in the act.

In reflexes, even under simple spinal or decerebrate conditions, interplay between excitation and inhibition is commonly induced even by the simplest stimulus. It need not surprise us therefore that variability of reflex result is met by the experimenter. Indeed, that it troubles him by being partly beyond his control, need not surprise him in view of the multiplicity and complicity of the sources of the inhibition and of the excitation. This variability seems underestimated by those who regard reflex action as too rigid to provide a prototype for cerebral behaviour. It is in virtue of their containing inhibition and excitation admixt that, in accord with central conditions prevailing for the time being, a limb-reflex provoked by a given stimulus in the decerebrate preparation can on one occasion be opposite in direction to what it is on another, e.g. extension instead of flexion («reversal»). Excitation and inhibition are both present from the very stimulus outset and are pitted against one another. The central circumstances may favour one at one time, the other at another. Again, if the quantity of contraction needed normally for a given act be reached by algebraic summation of central excitation and inhibition, it can obviously be attained by variously compounded quantities of those two. Hence when disease or injury has caused a deficit of excitation, a readjustment of concurrent inhibition offers a means of arriving once more at the normal quantity required. The admixture of inhibition and excitation as a mechanism for coordination thus provides a means of understanding the remarkable «compensations» which restore in course of time, and even quickly, the muscular competence for execution of an act which has been damaged by central nervous lesions. More than one way for doing the same thing is provided by the natural constitution of the nervous system. This luxury of means of compassing a given combination seems to offer the means of restitution of an act after its impairment or loss in one of its several forms.

Acknowledgments

We would like to thank Hannah Fisher, Nga Nguyen, and Robert Reinking for their help with many of the historical references, and Drs. Anders Lundberg, Arthur Prochazka, Uwe Proske, and Paul Stein for reading the final draft of this article. We would also like to thank the following colleagues

for their help with selected sections and with some historical and theoreti-
cal points: Drs. Marc Binder, David Burke, Roger Enoka, Simon Gandevia,
Eugene Gerner, Sid Gilman, Robert Gore, Allan Hamilton, Mollie Holman,
Larry Jordan, Richard Levine, Tim Neild, Bernado Odoriz, Serge Rossignol,
W. Zev Rymer, Thomas Sears, Nicholas Strausfeld, Lee Sweeney, Anthony
Taylor, Dirk Van Helden, Joel Vilensky, and Victor Wilson. The work was
supported, in part, by USPHS grants NS 20577 and NS 07309 (to D.G.S.)
and NS 01686 (to J.C.M.); a University of Newcastle Visiting Faculty Award
(to R.J.C. and D.G.S.); an Australian NH & MRC award #980382 (to R.J.C.);
and a New Staff Grant, University of Newcastle Research Management
Committee (to A.M.B.). The paper's contents are solely the responsibility
of the authors and do not necessarily represent the views of the awarding
agencies.

Endnotes

The following endnotes, besides containing the footnotes we have added
to Sherrington's original 1932 article, provide additional viewpoints with
the aim of highlighting several historical features and relating Sherrington's
ideas to modern-day motor control neuroscience.

[1] For brief historical accounts of the contributions of the Webers (Eduard and Ernst, 1845),
Rene Descartes,[2] Charles Bell,[3] Nicolai Bubnoff,[9] and Rudolph Heidenhain,[10] see Brazier
(1959, pp. 28 and 36).

[4-6] For the first definitive reports on peripheral, autonomic axons providing postsynaptic
(i.e., post-neuroeffector junction) inhibition to cardiac muscle, nonvascular smooth muscle,
and vascular smooth muscle, see Del Castillo and Katz (1955; frog heart[4]) and Burnstock
et al. (1963; smooth muscle of the taenia coli of the guinea pig;[5] see also Bulbring et al.
[1958; their Figure 12] and Bell [1969; guinea pig uterine artery[6]]). In addition, for the first
reports of neurohormonally mediated hyperpolarization of vascular smooth muscle and
its relative efficacy versus neuronally mediated responses, see Hermsmeyer (1982) and
Andriantsitohaina and Surprenant (1992). These various reports were all preceded by a
substantial amount of supportive, indirect 19th- and early-20th-century evidence (for review, see Wiggers, 1960).

[7] Here Sherrington is setting the stage for his subsequent discourse on central (spinal) inhibition. Originally he thought that skeletal muscle in vertebrates might well receive peripheral motor axons that provide post-neuromuscular junction inhibition to their muscle
fibers, as based on Biedermann's (1889) then-recent work on the claw of the *Astacus* crab
(Liddell, 1952). Peripheral post-neuroeffector junction inhibition is common in the neural
control of invertebrate skeletal muscle, the first definitive report being that of Van Harreveld
and Wiersma (1937) showing inhibition of a claw-opener muscle of the *Cambarus* crayfish
by stimulation of a slow nerve fiber. Shortly thereafter, Katz's laboratory (Katz, 1938, 1949;
Fatt and Katz, 1953) described two types of inhibition in muscle fibers of the *Eupagarus*
crab: "simple" or "beta" inhibition, which does not reduce post-neuroeffector junction
excitatory (postsynaptic) potentials (EPSPs) but nevertheless inhibits contraction; and
"supplemented alpha" inhibition, which indeed involves a reduction in the amplitude of
EPSPs. Somewhat later there was clear demonstration of both presynaptic and postsynaptic inhibition (Dudel and Kuffler, 1961).

[8] Here Sherrington is referring to a report of J. Setschenow, who was actually Ivan Sechenov
(1863a) (i.e., both Sechenov's first name and surname often appeared in different forms
and with different spellings). It would also have been appropriate for Sherrington to acknowledge the then-well-known essay by Sechenov (1863b), *Reflexes of the Brain*. Sechenov

was a particularly active and distinguished 19th-century neuroscientist and the true father of Russian neurophysiology (Brazier, 1959). He had long argued that there was a balance between active excitatory and inhibitory processes in the CNS. For example, in his essay, Sechenov (1863b) reasoned: "We therefore see that the cerebral mechanism which produces involuntary (reflex) movements of the body and the appendages, possess two apparatuses in the brain, one of which inhibits movements and the other, in the contrary, augments them" (p. 275 in the 1935 translation edited by Subkov). In the same essay, Sechenov also argued: ". . . Does the mechanism of inhibition, already known to us from the study of reflexes, play any role in originating voluntary movements? . . . in conscious life there are cases of inhibition both of movements generally regarded as involuntary, and of those known as voluntary. Since, however, voluntary movements develop in accordance with the basic laws of reflexes, we may, naturally, assume that the mechanism of inhibition in both cases is the same" (pp. 81-82 in the 1965 translation by Koshtoyants and Gibbons).

With regard to Pavlov, the following quote from Jeannerod (1985) is most revealing and provocative: "Sherrington . . . began with premises similar to those of Setchenov [i.e., Sechenov] and Pavlov, since he viewed the 'simple reflex' as the basic unit of neural function. His views differed radically from the Russian school, however, in the definition of this function. Sherrington did not seek to locate the role of the nervous system in some adaptation of the organism to its external environment. . . . To the contrary, this role must [i.e., according to Sherrington] be 'within,' as a force for ordering and organizing behavior. Sherrington's conception did, in fact, maintain that it was the nervous system which imposed its order on the environment, and not the inverse. One can thus understand the vehemence of his discussions with Pavlov, who had forbidden his students to read Sherrington's work. Sherrington, albeit less intolerant than Pavlov, nonetheless testified to the irreconcilable nature of the disagreement; and, when he visited Pavlov's laboratory in 1914 he told him: 'Your conditioned reflexes have little chance of being believed in England, because they have a materialistic flavor. . . .' In fact, E.G.T. Liddell, one of Sherrington's own students, did not even cite conditioned reflexes in his book regarding the discovering of reflexes—written in 1960" (p. 44). This exchange between Sherrington and Pavlov actually took place in London in 1912, and there are several different versions of the specific Sherrington quote (e.g., Volicer, 1973; p. 283) and of the encounter itself (e.g., Pavlov, 1938; p. 24).

Despite this particular difference between these two such influential neuroscientists, Sherrington apparently came away from his subsequent 1914 visit to St. Petersburg ". . . with a great enthusiasm for the leader of Russian neurophysiology" (Brazier, 1959; p. 56; see also Sherrington, 1953).

[9-10] See endnote 1.

[11] The specific reference (1892a) Sherrington cites here, one year after his first report (1891) on reflexes, was the forerunner to 13 reports between 1893 and 1908 on reciprocal innervation and to a 14th in 1909 on double reciprocal innervation. An example of this work is shown in figure 11.1. The presence of active inhibition in spinal reflex pathways was considered by Sherrington to be his best contribution to neuroscience (Granit, 1966; p. 50). In its entirety, it was an essential forerunner to the post-World War II advances in spinal cord neurophysiology made in the laboratories of Eccles, Granit, Lloyd, Renshaw, and Lundberg, using techniques that were far more advanced than the pre-electronic ones available to (and preferred by) Sherrington. In particular, these later techniques included intracellular (IC) recording, which was first accomplished in motoneurons by Eccles' group (Brock et al., 1951) and Woodbury and Patton (1952; see also Hoyle [1983] and Bretag [1983] for earlier use of the IC technique in nerve and other cells). For review of early post-World War II advances using IC and other post-Sherringtonian techniques, see the chapters of Eccles, Eldred, Granit, and Lloyd in Field et al. (1959-1960).

[12] Subsequent, far more recent IC recordings have revealed that reciprocal innervation is largely restricted, at least in the cat, to motoneurons (MNs) supplying muscles that operate almost exclusively as antagonists during forward overground locomotion (e.g., knee flexors vs. extensors, as commonly studied by Sherrington; figure 11.1). For example, MNs to thigh adductors and abductors are not linked by reciprocal innervation (see Table II in Jankowska and Odutola, 1980).

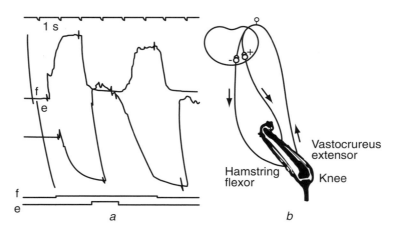

Figure 11.1
Examples of Sherrington's work and ideas on reciprocal inhibition. The terminology is that of
Granit (1966; his Figure 5). *(a)* Decerebrate cat, reciprocal effects of antagonistic muscles of
the knee—f: flexor of knee, *semitendinosus*; e: extensor of knee, *vastrocrureus*. Of the signal
lines (below), the upper (f) marks by its rise the period of stimulation of the ipsilateral
peroneal nerve; the lower marks similarly the stimulation of the contralateral peroneal nerve
(reprinted from Sherrington 1913d). *(b)* Diagram of cross-section of spinal cord to illustrate
innervation of knee extensor and knee flexor by the simplest possible circuit, explaining
reciprocal effects of ipsilateral muscular origin, excitatory (+) for extensor and inhibitory (−)
for flexor motoneurone. The same extensor muscular afferent has terminals on both types of
motoneurone. (reprinted from Granit 1966)

[13] Similarly, in post-1960s experiments, challenging IC-recording experiments have shown
that many primary sensory afferents have both excitatory and inhibitory di- and oligo (a
few)-synaptic connections with the same MN. The chosen postsynaptic effect depends on
the motor task under consideration, with the choice dictated by the CNS-controlled behavior of intercalated spinal interneurons in the alternative pathways (Stuart and
McDonagh, 1997).

[14] The most useful term, "motor unit," is now defined as a full MN (i.e., its cell body, dendrites, and axon) and all of the muscle fibers it supplies (Burke, 1981). The term was coined
by Liddell and Sherrington in 1924, and they then limited it to a MN's axon and the muscle
fibers innervated by that axon. The concept was established by several others somewhat
earlier, however. For example, Lewis (1984) has emphasized the 1913 report of Mines (see
also Lucas, 1905, 1909a).

[15] Much later work, using single-fiber EMG, has shown that unless subjected to ischemia or
fatigue, the action potential propagates along *all* the axon's collaterals. Likewise, the safety
factor for neuromuscular transmission is sufficiently high at all the axon collaterals' neuromuscular junctions to ensure that all the unit's muscle fibers are activated to contract
(Stålberg and Trontelj, 1994). To this extent, Sherrington's "all-or-nothing" phrase is still
correct, provided the length-tension relationship is also taken into account, as was well
known to him in the 1930s and indeed far earlier. More recent work has also shown, however, that the amount of force produced by a motor unit is highly dependent on the prior
activity level of the muscle, with factors like rest-shortening and rest-lengthening coming
into play (for review, see Hasan and Stuart, 1988).

[16] This issue was studied intensively in Sherrington's laboratory, a critical report of that period being that of Denny-Brown (1929).

[17] Much later, this technique (see endnote 25) was modified to gauge the elaboration of a
maximum voluntary contraction (Merton, 1954; Gandevia et al., 1995). Furthermore, other

modifications were exploited in the 1941-1957 work of Lloyd (see his 1960 review); in the 1940-1946 work of Renshaw (references in Eccles, 1964); and, of even wider impact, in Lundberg's post-1960 Goteborg laboratory, as a heroic means of unraveling the synaptic connectivity within spinal reflex pathways (for review, see Baldissera et al., 1981).

[18-19] "Liminal" (meaning "threshold") is a tricky term used in two ways by Sherrington in this lecture. Further on (footnote 21), he used the term more or less correctly to describe a stimulus barely above threshold for the activation of a single sensory axon in a muscle nerve. Here, as in most situations, however, Sherrington is speaking about a just-above-threshold stimulus that could bring a selected number of MNs into their "discharge zone" (latter term used in Creed et al., 1932). His idea was that such a stimulus level (strength) brought such MNs to firing (i.e., emitting repetitive action potentials). Other MNs received only subthreshold levels of excitation and constituted the "subliminal fringe." Still other cells within the potentially activatable MN pool (i.e., MNs innervating a single muscle and their close synergists) remained quiescent. As the sensory-reflex input to the pool was increased, MNs from the subliminal fringe could be recruited into the discharge zone, while other cells from the quiescent pool entered the subliminal fringe (for Lloyd's contributions to these ideas, see Lloyd, 1960; Patton, 1994).

"Threshold" itself is a clear-cut term: That is, in random fashion, MNs (and the membranes of other excitable muscle cells and neuron types) either discharge or they do not. To be just above this state, at the so-called threshold for repetitive discharge, was not quantitated in Sherrington's day; and, although studied valuably by Kernell from 1966 onward (e.g., his 1995 review), only recently has this latter threshold been addressed quantitatively (see, e.g., Binder and Jabre, 1999; chapters of Kudina, Matthews, and Piotrkiewicz).

[20] The decerebrate cat was a favorite preparation for Sherrington. The animal was prepared under ether anesthesia, and a cut was made between the midbrain and diencephalon (actually from between the superior and inferior colliculus dorsally to the posterior margin of the mammillary bodies ventrally). The anesthesia was then discontinued to provide an unanesthetized, pain-free preparation with lively reflexes, albeit favoring the extensor ones. The term "decerebrate rigidity" was coined by Sherrington in a paper read to the Royal Society in 1897 (full report in 1898). It is often used to describe the posture of the decerebrate preparation, but, as shown in figure 11.2, this is a misnomer, because the preparation's heightened extensor muscle activity can be obviated by the clasp-knife reflex. Hence the condition is one of decerebrate spasticity (for further details on this and allied issues in experimental animals and the relevance to humans, see Burke et al., 1972; Wetzel and Stuart, 1976; Rymer et al., 1979; Burke, 1988; Cleland and Rymer, 1990).

[21] See endnotes 18-19.

[22] After World War II, the selective activation of a single species of sensory afferent fibers with a mixed muscle nerve by use of electrical, mechanical, or both means became a very lively and often contentious field of study, and one about which remains many unresolved issues (see, e.g., Binder et al., 1982), particularly when applied to humans (for references, see Katz and Pierrot-Deseilligny, 1999).

[23-24] The terms "proprioceptives"[23] and "proprioceptive afferents"[24] are often misused or misunderstood in modern-day movement science. The terms should be used for the sensory receptors that respond to mechanical variables associated with muscles and joints and whose adequate stimuli arise from the actions of the organism itself. They include muscle spindles, Golgi tendon organs, and joint receptors in vertebrates and a variety of muscle-receptor and chordotonal organs in invertebrates. In contrast, and as Sherrington often discussed, exteroceptors (e.g., sensory tactile receptors) respond primarily to external stimuli. Confounding the precise definition somewhat is the fact that force-sensitive receptors in the exoskeleton of many invertebrates can function as proprioceptors (for further details on these issues and the role of proprioceptive input in motor control, see Hasan and Stuart, 1988).

[25] See endnote 12.

[26] It was largely for the extension of this idea by use of the IC-recording technique that Sherrington's former trainee, Sir John Eccles, was awarded his share (with Sir Andrew Huxley and Sir Alan Hodgkin) of the 1963 Nobel Prize in physiology or medicine.

[27] In modern-day terms, Sherrington meant that the inhibition caused by a MN's hyperpolarization does not propagate peripherally along the motor axon as does the action

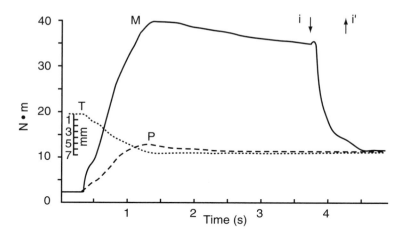

Figure 11.2

An example of Sherrington's work and ideas on the clasp-knife reflex of a decerebrate cat. Again, we have used Granit's own description (1966; his Figure 12). Whole quadriceps muscle is connected to the falling table that stretches it along curve (T), with inset ordinates in millimeters. The muscle responds with stretch reflex (M), which is inhibited by ipsilateral mixed nerve (n. peroneus and popliteus together) between (i) and (i'). After completion of the experiment on stretch reflex, the nerve is cut to demonstrate that without the added reflex contraction, stretch only causes the myographic response (P). Note that inhibition removes reflex completely so that the myograph level after inhibition actually coincides with (P) (reprinted from Liddell and Sherrington 1924).

potential. At the time of his Nobel Lecture, it would have been appropriate for Sherrington to cite Erlanger and Blair (1931) for the then-most-current views on cellular excitability. Sherrington first proposed "stationary" inhibition to have a neuronal membrane mechanism in 1925. His views differed from those of the more cellularly oriented Lucas and Adrian, who favored the idea of a CNS mechanism analogous to Wedensky inhibition (i.e., refractoriness in a nerve-muscle preparation following high-frequency stimulation of the nerve supply; that is, an inhibition subsequent to immediately preceding excitation) and from those of his former U.S. trainee, Forbes, who favored ". . . nerve-impulses travelling in 'delay paths' . . ." (Phillips, 1983; p. 338). The definitive proof of postsynaptic inhibition came much later (see Eccles, 1972).

[28-30] This paragraph on stepping is of major historical import because subsequently, and to this day, Sherrington has often been said to have favored a sensory-reflex rather than a central (interneuronal pattern-generator) control of rhythmical movements. In our opinion, he has been largely misquoted on this important issue, albeit due largely to his own ambivalent and obtuse statements. In his Nobel Lecture, which he must have regarded as of the utmost of importance, he generously acknowledged[29] that his former trainee (1910-1913) and subsequent collaborator, Graham Brown (see "Introduction"), was an authority on "the true rhythmic movement" of stepping. In this lecture, Sherrington mentions only one other of his own trainee/collaborators. This was Liddell, with whom he undertook the majority of his work on motor units, for which he was "officially" awarded a Nobel Prize. In this paragraph, Sherrington did not mention, however, that Graham Brown's 1911-1922 body of work (references in Wetzel and Stuart, 1976) had provided a de novo emphasis on an essentially spinal rather than sensory-reflex basis for the rhythmicity of mammalian stepping movements. All detailed, modern-day monographs, reviews, and symposium volumes on the neurobiology of locomotion and other forms of rhythmic automatic movement (e.g., Stein et al., 1997; Kiehn et al., 1998) emphasize that Graham Brown's work was a key forerunner of current work on central pattern generators for rhythmic movement in

both invertebrates and vertebrates (for further details on Graham Brown's important contributions, see Wetzel and Stuart, 1976).

This aspect of Sherrington's Nobel Lecture is quite puzzling because he himself had been the first to note that rhythmic scratching movements could operate in deafferented limbs (references in Creed et al., 1932), and he subsequently commented on similarities between the scratch reflex and spinal stepping (Sherrington, 1910a). In this latter classical paper, he extended earlier ideas by describing how spinal stepping continues in the decapitate cat during repetitive electrical stimulation of the cervical cord after deafferentation of the hindlimbs. Sherrington stated (1910a), "The rhythm is therefore central in its seat" (p. 87). That same year, he also stated (1910b), "It appears clear, therefore, that the rhythmic response of the musculature is referable to a rhythm not resident in the stimulus [presumably afferent] or in sense organs of the skin, but developed in the spinal centres occupied with the reflex action" (p. 6). According to Eccles (personal communication to D.G.S. in 1972), Sherrington felt that the time was not ripe in the 1910s to 1930s to focus on central pattern-generating mechanisms when so much systematic work was still required on spinal reflex contributions to movement. For example, in his 1913c report, although Sherrington conceded to Graham Brown's insistence that the rhythm of stepping is an intrinsic property of the spinal cord itself, he went on to say that this viewpoint ". . . demands careful attention, but, as it seems to remove stepping from the category of reflexes except in so far as concerns regulation, the present argument [i.e., concerning locomotion-induced reflexes; Sherrington, 1913a-c] proceeds on the assumption that the forms of stepping here dealt with are reflex would be led astray by its consideration now" (p. 207). This is precisely the strategy employed by Sherrington in his Nobel Lecture! Also strange is the late mention in this paragraph[30] of instigating rhythmic movement ". . . by stimulation of the <<stepping>>-point in the cut face of the lateral column of the cord. . . ." This procedure speaks to the central origin of the stepping rhythm, as should surely have been emphasized with due reference to Graham Brown. Nonetheless, in his earlier classical paper with Liddell (Sherrington, 1924) in which Philippson's (1905) measurements of muscle displacements during natural locomotion were used to quantify the potential magnitude of the stretch reflex during stepping, Sherrington warned against ". . . the supposition that the stretch-reflex or indeed the entirety of the proprioceptive arc is absolutely necessary for fundamental exhibition of 'stepping.' Graham Brown has advanced the view, and adduced considerable evidence in favour of it, that the essential nature of 'stepping' is central in origin, an autochthonous [i.e., intrinsic] rhythmic activity proper to the spinal cord" (p. 238). Finally, in one of the most influential pre-1950s books on spinal motor mechanisms, and one that summarizes much of his experimental work (Creed et al., 1932), Sherrington and his then far younger colleagues (albeit the relevant section was written by Sherrington alone) stated, "The nervous mechanism answerable for the essential rhythmicity of the scratch reflex and stepping seems a central spinal one, not requiring *rhythmic* impulsation from outside" (p. 146).

Despite these comments, and possibly partly because of a general widespread misinterpretation of this aspect of Sherrington's Nobel Lecture, the most valuable work of Graham Brown languished in most regrettable obscurity throughout the next 35 years. This oversight is also evident in Adrian's much later, puzzling 1966 biographical memoir of Graham Brown, which failed to even mention his contributions to locomotor neurobiology. For example, Adrian, who was Sherrington's companion 1932 Nobel laureate and a giant among pre-World War II cellular neurophysiologists, began his memoir of Graham Brown with the statement that he was ". . . well-known for the detailed studies of reflex movement and posture which he made by Sherrington's methods . . ." (p. 23). Continuing, Adrian states that ". . . the output of his work was disappointing . . ." (p. 25), then adding, "He had started well and had made his name as a scientist, but the route soon lost its direction" (p. 29). Nothing could be further from the true state-of-the-play! To be fair to Adrian, however, Graham Brown's independent, non-stepping segmental motor research (references in Adrian, 1966), while valuable at the time, lacked the imagination and prescience of his stepping research, and his published contributions after 1927 were indeed miniscule.

Despite this sorry fact, Graham Brown was restored to his rightful place in the history of movement science by Lundberg (a former trainee of Granit, and subsequent collaborator of Eccles) in his influential 1969a treatise on the neural control of stepping (for additional history on the neural control of locomotion, including Lundberg's own considerable contributions, see Wetzel and Stuart, 1976; Burke, 1985; Stuart and McDonagh, 1998).

[31] Hughlings Jackson (1835-1911) has contributed enormously to modern-day clinical and fundamental work in neurobiology, including its movement science component (for review of his extraordinary contributions, see Critchley and Critchley, 1998).

[32] The concept of extensor and flexor "half-centres" was that of Graham Brown, and again, it is puzzling that no such acknowledgment was made (for further details on this valuable and subsequently contentious concept, see Wetzel and Stuart, 1976; Lundberg, 1981; Grillner, 1981; Stein, 1985; Stein and Smith, 1997).

[33] This extrapolation of his work on the operation of active inhibition within spinal cord circuitry to the formulation of a general principle of motor control of relevance throughout the entire CNS was a distinguishing feature of Sherrington's research strategy. Indeed, Eccles and Gibson (1979) have suggested that this second-last paragraph of Sherrington's Nobel Lecture was ". . . an inspired summing up of the essence of his life's work on the nervous system . . ." (p. 72).

References

Note: Irrespective of first authorship, Sherrington's references are listed below under his name (such as the style used previously by Liddell, 1952).

Adrian, E.D. (1934) Cambridge 1904-14. In *Keith Lucas*, W.M. Fletcher (Ed.). Cambridge: Heffer, 88-108. (Note: Originally written in 1916 and edited by Walter Fletcher; published in original form after Fletcher's death.)

Adrian, E.D. (1966) Thomas Graham Brown. In *Biographical Memoirs of Fellows of the Royal Society*, Vol. 12. London: The Royal Society, 23-33.

Andersen, P., Lundberg, A. (1997) John C. Eccles (1903-1997). *Trends in Neuroscience*, 20: 324-325.

Andriantsitohaina, R., Surprenant, A. (1992) Acetylcholine released from guinea-pig submucosal neurones dilates arterioles by releasing nitric oxide from endothelium. *Journal of Physiology (London)*, 453: 493-502.

Baldissera, F., Hultborn, H., Illert, M. (1981) Integration in spinal neuronal systems. In *Handbook of Physiology, The Nervous System: Motor Control*, J.M. Brookhart, V.B. Mountcastle, V.B. Brooks (Eds.). Bethesda, MD: American Physiology Society, 509-595.

Beck, F., Eccles, J.C. (1998) Quantum processes in the brain: A scientific basis of consciousness. *Cognitive Studies* (Bulletin of the Japanese Cognitive Science Society), 5: 95-109.

Bell, C. (1969) Transmission from vasoconstrictor and vasodilator nerves to single smooth muscle cells of the guinea-pig uterine artery. *Journal of Physiology (London)*, 205: 695-708.

Bell, C., Bell, J. (1822) *The Anatomy and Physiology of the Human Body*, 4th American ed. New York: Collins.

Biedermann, W. (1889) Beitraege zur allgemeinen nerven- und muskelphysiologie. 21. mittheilung. ueber die innervation der krebsscheren. *Sitzungsberichte Oesterreichische Akademie der Wissenschaften, Mathematisch Naturwissenschaftliche Klasse*, 97: 49-82.

Binder, M.D. (Ed.) (1999) *Peripheral and Spinal Mechanisms in the Neural Control of Movement. Progress in Brain Research, vol. 123.* Amsterdam: Elsevier Science.

Binder, M.D., Heckman, C.J., Powers, R.K. (1996) The physiological control of motoneuron activity. In *Handbook of Physiology. Sec. 12, Exercise: Regulation and Integration of Multiple Systems*, L.B. Rowell, J.T. Shepherd (Eds.). New York: Oxford University Press, 3-53.

Binder, M.D., Houk, J.C., Nichols, T.R., Rymer, W.Z., Stuart, D.G. (1982) Properties and segmental actions of mammalian muscle receptors: An update. *Federation Proceedings*, 41: 2907-2918.

Binder, M.D., Jabre, J. (Eds.) (1999) Mechanisms underlying the control of firing in the healthy and sick motoneurone. *Journal of Physiology (Paris)*, 93: 1-182.

Binder, M.D., Mendell, L.M. (1990) *The Segmental Motor System*. New York: Oxford University Press.

Brazier, M.A.B. (1959) The historical development of neurophysiology. In *Handbook of Physiology, Neurophysiology*, Vol. I, J. Field, H.W. Magoun, V.E. Hall (Eds.). Washington, DC: American Physiological Society, 1-58.

Bretag, A. (1983) Who did invent the intracellular microelectrode? *Trends in Neuroscience*, 6: 365.

Brock, L.G., Coombs, J.S., Eccles, J.C. (1951) Action potentials of motoneurones with an intracellular electrode. *Proceedings of the University of Otago Medical School*, 29: 14-15.

Brownstone, R.M., Jordan, L.M., Kriellaars, D.J., Noga, B.R., Shefchyk, S.J. (1992) On the regulation of repetitive firing in lumbar motoneurones during fictive locomotion in the cat. *Experimental Brain Research*, 90: 441-445.

Bulbring, E., Burnstock, G., Holman, M.E. (1958) Excitation and conduction in the smooth muscle of the isolated taenia coli of the guinea-pig. *Journal of Physiology (London)*, 142: 420-437.

Bunge, M. (1989). From neuron to mind. *News in Physiological Sciences*, 4: 206-209.

Burke, D. (1988) Spasticity as an adaptation to pyramidal tract injury. In *Advances in Neurology*, Vol. 47: *Functional Recovery in Neurological Disease*, S.G. Waxman (Ed.). New York: Raven Press, 401-423.

Burke, D., Knowles, L., Andrews, C.J., Ashby, P. (1972) Spasticity, decerebrate rigidity and the clasp-knife phenomenon: An experimental study in the cat. *Brain*, 95: 31-48.

Burke, R.E. (1981) Motor units: Anatomy, physiology and functional organization. In *Handbook of Physiology, The Nervous System: Motor Control*, Sec. 1, Vol. II, Pt. 1, J.M. Brookhart, V.B. Mountcastle, V.B. Brooks (Eds.). Bethesda, MD: American Physiological Society, 345-422.

Burke, R.E. (1985) Integration of sensory information and motor commands in the spinal cord. In *Motor Control: From Movement Trajectories to Neural Mechanisms. Short Course Syllabus*, P.S.G. Stein (Ed.). Bethesda, MD: Society for Neuroscience, 44-66.

Burnstock, G., Campbell, G., Bennet, M., Holman, M.E. (1963) Inhibition of the smooth muscle of the taenia coli. *Nature*, 200: 581-582.

Cleland, C.L., Rymer, W.Z. (1990) Neural mechanisms underlying the clasp-knife reflex in the cat. I. Characteristics of the reflex. *Journal of Neurophysiology*, 64: 1303-1318.

Cooper, S., Adrian, E.D. (1924) The electric response in reflex contractions of spinal and decerebrate preparations. *Proceedings of the Royal Society of London Series B: Biological Science*, 96: 243-258.

Cooper, S., Eccles, J.C. (1930) The isometric response of mammalian muscles. *Journal of Physiology (London)*, 69: 377-385.

Cope, T.C., Clark, B.D. (1991) Motor-unit recruitment in the decerebrate cat: Several unit properties are equally good predictors of order. *Journal of Neurophysiology*, 66: 1127-1138.

Cope, T.C., Sokoloff, A.J. (1999) Orderly recruitment tested across muscle boundaries. In *Peripheral and Spinal Mechanisms in the Neural Control of Movement. Progress in Brain Research*, Vol 123, M.D. Binder (Ed.). Amsterdam: Elsevier Science, 177-190.

Creed, R.S., Denny-Brown, D., Eccles, J.C., Liddell, E.G.T., Sherrington, C.S. (1932) *Reflex Activity of the Spinal Cord*. Oxford: Clarendon Press. (Note: This book's 55-page chapter 7 was written solely by Sherrington and may be considered "his last purely scientific writing and . . . the crowning achievement of the Oxford School" [Eccles and Gibson, 1979], p. 65-66.)

Critchley, M., Critchley, E.A. (1998) *John Hughlings Jackson: Father of English Neurology*. Oxford: Oxford University Press, 224 pp.

Curtis, D.R., Andersen, P. (2000) John Carew Eccles (1903-1997). In *Biographical Memoirs of Fellows of the Royal Society*, Vol. 46. London: The Royal Society.

Davidoff, R.A. (1997) Glycine. In *Encyclopedia of Neuroscience* (CD-ROM also available), G. Adelman, B. Smith (Eds.). Amsterdam: Elsevier Science.

Del Castillo, J., Katz, B. (1955) Production of membrane potential changes in the frog's heart by inhibitory nerve impulses. *Nature*, 175: 1035.

Denny-Brown, D. (1929) On the nature of postural reflexes. *Proceedings of the Royal Society of London Series B: Biological Science*, 104: 252-301.

Denny-Brown, D. (1949) Interpretation of the electromyogram. *Archives of Neurology & Psychiatry*, 61: 99-128.

Denny-Brown, D., Pennybacker, J.B. (1938) Fibrillation and fasciculation in muscle. *Brain*, 61: 311-333.

Dudel, J., Kuffler, S.W. (1961) Presynaptic inhibition at the crayfish neuromuscular junction. *Journal of Physiology (London)*, 155: 543-562.

Eccles, J.C. (1964) *The Physiology of Synapses*. Berlin: Springer-Verlag.

Eccles, J.C. (1972) The ionic mechanism of postsynaptic inhibition. Nobel Lecture, December 11, 1963. In *Nobel Lectures: Physiology and Medicine, 1963-1970*. Amsterdam: Elsevier, 6-27.

Eccles, J.C. (1977) My scientific odyssey. *Annual Review of Physiology*, 39: 1-18.

Eccles, J.C., Gibson, W.C. (1979) *Sherrington: His Life and Thought*. Berlin: Springer-Verlag.

Eccles, J.C., Granit, R., Young, J.Z. (1932) Impulses in the giant nerve fibres of earthworms. *Journal of Physiology (London)*, 77: 23P-24P.

Enoka, R.M., Stuart, D.G. (1984) Henneman's "size principle": Current issues. *Trends in Neuroscience*, 7: 226-228.

Erlanger, J., Blair, E.A. (1931) The irritability changes in nerve in response to subthreshold constant currents, and related phenomena. *American Journal of Physiology*, 99: 129-155.

Fatt, P., Katz, B. (1953) The effect of inhibitory nerve impulses on a crustacean muscle fibre. *Journal of Physiology (London)*, 121: 374-389.

Ferrier, D. (1875) Experiments on the brain of monkeys. *Proceedings of the Royal Society of London*, 23: 409-430.

Fetz, E.E., Cheney, P.D., Mewes, K., Palmer, S. (1989) Control of forelimb muscle activity by populations of corticomotoneuronal and rubroneuroneuronal cells. *Progress in Brain Research*,80: 437-449.

Fetz, E.E., Perlmutter, S.I., Prut, Y., Meir, M.A. (1999) Primate spinal motoneurons: Muscle fields and response properties. In *Peripheral and Spinal Mechanisms in the Neural Control of Movement. Progress in Brain Research*, Vol 123, M.D. Binder (Ed.). Amsterdam: Elsevier Science, 323-330.

Field, J., Magoun, H.W., Hall, V.E. (Eds.) (1959-1960) *Handbook of Physiology, Neurophysiology*, Vols. I-III. Washington, DC: American Physiological Society.

Foster, M., Sherrington, C.S. (1897) *A Text Book of Physiology*, 7th ed., Pt. III, *The Central Nervous System and Its Instruments*. London: Macmillan.

Fulton, J.F., Liddell, E.G.T. (1926) Observations on ipsilateral contraction and "inhibitory" rhythm. *Proceedings of the Royal Society of London Series B: Biological Science*, 98: 214-227.

Gandevia, S.C., Allen, G.M., McKenzie, D.M. (1995) Central fatigue: Critical issues, quantification and practical implications. In *Fatigue: Neural and Muscular Mechanisms*, S.C. Gandevia, R.M. Enoka, A.J. McComas, D.G. Stuart, C.K. Thomas (Eds.). New York: Plenum Press, 281-294.

Gandevia, S.C., Burke, D. (1992) Does the nervous system depend on kinesthetic information to control limb movements? In Controversies in neuroscience 1: Movement control. *Behavioral and Brain Sciences*, 15: 614-632.

Georgopoulos, A.P. (1996a) On the translation of directional motor cortical commands to activation of muscles via spinal interneuronal systems. *Brain Research. Cognitive Brain Research*, 3: 151-155.

Georgopoulos, A.P. (1996b) Arm movements in monkeys: Behavior and neurophysiology. *Journal of Comparative Physiology [A]*, 179: 603-612.

Georgopoulos, A.P. (1997) Extrapersonal space, command, and control. In *Encyclopedia of Neuroscience* (CD-ROM also available), G. Adelman, B. Smith (Eds.). Amsterdam: Elsevier Science.

Getting, P.A. (1989) Emerging principles governing the operation of neural networks. *Annual Reviews of Neuroscience*, 12: 185-204.

Gillespie, C.C. (Ed.) (1971) Cushing, Harvey Williams. In *Dictionary of Scientific Biography*, Vol. III. New York: Scribner's, 516-519.

Gillespie, C.C. (Ed.) (1972a) Florey, Howard Walter. In *Dictionary of Scientific Biography*, Vol. V. New York: Scribner's, 41-44.

Gillespie, C.C. (Ed.) (1972b) Fulton, John Farquhar. In *Dictionary of Scientific Biography*, Vol. V. New York: Scribner's, 207-208.

Gillespie, C.C. (Ed.) (1972c) Gaskell, Walter Holbrook. In *Dictionary of Scientific Biography*, Vol. V. New York: Scribner's, 279-284.

Gillespie, C.C. (Ed.) (1973) Lucas, Keith. In *Dictionary of Scientific Biography*, Vol. VIII. New York: Scribner's, 532-535.

Golgi, C. (1880) Sui nervi dei tendini dell'uomo e di altri vertebrati e di unnuovo organo nervoso terminale musculo-tendineo. Reprinted in his *Opera Omnia*, 1903, Vol. 1. Milan: Ulrico Hoepli, 171-198.

Golowasch, J., Corey, D.P. (1997) Patch clamp. In *Encyclopedia of Neuroscience* (CD-ROM also available), G. Adelman, B. Smith (Eds.). Amsterdam: Elsevier Science.

Graham Brown, T. (1916) Die reflex functionen des zentralnerven mit besonderer berucksichtigung, der rhythmischen tatigkeiten bein sargeiter. *Ergebnisse der Physiologie*, 15: 480-490.

Graham Brown, T. (1947) Sherrington: The man. *British Medical Journal*, 2: 810-812. (Note: See Wetzel and Stuart [1976] for a full list of Graham Brown's contributions to spinal pattern generation.)

Granit, R. (1966) *Charles Scott Sherrington: An Appraisal*. London: Nelson.

Greenblatt, S.H. (1997) The crucial decade: Modern neurosurgery's definitive development in Harvey Cushing's early research and practice, 1900 to 1910. *Journal of Neurosurgery*, 87: 964-971.

Grillner, S. (1981) Control of locomotion in bipeds, tetrapods, and fish. In *Handbook of Physiology, The Nervous System: Motor Control*, J.M. Brookhart, V.B. Mountcastle, V.B. Brooks (Eds.). Bethesda, MD: American Physiological Society, 1179-1236.

Grillner, S. (1995) Ragnar Granit. In *Biographical Memoirs of Fellows of the Royal Society*, Vol. 41. London: The Royal Society, 185-197.

Grillner, S., Stein, P.S.G., Stuart, D.G., Forrsberg, H., Herman, R.M. (1986) *Neurobiology of Vertebrate Locomotion*. Basingstoke, U.K.: Macmillan.

Gross, C.G. (1997) Neuroscience, early history of. In *Encyclopedia of Neuroscience* (CD-ROM also available), G. Adelman, B. Smith (Eds.). Amsterdam: Elsevier Science.

Gurfinkel, V.S., Levik, Y.S., Kazennikov, O.V., Selionov, V.A. (1998) Locomotor-like movements evoked by leg muscle vibration in humans. *European Journal of Neuroscience*, 10: 1608-1612.

Gustafsson, B., Pinter, M.J. (1985) On factors determining orderly recruitment of motor units: A role for intrinsic membrane properties. *Trends in Neurosciences*, 8: 431-433.

Hasan, Z., Stuart, D.G. (1988) Animal solutions to problems of movement control: The role of proprioceptors. *Annual Review of Neuroscience*, 11: 199-223.

Henneman, E. (1957) Relation between size of neurons and their susceptibility to discharge. *Science*, 126: 1345-1347.

Henneman, E., Mendell, L.M. (1981) Functional organization of motoneuron pool and its inputs. In *Handbook of Physiology, The Nervous System: Motor Control*, Sec. 1, Vol. II, Pt. 1, J.M. Brookhart, V.B. Mountcastle, V.B. Brooks (Eds.). Bethesda, MD: American Physiological Society, 423-507.

Herman, R.M., Grillner, S., Stein, P.S.G., Stuart, D.G. (1976) *Neural Control of Locomotion*. New York: Plenum Press.

Hermsmeyer, K. (1982) The 27th annual Bowditch lecture. Electogenic ion pumps and other determinants of membrane potential in vascular muscle. *The Physiologist*, 25: 454-465.

Hornby, T.G. (2000) *Extrinsic Modulation of the Intrinsic Stimulus Current-Spike Frequency Relationship of Spinal Motoneurons in the Adult Turtle*. PhD dissertation, Tucson, AZ: University of Arizona.

Hoyle, G. (1983) Origins of intracellular microelectrodes. *Trends in Neuroscience*, 6: 163.

Ito, M. (1970) Neurophysiological aspects of the cerebellar control system. *International Journal of Neurology*, 7: 162-176.

Ito, M.,Yoshida, M. (1966). The origin of cerebellar-induced inhibition of Deiters neurones. I. Monosynaptic initiation of the inhibitory post-synaptic potentials. *Experimental Brain Research*, 2: 330-349.

Jankowska, E. (1992) Interneuronal relay in spinal pathways from proprioceptors. *Progress in Neurobiology*, 38: 335-378.

Jankowska, E., Lundberg, A. (1981) Interneurons in the spinal cord. *Trends in Neurosciences*, 4: 230-233.

Jankowska, E., Odutola, A. (1980) Crossed and uncrossed synaptic actions on motoneurons of back muscles in the cat. *Brain Research*, 194: 65-78.

Jasper, H.H. (1991) History of the development of electroencephalography and clinical neurophysiology at the Montreal Neurological Institute: The first 25 years 1939-1964. *Canadian Journal of Neurological Science*, 18, Suppl. 4: 533-548.

Jeannerod, M. (1985) *The Brain Machine: The Development of Neurophysiological Thought*, S. Belsky (Trans.). Cambridge, MA: Harvard University Press.

Jonas, P., Bischofberger, J., Sandkuhler, J. (1998) Corelease of two fast neurotransmitters at a central synapse. *Science*, 281: 419-424.

Jordan, L.M. (1998) Cholinergic interneurons involved in the control of locomotion. In *Peripheral and Spinal Mechanisms in the Neural Control of Movement*, Proceedings of an International Symposium, Tucson, AZ, Nov. 4-6, 1998, M.D. Binder, J.C. McDonagh, R.M. Reinking, P.A. Pierce (Eds.). Tucson, AZ: University of Arizona, 33.

Jung, R. (1975/92) Some European neuroscientists: A personal tribute. In *The Neurosciences: Paths of Discovery, I*, F.G. Worden, J.P. Swazey, G. Adelman (Eds.). Boston: Birkhäuser, 477-511 (first published by MIT Press in 1975).

Kandel, E.R., Schwartz, J.H., Jessell, T.M. (2000*) Principles of Neural Science*, 4th ed. New York: McGraw-Hill.

Katz, B. (1938) Neuromuscular transmission in crabs. *Journal of Physiology (London)*, 87: 199-221.

Katz, B. (1949) Neuromuscular transmission in invertebrates. *Biological Reviews*, 24: 1-20.

Katz, R., Pierrot-Deseilligny, E. (1999) Recurrent inhibition in humans. *Progress in Neurobiology*, 57: 325-355.

Kennedy, D. (1997) *Academic Duty*. Cambridge, MA: Harvard University Press.

Kernell, D. (1995) Neuromuscular frequency coding and fatigue. In *Fatigue: Neural and Muscular Mechanisms*, S.C. Gandevia, R.M. Enoka, A.J. McComas, D.G. Stuart, C.K. Thomas (Eds.). New York: Plenum Press, 135-145.

Kiehn, O., Harris-Warrick, R.M., Jordan, L.M., Hultborn, H., Kudo, N. (Eds.) (1998) *Neuronal Mechanisms for Generating Locomotor Activity. Annals of the New York Academy of Sciences*, 860: 1-573.

Kölliker, A. (1862a) Untersuchungen über die letzten Endigungen der Nerven. *Zeitschrift fuer Wissenschaftliche Zoologie*, 12: 149-164.

Kölliker, A. (1862b) On the terminations of nerves in muscles, as observed in the frog: And on the disposition of the nerves in the frog's heart. *Proceedings of the Royal Society of London*, 12: 65-84.

Kudina, L.P. (1999) Analysis of firing behaviour of human motoneurones within 'subprimary range'. In *Mechanisms Underlying the Control of Firing in the Healthy and Sick Motoneurone*, M.D. Binder and J. Jabre (Eds.). *Journal of Physiology (Paris)*, 93: 115-123.

Kühne, W. (1863a) Uber die endigung der nerven in den muskeln. *Virchow's Archiv fuer Pathologische Anatomie und Physiologie und fuer Klinische Medizen*, 27: 508-523.

Kühne, W. (1863b) Die muskelspindeln. Ein beitrag zur lehre von der entwickelung der muskeln und nervenfasern. *Virchow's Archiv fuer Pathologische Anatomie und Physiologie und fuer Klinische Medizen*, 28: 528-538.

Lassiera, P.A. (1979). Sixto Obrador. 1911-1978. *Surgical Neurology*, 11: 81-82.

Latash, M. (Ed.) (1998) *Progress in Motor Control: Bernstein's Traditions in Movement Studies*. Champaign, IL: Human Kinetics.

Leksell, L. (1945) The action potentials and excitatory effects of the small ventral root fibres to skeletal muscle. *Acta Physiologica Scandinavica*, 10, Suppl. 31: 1-84.

Lewis, D.M. (1984) Mammalian motor units. In *Handbook of the Spinal Cord*, Vols. 2 and 3: *Anatomy and Physiology*, R.A. Davidoff (Ed.). New York: Dekker, 269-314.

Liddell, E.G.T. (1952) Charles Scott Sherrington: 1857-1952. In *Obituary Notices of Fellows of the Royal Society*, Vol. 8, No. 21. London: The Royal Society, 241-270.

Liddell, E.G.T. (1960) *The Discovery of Reflexes*. London: Oxford University Press.

Liljestrand, G. (1962) *Nobel, the Man and his Prizes*. Stockholm: Nobel Foundation.

Lindsley, D.B. (1935) Electrical activity of human motor units during voluntary contraction. *American Journal of Physiology*, 114: 90-99.

Llinas, R. (1997) Cerebellum, network physiology. In *Encyclopedia of Neuroscience* (CD-ROM also available), G. Adelman, B. Smith (Eds.). Amsterdam: Elsevier Science.

Lloyd, D.P.C. (1960) Spinal mechanisms involved in somatic activities. In *Handbook of Physiology, Neurophysiology*, Vol. II, J. Field, H.W. Magoun, V.E. Hall (Eds.). Washington, DC: American Physiology Society, 929-949.

Lucas, K. (1905). On the gradation of contraction in a skeletal muscle fibre. *Journal of Physiology (London)*, 33: 125-137.

Lucas, K. (1909a) The "all or none" contraction of the amphibian skeletal muscle fibre. *Journal of Physiology (London)*, 38: 113-133.

Lucas, K. (1909b) The evolution of animal function. *Science Progress*, 20 cent., London, 3: 472-483.

Lucas, K. (1917) On summation of propagated disturbances in the claw of *Astagus* and on the double neuro-muscular system of the adductor. *Journal of Physiology (London)*, 50: 1-35.

Lundberg, A. (1969a) Reflex control of stepping. *The Nansen Memorial Lecture V.* Oslo: Universitetsforlaget, 1-42.

Lundberg, A. (1969b) Convergence of excitatory and inhibitory action on interneurones in the spinal cord. In *The Interneuron*, M.A.B. Brazier (Ed.). Los Angeles: University of California Press, 231-265.

Lundberg, A. (1981) Half-centres revisited. In *Regulatory Functions of the CNS: Motion and Organization Principles*, Vol. 1, J. Szentagothai, M. Palkovits, J. Hamori (Eds.). New York: Pergamon Press and Akademiai Kiado, 155-167.

Lundberg, A., Phillips, C.G. (1973) T. Graham Brown's film on locomotion in the decerebrate cat. *Journal of Physiology (London)*, 231: 90-91P.

Matsuyama, S., Mori, S. (1998) Lumbar interneurons involved in the generation of fictive locomotion in cats. In *Neuronal Mechanisms for Generating Locomotor Activity*, O. Kiehn, R.M. Harris-Warrick, L.M. Jordan, H. Hultborn, N. Kudo (Eds.). *Annals of the New York Academy of Sciences*, 860: 441-443.

Matthews, P.B.C. (1972) *Mammalian Muscle Receptors and Their Central Actions.* London: Arnold.

Matthews, P.B.C. (1977) Muscle afferents and kinaesthesia. *British Medical Bulletin*, 33: 137-142.

Matthews, P.B.C. (1999) Properties of human motoneurones and their synaptic noise deduced from motor unit recordings with the aid of computer modelling. In *Mechanisms Underlying the Control of Firing in the Healthy and Sick Motoneurone*, M.D. Binder and J. Jabre (Eds.). *Journal of Physiology (Paris)*, 93: 135-145.

McCrea, D.A. (1992) Can sense be made of spinal interneuron circuits? *Behavioral and Brain Sciences*, 15: 633-643.

McCrea, D.A. (1998) Neuronal basis of afferent-evoked enhancement of locomotor activity. In *Neuronal Mechanisms for Generating Locomotor Activity*, O. Kiehn, R.M. Harris-Warrick, L.M. Jordan, H. Hultborn, N. Kudo (Eds.). *Annals of the New York Academy of Sciences*, 860: 216-225.

McDonagh, J.C., Callister, R.C., Brichta, A., Reinking, R.M., Stuart, D.G. (1999) A commentary on the properties of spinal interneurons vs. motoneurons in vertebrates, and their firing-rate behavior during movement. In *Motor Control Today and Tomorrow*, G. Gantchev (Ed.). Sofia: Bulgarian Academy of Sciences, 3-29.

Merton, P.A. (1954) Voluntary strength and fatigue. *Journal of Physiology (London)*, 123: 553-564.

Messenger, J. (1997) John Zachary Young (1907-97). *Nature*, 388: 726.

Mines, G.R. (1913) On the summation of contractions. *Journal of Physiology (London)*, 169: 1-27.

Mizunami, M., Okada, R., Li, Y-S., Strausfeld, N.J. (1998a) Mushroom bodies of the cockroach: Activity and identities of neurons recorded in freely moving animals. *Journal of Comparative Neurology*, 402: 501-519.

Mizunami, M., Weibrecht, J.M., Strausfeld, N.J. (1998b) Mushroom bodies of the cockroach: Their participation in place memory. *Journal of Comparative Neurology*, 402: 520-537.

Modlin, I.M. (1998) Surgical triumvirate of Theodor Kocher, Harvey Cushing, and William Halsted. *World Journal of Surgery*, 22: 103-13.

Murphy, G. (1962) Robert Sessions Woodworth. 1869-1962. *American Psychologist*, 18: 131-133.

Palade, G.E., Palay, S.L. (1954) Electron microscope observations of interneuronal and neuro-muscular synapse (abstract). *Anatomical Record*, 118: 335-336.

Patton, H.D. (1994) David P.C. Lloyd. In *Biographical Memoirs*, Vol. 65. Washington: National Academy of Sciences, 197-209.

Pavlov, I.P. (1938) *Lectures on Conditioned Reflexes.* W. Horsley Gantt, G. Volborth (English trans.). New York: International Publishers.

Penfield, W. (1972) The electrode, the brain and the mind. *Zeitschrift fur Neurologie*, 201: 297-309.

Penfield, W. (1977) *No Man Alone. A Neurosurgeon's Life.* Boston: Little, Brown.

Philippson, M. (1905) L'autonomie et la centralisation dans le système nerveux des animaux. *Travaux de Laboratoire Instituts Solvay*, 7: 1-208.

Phillips, C.G. (1983) Edward George Tandy Liddell. In *Biographical Memoirs of Fellows of the Royal Society*, Vol. 29. London: The Royal Society, 333-359.

Piotrkiewicz, M. (1999). An influence of afterhyperpolarization on the pattern of motoneuronal rhythmic activity. In *Mechanisms Underlying the Control of Firing in Healthy and Sick Motoneurone*, M.D. Binder and J. Jabre (Eds.). *Journal of Physiology (Paris)*, 93: 125-133.

Porter, R., Lemon, R. (1993) *Corticospinal Function and Voluntary Movement*. Monographs of the Physiological Society, Vol. 45. New York: Oxford University Press. (Note: See historical section on pp. 1-34.)

Prochazka, A. (1996) Proprioceptive feedback and movement regulation. In *Handbook of Physiology. Sec. 12, Exercise: Regulation and Integration of Multiple Systems*, L.B. Rowell, J.T. Shepherd (Eds.). New York: Oxford University Press, 89-127.

Prochazka, A. (1999) Quantifying proprioception. In *Peripheral and Spinal Mechanisms in the Neural Control of Movement. Progress in Brain Research*, Vol. 123, M.D. Binder (Ed.). Amsterdam: Elsevier Science, 133-142.

Proske, U., Wise, A.K., Gregory, J.E. (2000) The role of muscle spindles in the detection of movements. *Progress in Neurobiology*, 60: 85-96.

Ramón y Cajal, S. (1933) Neuronismo o Reticularismo? Las pruebas objetivas de la unidad anatómica de las células nerviosas. *Archivos de Neurobiologia*, 13: 217-291. (Note: See also the following 1954 translation into English.)

Ramón y Cajal, S. (1954) *Neuron Theory or Reticular Theory? Objective evidence of the anatomical unity of nerve cells*, M.U. Purkiss, C.A. Fox (Trans.). Madrid: Consejo Superior de Investigaciones Cientificas, Instituto Ramón y Cajal.

Rothwell, J.C. (1994) *Control of Human Voluntary Movement*, 2nd ed. London/New York: Chapman and Hall.

Rymer, W.Z., Houk, J.C., Crago, P.E. (1979) Mechanisms of the clasp-knife reflex studied in an animal model. *Experimental Brain Research*, 37: 93-113.

Schäfer, E.A. (1900) *Text-book of Physiology*. New York: Macmillan.

Schieppati, M., Nardone, A. (1999) Group II spindle afferent fibers in humans: Their possible role in the reflex control of stance. In *Peripheral and Spinal Mechanisms in the Neural Control of Movement. Progress in Brain Research*, Vol. 123, M.D. Binder (Ed.). Amsterdam: Elsevier Science, 461-472.

Schultz, D.P., Schultz, S.E. (1992). *A History of Modern Psychology*, 5th ed. Fort Worth, TX: Harcourt Brace Jovanovich.

Sechenoff, I.M. (1863a) *Physiologische Studien uber die Hemmungsmechanismen fur die Reflexthatigkeit des Ruckenmarks im Gehirne des Frosches*. Berlin: Hirschwald. (Note: The name of Ivan Michailovich Setchenov [1829-1905] also appeared as Setschenow, Iwan S; Setchenow, J; Secheno, Ivan Mikhailovich; Secenov, Ivan Michajlovic; Setchenoff, Ivan Michailovich; Setschenov, J; and Setschenow, J.)

Sechenov, I.M. (1863b) *Reflexes of the Brain*. (Note: This essay was originally published in Russian by Medizinsky Vestnik [Moscow]. It subsequently became available in English in *Sechenov. Selected Works*, A. A. Subkov [Ed.], Moscow/Leningrad: State Publishing House, 1935, pp. 263-336. See also 1965 translation by K. Koshtoyants [Russian ed.], G. Gibbons [English ed.], Cambridge, MA: MIT Press.)

Seyffarth, H. (1940) The behaviour of motor-units in voluntary contraction. *Av Norske Videnskap Akad Oslo. I. Matematisk-Natur Klasse*, 4: 1-63.

Sherrington, C.S. (1884a; with Langley, J.N.) On sections of the right half of the medulla oblongata and of the spinal cord of the dog which was exhibited by Professor Goltz at the International Medical Congress of 1881. Proceedings of the Physiological Society. *Journal of Physiology (London)*, 5: vi.

Sherrington, C.S. (1884b; with Langley, J.N.) Secondary degeneration of nerve tracts following removal of the cortex of the cerebrum in the dog. *Journal of Physiology (London)*, 5: 49-65.

Sherrington, C.S. (1889) On nerve-tracts degenerating secondarily to lesions of the cortex cerebri. (Preliminary.) *Journal of Physiology (London)*, 10: 429-432.

Sherrington, C.S. (1891) Note on the knee jerk. *St. Thomas's Hospital Report*, 21: 145-147.

Sherrington, C.S. (1891; with Langley, J.N.) On pilo-motor nerves. *Journal of Physiology (London)*, 12: 278-291.

Sherrington, C.S. (1892a) Note toward the localization of the knee jerk. *British Medical Journal*, 1: 545. Addendum to note on the knee jerk. *British Medical Journal*, 1: 654.

Sherrington, C.S. (1892b) In memorium. W.B. Hadden. M.D. (Lond), F.R.C.P. *St. Thomas's Hospital Report*, 22: xix-xxi.

Sherrington, C.S. (1893) Note on the knee-jerk and the correlation of action of antagonistic muscles. *Proceedings of the Royal Society of London Series B: Biological Science*, 52: 556-564.

Sherrington, C.S. (1894) On the anatomical constitution of nerves of skeletal muscles; with remarks on recurrent fibres in the ventral spinal nerve-root. *Journal of Physiology (London)*, 17: 211-258.

Sherrington, C.S. (1895; with Mott, F.W.) Experiments upon the influence of sensory nerves upon movement and nutrition of the limbs. Preliminary communications. *Proceedings of the Royal Society of London Series B: Biological Science*, 57: 481-488.

Sherrington, C.S. (1897; with Foster, M.) The central nervous system. In *A Text Book of Physiology*, 7th ed., Pt. III, M. Foster (Ed.). London: Macmillan, pp. 915-1252.

Sherrington, C.S. (1898) Decerebrate rigidity, and reflex co-ordination of movement. *Journal of Physiology (London)*, 22: 319-332.

Sherrington, C.S. (1899) On the spinal animal. (Marshall Hall lecture.) *Medico-Chirurgical Transactions*, 82: 449-477.

Sherrington, C.S. (1900) The spinal cord. In *Textbook of Physiology*, Vol. 2, E.A. Schäfer (Ed.). London: Pentland.

Sherrington, C.S. (1901; with Grunbaum, A.S.F.) Observations on the physiology of the cerebral cortex of some higher apes. *Proceedings of the Royal Society of London Series B: Biological Science*, 69: 206-209.

Sherrington, C.S. (1903; with Grunbaum, A.S.F.) Observations on the physiology of the cerebral cortex of the higher anthropoid apes. *Proceedings of the Royal Society of London Series B: Biological Science*, 72: 152-155.

Sherrington, C.S. (1904) The correlation of reflexes and the principle of the common path. *Report of the British Association for the Advancement of Science*, 74: 1-14.

Sherrington, C.S. (1906a) *Integrative Action of the Nervous System*. New Haven, CT: Yale University Press (republished by Cambridge University Press in 1947).

Sherrington, C.S. (1906b) Observations on the scratch reflex of the spinal dog. *Journal of Physiology (London)*, 34: 1-50.

Sherrington, C.S. (1908) On the reciprocal innervation of antagonist muscles. Thirteenth note. On antagonism between reflex inhibition and reflex excitation. *Proceedings of the Royal Society of London Series B: Biological Science*, 80: 565-578.

Sherrington, C.S. (1909) On the reciprocal innervation of antagonist muscles. Fourteenth note. On double reciprocal innervation. *Proceedings of the Royal Society of London Series B: Biological Science*, 81: 249-268.

Sherrington, C.S. (1910a) Flexion-reflex of the limb, crossed extension-reflex, and reflex stepping and standing. *Journal of Physiology (London)*, 40: 28-121.

Sherrington, C.S. (1910b) Remarks on the reflex mechanism of the step. *Brain*, 33: 1-25.

Sherrington, C.S. (1910c) Notes on the scratch reflex of the cat. *Quarterly Journal of Experimental Physiology*, 3: 213-220.

Sherrington, C.S. (1913a) Reciprocal innervation and symmetrical muscles. *Proceedings of the Royal Society of London Series B: Biological Science*, 86: 219-232.

Sherrington, C.S. (1913b) Nervous rhythm from rivalry of antagonistic reflexes: Reflex stepping as a result of double reciprocal innervation. *Proceedings of the Royal Society of London Series B: Biological Science*, 86: 233-261.

Sherrington, C.S. (1913c) Further observations on the production of reflex stepping by combination of reflex excitation with reflex inhibition. *Journal of Physiology (London)*, 47: 196-214.

Sherrington, C.S. (1913d) Reflex inhibition as a factor in the co-ordination of movements and postures. *Quarterly Journal of Experimental Physiology*, 6: 251-310.

Sherrington, C.S. (1915; with Sowton, S.C.M.) Observations on reflex responses to single break-shocks. *Journal of Physiology (London)*, 49: 331-348.

Sherrington, C.S. (1917; with Leyton, A.S.F.) Observations on the excitable cortex of the chimpanzee, orang-utan and gorilla. *Quarterly Journal of Experimental Physiology*, 11: 135-222.

Sherrington, C.S. (1918). Observations on the sensual role of the proprioceptive nerve-supply of the extrinsic ocular muscles. *Brain*, 41: 332-343.

Sherrington, C.S. (1919) *Mammalian Physiology: A Course of Practical Exercise*. Oxford: Clarendon Press.

Sherrington, C.S. (1921; with Sassa, K.) On the myogram of the flexor-reflex evoked by a single break-shock. *Proceedings of the Royal Society of London Series B: Biological Science,* 92: 108-117.

Sherrington, C.S. (1923; with Liddell, E.G.T.) Recruitment type of reflexes. *Proceedings of the Royal Society of London Series B: Biological Science,* 95: 407-412.

Sherrington, C.S. (1924) Problems of muscle receptivity. *Nature,* 113: 732, 892-894, 929-932. (Note: Sherrington's Linacre Lecture.)

Sherrington, C.S. (1924; with Liddell, E.G.T.) Reflexes in response to stretch (myotatic reflexes). *Proceedings of the Royal Society of London Series B: Biological Science,* 96: 212-242.

Sherrington, C.S. (1925a) Remarks on some aspects of reflex inhibition. *Proceedings of the Royal Society of London Series B: Biological Science,* 97: 519-545.

Sherrington, C.S. (1925b; with Liddell, E.G.T.) Further observations on myotatic reflexes. *Proceedings of the Royal Society of London Series B: Biological Science,* 97: 267-283.

Sherrington, C.S. (1925c) J.N. Langley, Obituary. *British Medical Journal,* 2: 925.

Sherrington, C.S. (1927) Lucas, Keith (1876-1916). In *Dictionary of National Biography, 1912-1921* (Suppl. 3), H.W.C. Davis, J.R.H. Weaver (Eds.). London: Oxford University Press, 347.

Sherrington, C.S. (1929a) Some functional problems attaching to convergence. Ferrier lecture. *Proceedings of the Royal Society of London Series B: Biological Science,* 105: 332-362.

Sherrington, C.S. (1929b; with Eccles, J.C.) Improved bearing for the torsion myograph. Proceedings of the Physiological Society. *Journal of Physiology (London),* 69: i.

Sherrington, C.S. (1930; with Eccles, J.C.) Numbers and contraction-values of individual motor-units examined in some muscles of the limb. *Proceedings of the Royal Society of London Series B: Biological Science,* 106: 326-357.

Sherrington, C.S. (1931) Quantitative management of contraction in lowest level co-ordination. Hughlings Jackson Lecture. *Brain,* 54: 1-28.

Sherrington, C.S. (1931; with Eccles, J.C.) The flexor reflex. I-VI. *Proceedings of the Royal Society of London Series B: Biological Science,* 107: 511-534, 535-556, 557-585, 586-596, 597-605; 109: 91-113.

Sherrington, C.S. (1932) Inhibition as a coordinative factor. Nobel Lecture, December 12, 1932. In *Les Prix Nobel.* Stockholm: Nobel Foundation, 278-289.

Sherrington, C.S. (1934) Reflex inhibition as a factor in co-ordination of muscular acts. *Revista de la Sociedad Argentina de Biologia,* 10: 510-513.

Sherrington, C.S. (1935) Santiago Ramon Y Cajal 1852-1934. In *Obituary Notices of Fellows of the Royal Society,* 1932-1935. Vol. 1, Pt. 2. London: The Royal Society, 425-441.

Sherrington, C.S. (1939) Note on Harvey Cushing. *British Medical Journal,* 2: 831-832.

Sherrington, C.S. (1948) Introduction to BBC Third Program series entitled *The Physical Basis of Mind.* Recording (14 min) on three sides of 78 rpm discs. Copies available on request from the British National Sound Archive and the Wellcome Institute for the History of Medicine.

Sherrington, C.S. (1951) *Man on His Nature,* 2nd ed. Cambridge: Cambridge University Press.

Sherrington, C.S. (1953) *Marginalia.* In *Science Medicine and History, Vol. 2,* E.A. Underwood (Ed.). London: Oxford University Press, 545-553. (Note: Sherrington submitted this essay in 1946 and corrected its proof shortly before his death in 1952.)

Smith, O.C. (1934) Action potentials from single motor units in voluntary contraction. *American Journal of Physiology,* 108: 629-638.

Stålberg, E., Trontelj, J.V. (1994) *Single Fiber Electromyography: Studies in Healthy and Diseased Muscle,* 2nd ed. New York: Raven Press.

Stein, P.S.G. (1985) Neural control of the vertebrate limb: Multipartite pattern generators in the spinal cord. In *Comparative Neurobiology: Modes of Communication in the Nervous System,* F. Strumwasser, M. Cohen (Eds.). New York: Wiley, 245-253.

Stein, P.S.G. (1995) A multi-level approach to motor pattern generation. In *Neural Control of Movement,* W.R. Ferrell, U. Proske (Eds.). New York: Plenum Press, 159-165.

Stein, P.S.G. (1997) Scratch reflex. In *Encyclopedia of Neuroscience* (CD-ROM also available), G. Adelman, B. Smith (Eds.). Amsterdam: Elsevier Science.

Stein, P.S.G., Grillner, S., Selveston, A., Stuart, D.G. (Eds.) (1995). *Neurons, Networks, and Motor Behavior,* Proceedings of an International Symposium, Tucson, AZ, Nov. 8-11, 1995. Tucson, AZ: University of Arizona, 87 pp. (See also **http://server.physiol.arizona.edu/CELL/ Department/Conferences.html**.)

Stein, P.S.G., Grillner, S., Selverston, A.I., Stuart, D.G. (Eds.) (1997) *Neurons, Networks, and Motor Behavior.* Boston: MIT Press.

Stein, P.S.G., Smith, J.L. (1997) Neural and biomechanical control strategies for different forms of vertebrate hindlimb motor tasks. In *Neurons, Networks, and Motor Behavior,* P.S.G. Stein, S. Grillner, A.I. Selverston, D.G. Stuart (Eds.). Boston: MIT Press, 61-73.

Strausfeld, N.J., Li, Y., Gomez, R., Kei Ito, K. (1998) Evolution, discovery, and interpretations of arthropod mushroom bodies. *Learning and Memory,* 5: 11-37.

Strauss, R., Hanesch, U., Kinkelin, M., Wolf, R., Heisenberg, M. (1992) No-bridge of *Drosophilia melonogaster:* Portrait of a structural brain mutant of the central complex. *Journal of Neurogenetics,* 8: 125-155.

Stuart, D.G. (Ed./Org.) (1998) *Paths of Discovery in Motor Control Neurobiology.* Graduate colloquium course offered by the University of Arizona/Barrow Neurological Institute/Arizona State University Motor Control Group. See **http://server.physiol.arizona.edu/Physiology/Instruct/695a/695aSched.html**.

Stuart, D.G. (1999) The segmental motor system: Advances, issues, and possibilities. In *Peripheral and Spinal Mechanisms in the Neural Control of Movement. Progress in Brain Research,Vol. 123,* M.D. Binder (Ed.). Amsterdam: Elsevier Science, 3-28.

Stuart, D.G., Enoka, R.M. (1983) Motoneurons, motor units, and the size principle. In *The Clinical Neurosciences, Neurobiology,* Sec. 5, R.N. Rosenberg, W.D. Willis (Eds.). New York: Churchill Livingstone, 471-517.

Stuart, D.G., Enoka, R.M. (1990) Henneman's contributions in historical perspective. In *The Segmental Motor System,* L.M. Mendell, M.D. Binder (Eds.). New York: Oxford University Press, 3-19.

Stuart, D.G., McDonagh, J.C. (1997) Muscle receptors, mammalian, spinal actions. In *Encyclopedia of Neuroscience* (CD-ROM also available), G. Adelman, B. Smith (Eds.). Amsterdam: Elsevier Science.

Stuart, D.G., McDonagh, J.C. (1998) Reflections on a Bernsteinian approach to systems neuroscience: The controlled locomotion of high-decerebrate cats. In *Progress in Motor Control: Bernstein's Traditions in Movement Studies,* M. Latash (Ed.). Champaign, IL: Human Kinetics, 21-49.

Swazey, J.P. (1969) *Reflexes and Motor Integration: Sherrington's Concept of Integrative Action.* Cambridge: Harvard University Press.

Taylor, A., Gladden, M.H., Durbaba, R. (Eds.) (1995) *Alpha and Gamma Motor Systems.* New York: Plenum Press.

Taylor, A., Prochazka, A. (Eds.) (1981) *Muscle Receptors and Movement,* London: Macmillan.

Thorne, F.C. (1976) Reflections on the golden age of Columbia psychology. *Journal of the History of the Behavioral Sciences,* 12: 159-165.

Van Harreveld, A.V., Wiersma, C.A.G. (1937) The triple innervation of crayfish muscle and its function in contraction and inhibition. *Journal of Experimental Biology,* 14: 448-461.

Vilensky, J.A., Gilman, S., Dunn, E. (1998) Derek E. Denny-Brown (1901-1981): His life and influence on American neurology. *Journal of Medical Biography,* 6: 73-78.

Volicer, L. (1973) Relationship between physiological research and philosophy in the work of Pavlov and Sherrington. *Perspectives in Biology and Medicine,* 16: 381-392.

Waller, A. (1850) Experiments on the section of the glossopharyngeal and hypoglossal nerves of the frog, and observations of the alterations produced thereby in the structure of their primitive fibres. *Philosophical Transactions of the Royal Society,* 140, Pt. II: 423-429.

Weber, E.F., Weber, E.H. (1845) Experimenta, quitus probatur nervos vagos rotatione machinae galvano-magneticae irritatos motum cordis retardare et adeo intercipere. *Annali Universali di Medicina Campilatidal Dottore Annibale Omodei, Milano,* 3s. 20: 227-233.

Wetzel, M.C., Stuart, D.G. (1976) Ensemble characteristics of cat locomotion and its neural control. *Progress in Neurobiology,* 1-98.

Wiesendanger, M. (1997a) Pyramidal tract. In *Encyclopedia of Neuroscience* (CD-ROM also available), G. Adelman, B. Smith (Eds.). Amsterdam: Elsevier Science.

Wiesendanger, M. (1997b) Paths of discovery in human motor control: A short historical perspective. In *Perspectives of Motor Behavior and Its Neural Basis.* M.-C. Hepp-Reymond, G. Marini (Eds.). Basel: Karger, 103-124.

Wiggers, C.J. (1960) Some significant advances in cardiac physiology during the nineteenth century. *Bulletin of the History of Medicine,* 34: 1-15.

Wise, S.P. (1997) Motor cortex. In *Encyclopedia of Neuroscience* (CD-ROM also available), G. Adelman, B. Smith (Eds.). Amsterdam: Elsevier Science.

Woodbury, J.W., Patton, H.D. (1952) Electrical activity of single spinal cord elements. *Cold Spring Harbor Symposia on Quantitative Biology,* 17: 185-188.

Worden, F.G., Swazey, J.P., Adelman, G. (Eds.) (1992) *The Neurosciences: Paths of Discovery, I.* Boston: Birkhäuser (first published by MIT Press in 1975).

Young, J.Z. (1992) Sources of discovery in neuroscience. In *The Neurosciences: Paths of Discovery, I,* F.G. Worden, J.P. Swazey, G. Adelman (Eds.). Boston: Birkhäuser, 15-46 (first published by MIT Press in 1975).

Young, R.R. (1997) Elwood Henneman—1915-1996. *Muscle & Nerve,* 20: 133-135.

Zigmond, M.J., Bloom, F.E., Landis, S.C., Roberts, J.L., Squire, L.R. (1999) *Fundamental Neuroscience.* New York: Academic Press.

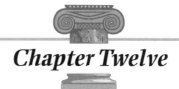
Kurt Wachholder: Pioneering Electrophysiological Studies of Voluntary Movements

Dagmar Sternad
The Pennsylvania State University

Revisiting the work of Kurt Wachholder

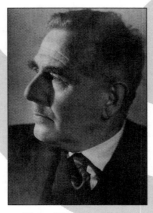

Kurt Wachholder
Reprinted from Weisendanger 1997.

In the literature of the 1970s and 1980s on electromyographic (EMG) activity during discrete single-joint movements, one can find an occasional reference to Wachholder's *Willkürliche Haltung und Bewegung, insbesondere im Lichte elektrophysiologischer Untersuchungen*, published in 1928. For the Anglo-American reader who is not versed in the German language, this title is obviously not very illuminating; and one looks in vain for a translation of this monograph, *Voluntary Posture and Movement, From the Perspective of Electrophysiological Studies*. Wachholder's work is only one example from an era of remarkable scientific achievements in the biological and behavioral sciences—biology, psychology, physiology, and neurology—in the Germany of the 1920s and 1930s. This was the prosperous but short time following the first World War that was soon overshadowed by Hitler's political reorganization in the early 1930s and radically terminated by the ensuing World War II in 1939. The legacy of most of these eminent scientists falls short of their remarkable achievement, especially in the Anglo-American-dominated world of science today. Barriers to an appreciation and continuation of their work were the extended political aftermath in postwar Germany and Europe in general and the dramatic depletion of the German academic community of scientists of Jewish descent that curtailed regular academic activity for a long time. Driven by political circumstances, German postwar scientists reoriented their attention to the United States; and in conjunction, their scientific language switched from German to English. If there was no direct continuation of German prewar research, the newly prevailing English language has prohibited easy access to this large body of work in the German archives ever since. One purpose of this chapter is to raise the awareness of readers, or to remind them, of at least one representative of this era who produced remarkable work in the field of motor control. As will be seen, the quality of scientific inquiry and methodology meets the standards of present-day research. Moreover, the reported results are well worth publishing again since they present an interesting and still relevant piece of research in their own right.

In the neurophysiological literature on movement coordination, Kurt Wachholder is known for his pioneering work on the electrical activity in muscles involved in the generation of voluntary movements. Wachholder was the first to perform extensive studies using the new technology of needle-electrode recording with string galvanometers to measure "action currents" (*Aktionsströme*) in agonist and antagonist muscles during voluntary single-joint movements. Before their discovery, insights into the nature of coordinated muscle contractions could be obtained only through the study of animal preparations or from static contractions in humans where muscle contractions were measured mechanically by palpation. Obviously, any transfer to movement coordination in healthy humans was highly problematic. With the advanced technology of silver or platinum electrodes together with string galvanometers, Wachholder could address a series of open questions raised by neurophysiologists of the time—ranging from the nature of innervation signals to the coordination of agonist, synergist, and antagonist muscles, from the relative contribution of reflex and central commands to the interaction of passive and active forces. Although Wachholder's investigations focused on the peripheral signature of innervation patterns in controlled monoarticular movements, because these were accessible to objective measurement, his ultimate interest always lay in understanding the nature of the central nervous system and its role in producing goal-directed actions.

Wachholder is best known for his discovery of the triphasic EMG pattern in agonist and antagonist muscles during single-joint movements. However, it is indicative of this era of research that this phenomenon was lost in the archives and had to be rediscovered twice before Wachholder's pioneering insight was acknowledged (see Wiesendanger, 1997). In a 1926 publication, Wachholder described the triphasic burst pattern as a function of movement frequency and discussed this finding as an interaction among voluntary activation, reflex activity, passive forces, and a braking function assigned to the agonist burst (Wachholder & Altenburger, 1926c). It took a series of publications in the 1970s and 1980s to arrive at the same conclusions again! For the present volume, I selected a lesser-known paper by Kurt Wachholder and his research assistant Hans Altenburger, which is the ninth paper in his remarkable series of 11 papers in *Pflüger's Archive* published between 1923 and 1927. The selected study on electromyographic (EMG) activity—or in Wachholder's terminology *action currents*—in rhythmic movements is no less important, and it complements his insights about generative principles in discrete movements.

Some Milestones in Wachholder's Life

Kurt Wachholder was born on March 23, 1893, in Oberhausen in the German Rhineland. After finishing the gymnasium in 1912, he took up studies in medicine at the University of Freiburg. After only two semesters he changed universities to continue his studies in Bonn, which had one of the leading institutes for physiology. After a forced interruption of his studies by World War I, Wachholder graduated and received his doctoral degree in 1919 in Bonn, with Max Verworn as his advisor. Wachholder's academic education and career coincided with a thriving scientific era in Germany in the early 1920s and 1930s when the German universities were at the height of their scientific achievement. Particularly in the still relatively young field of physiology, or the newly forming discipline named neurophysiology, major new research directions were opening up: As early as 1910 Paul Hoffmann in Freiburg had discovered the phasic reflex in response to electrical stimulation of the muscle nerve ("Eigenreflex"), which has become known as the H-reflex in his honor; Hans Berger introduced electroencephalography in Jena in 1924; Albrecht Bethe was a leading figure in Frankfurt for more than 30 years, arguing for functional plasticity of the central nervous system as opposed to the prevailing hypothesis of a static structural mapping; and Erich von Holst published his work on the endogenous generation of basic rhythmic patterns in the spinalized fish in 1937, countering the predominant emphasis on the reflex-based nature of actions. These are only a few of the distinguished names that contributed to the scientific productivity in the period between World Wars I and II (see Jung, 1973 for a personal report about this period in science).

Before Wachholder came to Bonn, the physiology institute had been led by E.F.W. Pflüger, who had founded the *Pflüger's Archive für die Gesamte Physiologie der Menschen und Tiere* in 1868. Commonly abbreviated as *Pflüger's Archive*, it quickly became the most reputable German journal promoting a comprehensive physiology. As the title *Pflüger's Archives for the Entire Physiology of Humans and Animals* signaled, it was to become the major outlet for an integrated physiology, comprising respiratory, metabolic, and neurological lines of inquiry in animals and humans. Max Verworn, mentor of Wachholder and many other leading German physiologists, had taken over the editorship of *Pflüger's Archive* in 1910 from Pflüger himself. Verworn's own research on the interrelation of inhibitory and excitatory effects in muscle activation provided the main source of inspiration for Wachholder's studies. Wachholder's dissertation was on the coordination of muscular contractions in the spinal frog's wiping reflex. The study, published in 1923 in Verworn's second journal, *Zeitschrift für Allgemeine Physiologie*, included detailed myographic analyses of the coordination of synergistic and antagonistic muscles during the flexion and extension phases in the frog leg's wiping action. Already foreshadowing his fastidious style of working, Wachholder clarified contradictory findings in the literature and revealed the complicated activation patterns involving maximal contractions and stabilizing contractions in the mostly biarticular muscles of the frog's leg (Wachholder, 1922; Wachholder, 1923a).

After completing his dissertation in 1920, Wachholder took up a position as university lecturer (*Privatdozent*) in Breslau in the eastern part of Germany. It was in this new environment that he turned his attention from the study of reflexes in the frog to the investigation of voluntary movements and postures in humans. Only three years later in Breslau, he completed his *Habilitation*, the second and final qualification for becoming a full professor, and in 1928 he was appointed full professor in Breslau. These studies on movements in healthy humans became possible as a result of considerable advances in the technology of electromyography. Wachholder had fine needle electrodes and very sensitive string galvanometers that he used to measure the detailed progression of "action currents" in isolated muscles. The reader should note that amplification technology was introduced only in 1934. The expensive experimental equipment was financed by the distinguished Rockefeller Foundation located in New York, which promoted international communication at a time when research was still largely confined within national boundaries.

From 1923 to 1928 Wachholder published in *Pflüger's Archive* a series of 11 articles on muscle activity in voluntary movements; some of these were joint publications with Hans Altenburger. These outstanding investigations culminated in an extensive review volume, published in 1928 in the series of *Ergebnisse der Physiologie* (*Results in Physiology*), as well as a contribution in the *Handbuch der Neurologie (Handbook of Neurology)* in 1937 (Wachholder, 1937). With recordings from isolated muscles involved in unconstrained voluntary performance, Wachholder pioneered an objective muscle physiology that could yield more direct answers to long-standing questions on sensorimotor control.

In 1929 Wachholder was called to the University of Zürich to occupy the chair of physiology. In 1933, he returned to Germany, where he was appointed director of the Physiological Institute at the University of Rostock. With this promotion in Rostock, which was one of the oldest institutes for physiology and anatomy in Germany, Wachholder began to redirect his line of research to questions on the physiology of nutrition. His inaugural address in Rostock on the internal production of vitamin C reflected this change. The ensuing years were tainted by the tumultuous political climate of Hitler Germany; and Wachholder's leadership of a large institute through this turmoil was not easy, especially as he never became a member of the Nazi party. With the beginning of the war in 1939, he was drafted into the medical staff of the army with the order to supervise research on the nutrition of soldiers. Only one year later, he was allowed to return to his teaching position at the University of Rostock, where he continued this line of research throughout the rest of his career. Wachholder never became a member of the Socialist party in postwar East Germany. This apolitical position in a high administrative post became particularly problematic during the Stalinist period, and his "nondemocratic attitude" led to problems that finally made him accept a position at his alma mater in Bonn, West Germany. In 1953, before the Iron Curtain came down, he took over the position as chairman of the Physiological Institute, handed down directly from his former mentor Max Verworn.

Kurt Wachholder continued his active research in various fields, ranging from the production and utilization of vitamin C in the human organism to questions of optimal caloric uptake, rhythm and variability in biological systems, and the hormonal and nervous regulation of white blood cells. He never returned to his initial field of research on movement coordination and muscle physiology. Wachholder died at the age of 68 years on August 7, 1961, in Bonn. Before his death he had been working on a paper on the vegetative nervous system for the *Handbook of Ergonomic Medicine*. His work had resulted in 150 contributions in books and journals.

Overview of Wachholder's Work on Movement Coordination

To provide context for the article selected for this volume, a brief summary of Wachholder's perspective on movement coordination and the kinds of questions he addressed precedes the translated paper. An appreciation of the selected study with a link to more recent research concludes this chapter. A good sense of Wachholder's style of inquiry is obtained from the impressive series of 11 articles in *Pflüger's Archive,* while his conceptual framework is best laid out in the 1928 monograph. To appreciate the following summary, which in the main follows the progression of the 11 articles, keep in mind that much of what is now basic textbook knowledge—from the concept of a motor unit, Renshaw cells, and the Henneman size principle to the formation of cross-bridges in the myofibrils during contraction—had not been discovered then. Hence, some questions and conclusions are outdated now. Not outdated, though, is Wachholder's systematic strategy of posing questions, his careful manipulation of independent variables, and the extensive integration of facts from the literature, as well as his balanced argumentation.

Asserting that movement coordination should be an independent field of research in his 1928 monograph, the physiologist Wachholder set out to emphasize that coordination was not defined simply by a set of physiological mechanisms—rather that a coordinated action could be understood only in the light of its movement goal and the actor's intention. If a physiological study of movement coordination were to render useful results that contributed to the understanding of everyday actions, it had to turn away from what he called a mechanistic physiology, which searched for elementary preestablished schemata or programs in muscular activity. Building on earlier views of Foerster and Kohnstamm, he endorsed an organismic physiology that interpreted coordination as a unitary purposeful action constrained by its goal (Foerster, 1902; Kohnstamm, 1901). By definition, coordination was therefore as varied as the intentions that humans could have. Despite the functional and semantic emphasis in the definition, an objective approach was possible. To paraphrase Wachholder's strategy, the aim of research was to systematically vary as many as possible *objective* conditions (e.g., speed, load), as well as *subjective* conditions (e.g., intentions), to investigate the variations in coordination of voluntary movements and thereby to extract *laws* of coordination from the *changes* that are induced by these conditions (Wachholder, 1928, p. 583 [italics by author of this commentary]).

In his opening article, Wachholder introduced his experimental method and critically discussed the nature and limitations of the electrical signal recorded in the muscle. The hallmark of his methodology was the combined recording of electrical signals and continuous position curves (using a high-speed kymograph camera) all aligned to a common time base (using a Jaquet clock)—a technology remarkably advanced for the early days of movement analysis, especially when compared to the predominance of outcome measures in the revival period of motor behavior research in the 1960s and 1970s. The real leading edge, though, was in his use of silver or platinum needle electrodes with very sensitive string galvanometers to measure the isolated activity of single muscles or even motor units during voluntary movements performed by healthy humans. In his first investigations he used one pair of needle electrodes that were inserted 1 to 2 cm (0.4 to 0.8 in.) apart following the direction of the muscle fibers. The measures recorded were therefore not from single muscle fibers, as he surmised, but rather reflected the collective activity of typically a set of motor units. His signals therefore showed different amplitude and frequency patterns, similar to those of surface-electrode measurements. In a critical evaluation of his measurements, he was well aware that the activity patterns were not proportional to muscle forces but that they could give information only about the temporal duration of muscle activity and, at best, about relatively weak or strong muscle activity. Also well aware of the complexity of functional tasks in a natural context, Wachholder designed tightly controlled laboratory movements, such as single-joint rotations of the elbow, wrist, and foot. Unless specifically in focus, all movements were performed in the horizontal plane to avoid the external changing resistance imposed by gravity.

Wachholder's initial goals were to clarify basic issues around the nature and the interpretation of the recorded signal: What were the frequency and amplitude characteristics of the action currents? Is there electrical activity during static postures? Did the measured frequency and amplitude of action currents reflect the innervation frequency coming from the higher nervous centers or motor centers in the spinal cord, or were there specific transformations between central processes and actuator properties, such as resonance? By performing experiments on static postures and dynamic movements, Wachholder rejected Piper's earlier hypothesis of a fixed innervation frequency of 50 Hz (Piper, 1913). Instead, he found two predominant frequency ranges, one between 5 and 75 Hz and a second one at around 150 Hz. In the light of more recent work, both results appear to have been an artifact of his measurements; but it is important that he emphasized the variations that the central nervous system seemed to display. More important and relevant, however, was his exhaustive preparation of basic methodological issues before entering into more complex problems of coordination (Wachholder, 1923b).

With the objective of shedding light on the coordination of muscles involved in discrete movements, the activities of agonist, antagonist, and synergist were recorded under isotonic conditions and different degrees of resistance. While some researchers, such as Hering (1865), had argued that antagonists were totally relaxed during contraction, others claimed that their elongation due to agonist contraction activated a reflexive contraction. Alternatively, Sherrington argued that reciprocal inhibition and reflex excitation acted in an additive fashion (Sherrington, 1906). Resolution of this bone of contention became possible only with the use of needle electromyography since previous measurement techniques, such as palpation of thickness and hardness of muscle bellies or the use of isolated muscle preparations, had been unsuccessful. As a first general result Wachholder pointed out that the interrelation of antagonists' activity patterns was highly variable in different task conditions and that no preestablished pattern could be identified. He found that in movements with no added loads the antagonist activity was minimal, although small bursts led to small decelerations in slow movements. For movements against external resistance, the antagonists showed higher-amplitude activity, and Wachholder discussed their braking function. Given that in the 1970s the nature and origin of the triphasic burst pattern were still a research topic, his discussion of the mechanisms involved, ranging from the stretch reflex and reciprocal inhibition to central coactivation, is remarkable (Wachholder, 1923c).

In a series of further experiments, Wachholder detailed the picture of antagonistic activity in discrete movements. Using an exemplary systematic mechodology, he manipulated experimental conditions and measured antagonist activity for different movement speeds, for different levels of voluntary tension, for different movement amplitudes, for movements against and without the influence of gravity, and on biarticular muscles that served in agonistic and antagonistic functions simultaneously. While the results again showed many variations across subjects and seemingly incoherent patterns for different manipulations (evidence for his antimechanistic view of coordination), Wachholder crystallized two invariant activity types for agonist-antagonist coordination. First, for a single-direction movement the agonist was active in an alternating fashion: once before the onset of the overt movement and a second time at the end of or after the overt movement. The phasing of antagonist activity in relation to the kinematic movement phases varied systematically with movement speed. Second, a continuous low level of agonist and antagonist activity was observed throughout the movement and was especially noticeable in phases in which no high-amplitude activity in the agonist was present. Although Wachholder still had to rely on only one galvanometer, and several measurements on different muscles of the "same" movement were in fact conducted on successive movements, he had already arrived at the conclusion that the two opposing muscles appeared to act in alternation (Wachholder, 1923d).

Turning next to the synergists,[1] Wachholder examined various movements such as abduction of the arm or closing of the hand to a fist at different frequencies and against different resistances. Results demonstrated that phasic activity of synergists was always present and showed patterns similar to those of the agonist: Intervals of activity were observed before onset and prior to termination of the kinematic trace. For a range of movements, the action currents were also shown to consist of successive bursts. Additionally, this polyphasic pattern was shown to influence the kinematic trace, giving it a fine-grained, intermittent structure. However, the activity patterns could not be systematically related to the specific role of the synergists, like joint fixation or additional support to the main movement direction. Under certain conditions, such as in the absence of external load, synergist activity could be weakened, but it could not be intentionally suppressed (Wachholder & Altenburger, 1925a).

The aim of the second paper coauthored by Wachholder and Altenburger was to shed light on the controversy about whether the individual muscle fibers of one muscle acted in synchrony during a contraction, or whether asynchrony or alternation of muscle fiber contractions was the mechanism by which force was graded. The latter conjecture is based on the all-or-none principle for contraction. Using two pairs of needle electrodes for the first time, the authors were able to record two separate activity patterns within the same muscle, measured at different distances and for different movements and postures. Note the methodological comment made earlier, that the recordings actually did not measure individual muscle fibers. Therefore, the recording addressed whether different compartments of muscles act synchronously. The overall results spoke in favor of the synchronous firing of different parts of one muscle during movement: Only during postural tasks did bursts with different spike amplitudes document a significant degree of independence. The result showing that a muscle acted as a functional unit was a prerequisite for the subsequent studies in which the authors examined the temporal relations between bursts in different muscles, measured by single electrode probes. Further, the agreement between neighboring "fibers" was interpreted as evidence that the recorded rhythmic activity reflected an innervation signal from the central nervous system, as opposed to the conjecture that the muscle properties transformed the frequencies (Wachholder & Altenburger, 1925b).

Do central commands that originate from the motor cortex activate both agonists and synergists, or are synergists activated as secondary reflexes triggered by agonist stimulation? Wachholder and Altenburger addressed this question in a study that used two simultaneous recordings. Results showed that the temporal onset and the duration of agonist and synergist were largely coincident. On the other hand, periodicity and amplitudes of bursts suggested that they were independent of each other. The temporal differences in onset were of the order of 10 to 25 ms, which was shorter than reflex activation would allow. Even more convincing and in favor of central coactivation were the cases in which the temporal onset of synergists occurred even earlier than that of the agonist. While this ruled out the sole dependency of synergistic activity on reflex activation, other results were discussed that favored the concomitant involvement of reflexes (Wachholder & Altenburger, 1925c).

For static postures and movements executed under different degrees of voluntary "stiffening" (i.e., subjects cocontracted muscles intentionally), Wachholder and Altenburger measured the concurrent activity within one agonist muscle as well as in both synergist and antagonist. With the exception of postures that were maintained against very high loads, the authors found no congruent activity patterns. With such independence of innervation, any conclusions about the descending signals and organization of the central nervous system were circumspect; and, according to Wachholder and Altenburger, Graham Brown's half-center theory about antagonistic muscular innervation could be valid only for a limited set of conditions (Wachholder & Altenburger, 1926a).

The follow-up study examined the congruence of activity patterns in different parts of the agonist as well as in different synergists and antagonists during relaxed and voluntarily "stiffened" movements. The results showed that in relaxed movements similar activity patterns were observed in different parts of the agonist and in the synergists, whereas in stiffened movements only the general temporal features of the activity were comparable. With this result taken together with the previous findings on postural tasks, the conclusion was that posture and unimpeded movements were governed by two different innervation types. While the similarity in muscle activity in movements was interpreted as indication for a central mechanism, postural tasks did not show such signs (Wachholder & Altenburger, 1926b).

The 10th publication in this series revisited the issue of the alternating action pattern of agonist and antagonist, now however using two electrode pairs to better determine the temporal relationships across muscles. When the antagonist muscle activation was measured in discrete movements performed at different speeds and different levels of voluntary "stiffening," a systematic coactivation pattern appeared: Whereas in slow movements it was only the agonist that appeared to produce the movement, the antagonist was progressively included when movement speed was increased. When over- and undershoot at the end of the movement ("rebound") occurred, a continued alternating activity of the antagonists was observed. Here, as in the translated paper presented in this chapter, a major concern was to determine the active and passive forces involved in the generation of movement. From this observation Wachholder and Altenburger concluded that the antagonist had to cancel inertial forces and elastic forces arising at the end of the movement that led to the rebound. The coactivation was interpreted as the additive result of reciprocal inhibition in conjunction with the common alternating activation of antagonists. From the elastic forces and the dominant periodic antagonist activity in the second half of the movement, the authors concluded that rhythmic movements were the more "natural" form of movements since passive forces were exploited best (Wachholder & Altenburger, 1926c; Wachholder & Altenburger, 1927).

The discussion of the contribution of active and passive forces as extracted from kinematic and electrical signals, as well as the concern about the most "natural form" of movement, is a recurring theme in Wachholder's 1928 review. The following unabridged translation of a study on rhythmic movements again revolves around the conjoint contribution of active and passive forces. In the experimental manipulations, it also emphasizes the role of subjective accentuations, which is a good example of Wachholder's concern about the voluntary contributions to the physiological patterning in coordination.

Contributions to the Physiology of Voluntary Movements
IX. Article
Continuous Rhythmic Movements[2]

K. Wachholder and H. Altenburger

Translation
(From the Physiological Institute of the University Breslau)
Including 8 figures
(Received July 19, 1926)

Contents

Introduction: Objective of the study and criticism of the methodology

- Particular features of continuous forth and back movements
- Types of activities deduced from action currents recorded in agonists and antagonists
  a) Complementary activity of antagonistic muscles
  b) Muscle activity and its relation to the phases in the displacement signal
- Reconstruction of the movements' generating forces

Summary

Objective and criticism of the methodology

As we are going to record the displacements and the action currents[3] of agonist and antagonist simultaneously with the objective to elucidate the forces and their interrelation in generating simple voluntary movements, we are well aware of the limitations of our methods. It seems therefore necessary to briefly discuss the limitations of these measurement methods:

Investigations by Fulton[4] on nerve-muscle preparations of the frog and research by Haas[5] on normal voluntary innervation demonstrated that the magnitude of the action currents in muscles is to a large degree, but not completely, proportional to its tension. Tension, on the other hand, is also a function of the muscle length and of the synchronous or asynchronous activity of the individual muscle fibres. It is therefore impossible to determine the magnitude of the individual muscle forces and to calculate the torques on the basis of the action currents alone. However, as our previous publications have shown, it is very well possible to determine not only whether a muscle is active or inactive during a particular movement, but also at what times it is active, whether the activity is weak, moderate or high, and when this activity increases and decreases.

A second difficulty is to determine whether and to what degree there are, in addition to active muscle activity, also significant passive forces like friction, inertia and elasticity since these forces are not accompanied by fluctuations in the action currents. Despite these shortcomings, we believe that the measured action currents can under certain conditions provide insight into the nature and contribution of elastic and inertial forces.

If we can see that the action currents continue with the same magnitude throughout a continuous movement in one direction, we can conclude that the movement is, in essence, generated by this muscular activity and that inertial forces are hardly relevant. On the other hand, if currents in the agonist cease significantly before the end of the movement, we must conclude that the movement is generated by inertial torques. These can be assumed to be rather large, especially if there are simultaneous currents in the antagonist, i.e., the movement must be slowed down by an antagonist contraction before the movement can be reversed.

Furthermore, if the movement direction is reversed without noticable action currents, we must assume that the reversal is effected by the elastic properties of the tissues (muscles, etc.) that are stretched prior to the reversal. If we can provide evidence for the existence of elastic forces, whose role in voluntary movements is still controversial, it can be concluded that these are also significant contributors in other conditions, such as different movement speeds, in which action currents exist but conceal the contribution of elastic forces.

This method to infer elastic and inertial forces from the absence of action currents is contingent upon: a) that no other agonist or antagonist is active besides the one that is recorded, and b) that the measurement of the currents is sensitive enough[6] to detect weak active tensions in the muscle. The first contingency was satisfied because we chose movements in joint positions in which, according to our experience, the measured muscle was the major agonist or antagonist, for instance, the extensor carpis radialis in wrist movements with flexed fingers. To satisfy the second requirement, we showed that our technology could record action currents in flexors or extensors of the (supported) hand when the hand held weights of as little as 30g.

While our method can reliably determine the effect of elastic and inertial forces under certain conditions, the third type of passive force, friction, is not as easily accessible. Although one can safely assume that there are passive forces in all those cases where the movement slows down or comes to a halt without antagonist activity, there is no possibility to distinguish between frictional or elastic forces. Yet, to anticipate our experimental results, under certain conditions, elastic forces significantly contribute to reversal movements. As in these movements frictional forces must be overcome as well, we have come to believe that the latter forces are only small and can normally be neglected compared to other forces. This has already been emphasized by Wagner.[6]

A third limitation of our method is that, due to external reasons, we are not able to simultaneously record action currents of more than two of the many muscles that are involved in a voluntary movement. Therefore, we cannot provide a complete but rather a restricted picture of the muscular activity. This shortcoming, however, is not too severe because we found in previous studies that not only the activity of different parts of the same muscle but also of the different agonists and antagonists are to a large degree congruent. This finding holds at least for relaxed unimpeded movements. It is therefore feasible and safe to generalize from action currents taken from one restricted muscle part to the activity of the whole muscle as well as to all agonists and antagonists involved in this movement. This congruence only deteriorates if there is an additional impulse directed to obtain a certain posture as, for instance, when movements are voluntarily stiffened, when weights are lifted or lowered, or during a voluntary posture before or after an isolated flexion or extension.[7]

Therefore it appears appropriate to start this study with a type of movement in which such voluntary postures do not play a role, as is the case in continuous forth and back movements in which the individual flexions and extensions follow each other without pause in a fluent progression. The execution of such "unified" forth and back movements is only possible if the respective joint is not intentionally stiffened and remains as relaxed as possible. We are therefore going to investigate only such relaxed forth and back movements. On the basis of these insights we intend to examine more complex movements in the following study where isolated flexions and extensions are complicated by including static postural components.

In the following we will discuss the detailed features of continuous forth and back movements, and the activity patterns of agonist and antagonist in their interrelation during phases of the displacement curve. Lastly, an attempt will be made to evaluate the role of the different active and passive forces that are involved in the generation of these movements.

This objective is notably different from Wagner's extensive investigations.[8] He was interested in the question of how the muscles' coactivation changes under changing external circumstances. He therefore examined the possible limiting cases where the movements were influenced exclusively by frictional forces (as in the stirring of a viscous fluid), or exclusively by inertial forces (as in moving a heavy weight), or exclusively by inertial forces (as in the pulling of a stiff spring). He is of the opinion that "the movements of terrestrial animals are predominantly determined by inertia and, of course, gravity; consequently, he did not appear to consider normal relaxed movements, which are not dominated by such external forces. In contrast, the following study focusses exclusively on such uninfluenced movements which are predominantly determined by inner forces.

Our movements further differ from Wagner's in that he was not interested in the velocity at which the movements were performed, and, hence, only measured slow movements of a duration of 1-2 seconds. According to our earlier results, however, movement velocity is one, if not the central property which determines muscle activity.

Consequently, we did not, like Wagner, manipulate the external factors, such as friction, gravity and resistance of different sorts, but kept them constant or tried to eliminate them. We focussed on how, under these simplified external conditions, the interrelation of the inner forces varied as a function of increasing movement frequency.

I. Specific properties of continuous forth and back movements

Some specific features in the form of simple forth and back movements have been described several times already, particularly by Pfahl.[9] In agreement with earlier results, he found that slow movements do not occur smoothly as one single flow, but rather in steps which is seen as several small accelerations and delays. These irregularities become less frequent and less distinct when the movement is accelerated. At some intermediate tempo the curves become smooth and approximately sinusoidal. He regarded this tempo as especially economical and believed that these movements are largely generated by elastic forces—which is the reason why he called this tempo the "elasticity tempo". This tempo is obtained when the passive limb is pushed and the person then voluntarily continues the wavelike motion at this rhythm. For forearm movements he determined an average frequency of 1 cycle per second, for hand movements 3 cycles per second, and for finger movements 6 cycles per second.

When repeating these experiments we found slightly smaller frequency values which are for the forearm slightly below 1 cycle, for the hand around 2-2.5 cycles [*figure 12.1*], and for the finger around 3-4 cycles per second.

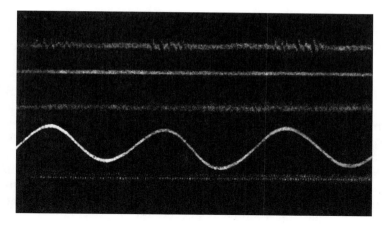

Figure 12.1
Movement of the hand in the tempo following passive pushing (so-called elastic tempo). Extension ↑. Signal at the top: flexor carpis radialis; third signal from the top: extensor carpis radialis. In all figures the second line is the separation between the two signals of action currents. The bottom line shows time in hundredths of seconds.

However, the amplitudes of our movements were significantly larger than those of Pfahl, an observation that is not irrelevant according to our experience. In general, the so-called elasticity tempo is not a narrowly defined and numerically fixed tempo. Rather, we found that, when subjects performed forth and back movements with gradually increasing frequency, they have smooth sine-like forms at significantly slower velocities than found by Pfahl (Figure 3 [*figure 12.3 here*]: a full cycle of a forth and back movement of the hand lasting 62/100 seconds). Also, the irregularities of slow movements are less pronounced, the more the movement is performed in a relaxed fashion. When movements are performed extremely slowly, such that each single phase lasts at least one second, these irregularities are always there, even in people who are well practiced in performing relaxed movements.

If the frequency is increased beyond the elasticity tempo the curves remain smooth but the sinusoidal shape gradually disappears and gives way to a curve with steep straight segments and sharp turning points (Figure 4 [*figure 12.4 here*]). Precise measurements of the curves show that at a frequency of one cycle per second, the gradual deceleration, reversal and renewed acceleration take up 840 ms of the movement time, while the middle portions with maximal velocity only take 160 ms. At a movement frequency of a little less than 2 cycles per second (duration 620 ms), the distribution is 500 ms for the reversal and 120 ms for the middle portions; at a frequency of 4 cycles per second (duration 250 ms) it is 140 and 110 ms [*figures 12.2-12.4*]. The increase in frequency in these moderately fast forth and back movements is therefore only brought about by a shortening of the time needed for the reversal of the movements. At the higher frequencies of 5 cycles per second, the middle portions become smaller due to the involuntary decrease of movement amplitudes; at the highest possible frequencies, the whole movement consists of a sequence of concatenated reversals. Hence, the maximal frequency for forth and back movements of a limb appears to be dependent on the speed at which a reversal can be executed.

On the other hand, there is also a lower frequency boundary to which smooth uniform forth and back movements can still be executed. In extremely slow movements the reversal of movement direction rarely happens in a smooth continuous fashion. Very often there is a sharp discontinuity or a plateau, which is not continuous with the overall rhythm. This observation is in line with the subjective impression that during slow movements, single flexions and extensions are concatenated together, and only when movements are performed at a medium tempo do the forth and back movements become integrated and flowing.

But even for movements performed at these intermediate speeds, closer observation reveals that the two movement directions differ from each other (*Isserlin*).[10] If we turn our attention to such a movement, we can feel that the impulses in the one direction are more noticeable than in the other; or that they even appear to occur in this one direction only. According to our experience, the direction at which this involuntary emphasis takes place is always the same, and this not only holds for the same movement but also for different movements performed by one person with the same joint. For wrist movements some of our subjects always place the emphasis on the extension phase, while others on the flexion phase; for finger movements, all subjects accentuate the same direction. Whether these subjects place an emphasis in the same direction in all other joint movements as well, and whether there are flexion or extension types among people, must remain an open question.

These subjectively different accentuations of flexion and extension, however, do not always show differences when the two movement phases are analyzed objectively. Differences, however, become pronounced if the subject puts a *voluntary* emphasis on the impulse in the one direction. In this case, the movement in the accentuated direction is shorter and steeper than in the unaccentuated one (Figures 6 and 7 [*figures 12.6 and 12.7 here*]). Moreover, it frequently begins with a more or less distinct discontinuity, which either lies at the reversal point or shortly thereafter, while the transition into the other direction occurs smoothly (Figure 7 [*figure 12.7 here*]). The same differences between the two movement directions can also be observed in relaxed, non-accentuated movements, but they are far less pronounced.

Voluntarily accentuated movements of one joint can only be performed smoothly and fluently in one direction, which is the one that the subject would also accentuate involuntarily. If the subject attempts to emphasize the opposite direction, there will be irregularities in the movement, besides the subjective difficulty in doing so. Figures 6 and 7 [*figures 12.6 and 12.7 here*] are taken from a subject who is inclined to involuntarily accentuate the extension direction of the wrist movement. Therefore, the voluntarily accentuated extension movement (Figure 6 [*figure 12.6 here*]) is fairly regular and without differences between flexion and extension. In contrast, the movement which accentuates flexion (Figure 7 [*figure 12.7 here*]) is noticably more irregular. Such differences can be used to objectively determine the direction of involuntary emphasis.

II. Types of activity in the agonist and antagonist as determined from action current recordings

a) Complementary behavior of antagonistic muscles

Inspecting Figures 1-7 [*figures 12.1-12.7 here*], which show forth and back movements of the hand at different frequencies, a clear alternating activity of the two antagonist muscles, flexor and extensor carpi radialis, can be discerned. Very rarely, there is temporal overlap of the activity intervals of the two muscles, and if there is overlap, it is very small. At intermediate movement frequencies, close to the elasticity tempo, the two activity periods do not directly follow each other in time, so that there are phases where both muscles are completely free of action currents (Figures 1, 2, and 3 [*figures 12.1, 12.2, and 12.3 here*]). These pauses typically only last a few hundredths of seconds, and they are longer if the movement is performed in a more relaxed fashion. For extremely relaxed movements, these pauses can take up as much as 1/3 of the total movement duration. In other signals, as for instance seen in Figure 6 [*figure 12.6 here*], there are invariably longer pauses between extensor and flexor currents than between flexor and extensor currents. Another case is exemplified in Figure 7 [*figure 12.7 here*], where extensor and flexor activity is separated by a short pause while the flexor and extensor activities directly connect to each other, or even overlap. Besides these observations, there are also differences between the duration and magnitude of the two muscles' currents. Typically, there is a longer interval between the end of the strong activity and the beginning of the weak activity. All these differences are characteristic for distinctly accentuated movements, regardless of whether the accentuation is voluntary or involuntary. In trials with voluntary emphasis it is evident that the longer and stronger activity is seen in the muscle performing the accentuated movement and the pause lies prior to the unaccentuated muscle activity. This latter finding has most likely implications for a theory of the central nervous coupling of agonists and antagonists (rebound).[11]

The evidently reciprocal behavior of the agonists and antagonists is most clearly seen at intermediate movement frequencies; if the movements are sufficiently relaxed, the antagonist is always completely quiescent during the agonist activity (Figures 2 and 3 [*figures 12.2 and 12.3 here*]). In very slow movements, where the forth and back movement lasts 2 seconds or more, there are almost always weak action currents in the antagonist which are typically separated into single currents or groups of currents; after a short interval these are, in turn, followed by small irregularities (delays) that are characteristic for slow movements. To better understand how slow movements are generated, it is important to recognize that these movements sometimes show clearly distinguishable steps which are not accompanied by action currents in the antagonist. In this case, the action currents in the agonist are not of equal magnitude, rather, they become weaker before each deceleration of the movement and stronger shortly before each acceleration. Such curves without antagonistic activity are only obtained when the subject is able to perform very relaxed movements. In general, the magnitude of the action currents in the antagonist is dependent on how relaxed the movement is. The violation of this strictly reciprocal behavior of the antagonists is most likely due to a stiffening of the joint, which is difficult to avoid during the execution of a very slow movement.

The same reasoning probably also applies to fast forth and back movements where, even when the muscle functions as an antagonist, the galvanometer is never completely still. With the gradual increase in movement frequency fluctuations between the intervals with strong action currents become visible; this typically happens first in the muscle that acts in the direction of the accentuated (voluntarily or involuntarily) movement direction (Figure 5 [*figure 12.5 here*]). With increasing movement frequency these fluctuations become stronger and gradually become also visible in the other muscle such that the antagonists no longer alternate between silence and activity but between strong and weak activity. Close to the maximal movement frequency the rhythmically alternating activity gives way to a cramp-like contraction of both antagonists as can otherwise be found during voluntary strong joint stiffening. This means that here, similar to what was already noted for slow forth and back movements, the simultaneous activity of antagonists must be ascribed to an involuntary stiffening. The principle of reciprocity is therefore not violated in voluntary movements (H.E. Hering). In fact, the more relaxed the movement is, the later does this cramped state set in and the higher is the maximal frequency that can be obtained. One last thing to add is that in the elbow joint the stiffening starts at lower frequencies than in the hand and finger joints, and it starts earlier in all joints when the movements are performed with large amplitudes.

b) Muscle activity and its relation to the phases of the displacement

The temporal relation between the activity intervals of the two antagonists and the phases of the displacement curve are highly dependent on the frequency of the rhythmic movements. Figure 2 [*figure 12.2 here*] shows a typical picture for slow movements. One can see that the weak action currents of the extensor carpi radialis do not begin at the same time, but only 20-30 milliseconds *after* the beginning of the extension movement. These last throughout the entire extension movement with gradually increasing frequency and magnitude; they decrease towards the end, however, without ever completely ceasing at the reversal, and weak activity remains throughout the reversal right into the beginning of the flexion phase. During this phase the string galvanometer of the flexor carpi radialis is completely quiescent. Analogously, the action currents of the flexor carpi radialis only start after the beginning of the flexion and last into the extension phase of the movement (Figure 2, left [*figure 12.2 here*]).

Another feature is that in slow movements the individual flexion and extension phases and the respective activity of the agonists are shifted in time against each other so that the latter lags the former by 20-30 milliseconds. With increasing movement frequency, however, the activity intervals of the respective movement phases move forward in time. At intermediate frequencies the action currents no longer set in after the beginning of the movement but at the points of reversal of direction (Figure 3 [*figure 12.3 here*]). Similarly, the end of the activity interval moves forward in time and does no longer extend into the following movement phase (Figure 2, right [*figure 12.2 here*]). Indeed, when the beginnings of the movement and the action current coincide, then the currents end significantly before the respective movement phase (Figure 3 [*figure 12.3 here*]). The faster the movement frequency, the more the action currents lead the respective movement phase in time. For instance, the currents in the extensor already begin during the second half of the flexion and last

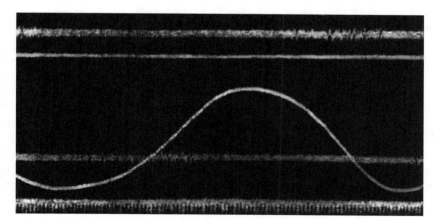

Figure 12.2
Slow movement. Action currents set in after the reversal. Figures 12.2-12.4 are sections of one continuous forth and back movement which is gradually accelerated.

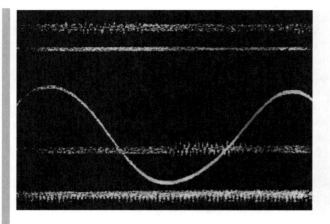

Figure 12.3
Moderately fast move-
ment. Action currents
start at the reversal.

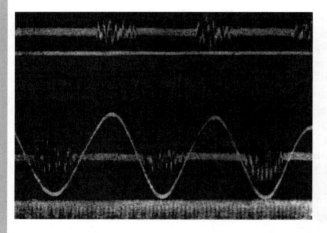

Figure 12.4
Fast movement. Action
currents start before
the reversal.

throughout the reversal into the first half of the extension, to be followed
by action currents in the flexors (Figure 4 [*figure 12.4 here*]). At maximal
movement frequency with small amplitude it is even observed that the
activity intervals fall entirely into the preceding movement phase (Figure 5
[*figure 12.5 here*]). Simultaneous with this increasing shift in time, the currents
become significantly stronger than the ones recorded at slow frequencies.

If the movement is accentuated in one direction, be it voluntarily or
involuntarily, then the accentuated activity always starts earlier than the
unaccentuated one. This is seen in addition to the differences between the
agonists in the accentuated versus unaccentuated direction. In the extension-
emphasized movement (Figure 6 [*figure 12.6 here*]) the action currents of
the extensors begin 100 milliseconds before the extension phase, while the
flexor activity only begins at the moment of reversal to the flexion phase.
At slow movement frequencies it often happens that the action currents in

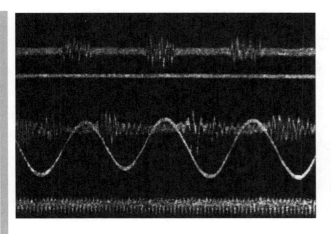

Figure 12.5
Very fast movement. Extension ↑. Top: flexor carpis radialis; bottom: extensor carpis radialis.

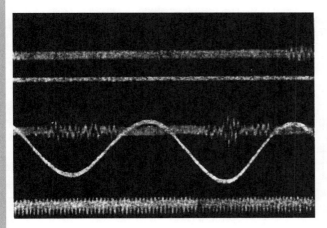

Figure 12.6
Movement with intentional accentuation on extension (↑). Top: flexor; bottom: extensor. Figures 12.5-12.7 are taken from the the same trial.

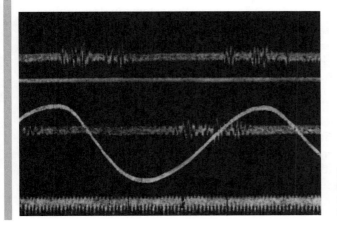

Figure 12.7
Movement with intentional accentuation on the flexion.

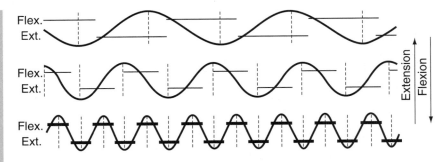

Figure 12.8
Schematic pattern of action currents and phases of displacement for slow, intermediate, and fast movements.

Table 12.1   Average Duration of a Forth and Back Movement on Seconds Where the Action Currents Set in Before, Simultaneously, or After the Beginning of the Respective Movement Phase

Start of action currents in relation to the beginning of the movement	Movement duration		
	Finger	Wrist	Elbow
After	–	Above 0.6	Above 1.5
Simultaneous	0.3-0.4	0.5-0.6	1.3-1.5
Before	0.25 and less	0.5 and less	Below 1.2

the accentuated direction set in with the beginning of the movement while in the unaccentuated direction they set in significantly later.

The typical pattern of action currents and phases of the displacement curve for slow, intermediate and fast movements is summarized schematically in Figure 8 [*figure 12.8 here*]. Table 1 [*table 12.1 here*] shows quantitative data of the average durations of upper extremity movements together with the phasing of the action currents (before, simultaneously and after). One can see that in the elbow joint the start of muscle activity coincides with the start of the movement phase for a movement duration of approximately one cycle per second, in the wrist joint of approximately two cycles per second, and in the finger joint at 2 1/2-3 forth and back movement cycles per second; at higher frequencies the activity intervals are shifted significantly forward. The more proximal the joint is, the earlier the forward shift begins. In contrast to these systematic results, we did not find any dependency on the amplitude.

III. Derivation of the generating forces

From the preceding results it can be concluded that, under certain conditions, such as higher movement velocities, the movement is continued after the agonist has stopped its activity, and that for slower movement velocities the change of direction happens without the influence of the antagonist. It can therefore be concluded, in line with the arguments developed in the introduction that, besides the active muscle forces, there are also passive inertial and elastic forces which participate in the generation of voluntary forth and back movements. On the basis of the reported results, a number of conclusions can be drawn about the role that these passive forces play at different movement frequencies and about how active and passive forces act together.

Slow movements are generated with a weak continuous activity of the agonist in the respective phase of the movement. As each temporary weakening of the action currents is immediately followed by a slowing down of the movement, it can be assumed that this muscle activity is just strong enough to maintain the movement and that no significant inertial forces are developed. Furthermore, without support from antagonists, and even despite the continued agonistic activity, the movement not only comes to a halt but reverses its direction. Consequently, the slowing down and reversing of movement direction in slow movements happens completely passively: the muscles that are stretched during the flexion develop significant elastic forces. Only after the reversal the activity of the respective muscles sets in so that the movement does not subside, as it would if there were only elastic forces and it therefore continues with full amplitude to the next reversal of direction. In many displacement profiles this late beginning is marked by a clearly visible sudden acceleration approximately 100 milliseconds after movement reversal.

At *intermediate movement frequencies* the activity of the agonist stops significantly before the movement reversal. The remaining movement, and predominantly the slowing down, happens passively. Therefore, inertial forces of considerable magnitude must have been generated which continue the movement. These are cancelled out by the elastic forces of the stretched antagonists which leads to a breaking of the movement. The elastic forces presumably also play a significant role in the generation of the reversal movements; but the proportional contribution is difficult to estimate because the muscles, which are now agonists, contract immediately at the beginning of the reversal movement.

In *fast movements* the agonist is already strongly contracted at the beginning of a movement phase. This contraction, however, already stops in the middle of the movement so that the second half is carried out entirely by inertial forces that have been generated in the first half. Yet, they cannot be fully exploited because otherwise the movement would last longer than the desired tempo permits. Rather, in the second half of the movement, a strong contraction of the antagonist sets in rather abruptly which cancels all inertial forces and reverses the direction of the movement. It is most likely that these elastic forces are also participating in the slowing down and the reversal of movement direction. However, they presumably play only a minor role in relation to the strong active forces which are required here. To make use of them in a similar fashion as in slow movements, a considerably longer time would be needed.

If a slow forth and back movement is gradually accelerated to its maximal frequency, then this happens mainly through an acceleration of the reversal phases, as was already described above. At the transition from slow to moderately fast movements this becomes possible because the elastic forces, which slow down the first movement phase, do not have to fight against a continuous contraction of the antagonist, but only against relatively small inertial forces which are easily overcome. The reversal is further accelerated because the reversal is from the beginning not only caused by elastic effects but is accelerated by muscular contraction. At the transition from intermediate to fast movements, the reversal phase continues to be shortened, but it is now the increasingly stronger sudden contractions of the antagonists which replace the relatively slow elastic forces and effect the slowing down. As the inertial forces, which need to be cancelled out, increase with the square of the speed, and as the reversed movement also needs to be accelerated, considerable muscle forces are required. This explains the remarkably fast increase of the action currents when the movement speed is increased from moderately fast to fast rhythmic movements. Accordingly, the maximal frequency that an individual can attain is dependent on the degree with which he is able to contract his muscle quickly and maximally. Of probably equal importance is the ability to quickly relax the muscle, as otherwise the continuous forth and back movements are terminated by a general muscle cramp.

From the preceding analysis of the interaction of forces at different movement speeds the following points are worth noting: During slow movements, active forces are consumed by the fact that the movement is executed against the opposing elastic forces of the stretched antagonist; this is the case throughout its full amplitude and across the reversal. During fast movements active forces of the antagonist have to oppose strong inertial forces. In contrast, at an intermediate speed the inertial and elastic forces are exploited for the execution and the deceleration of the movement, and the only function of active forces is to sustain the movement by repeated impulses of similar magnitude. This is the case when the action currents of the agonist set in at the beginning of the movement and cease shortly before the movement comes to a halt. For the elbow joint, this frequency is approximately 1.3-1.5 seconds per cycle, for the wrist joint at 0.5-0.6 seconds per cycle, and for the finger at 0.3-0.4 seconds per cycle. These differences in frequency are understandable if one considers that the inertial forces, which have to be opposed, are a function of the moving mass which, for comparable speeds, is largest for the elbow joint. Therefore, a contraction of the antagonist in the elbow has to contribute to the deceleration already at slow speeds, whereas for the wrist and finger joint, this contribution is only needed at higher speeds.

The analysis of the cooperation of forces leads to the conclusion that the performance of rhythmic movements at an intermediate tempo is most economical because a great proportion of the work is done by passive forces.[12] Pfahl was the first to direct attention to the fact that at an intermediate tempo the mechanical relations are most favorable for rhythmic forth and back movements. In contrast, though, he arrived at this conclusion in a purely deductive fashion, based entirely on the analysis of the displacement profile.

The tempi that our studies identified as most favorable for the economical cooperation of active and passive forces are not identical to the ones that Pfahl reported as most economical when he used the method of pushing the passive limb. His frequencies are considerably faster, even if we compare them to our fastest estimates. When replicating his experimental conditions, we found that in most cases the action currents did not set in exactly at, but rather well before the reversal point (Figure 1 [*figure 12.1 here*]). Thus, muscular activity supported not only the phase after the reversal, but also the deceleration phase of the movement, at least at the very end of the first movement phase. We never found for these movement conditions that the action currents set in after the reversal. Therefore, we could not confirm Pfahl's[13] results on elastic tempi where he claimed that movements would be effected only by elastic forces.

The question whether Pfahl's elastic tempi, which he found by using his passive pushing method, are the most economical ones, or our intermediate tempi, in which the action currents set in exactly at the reversals of the movement, but which are slightly slower than Pfahl's tempi, has to remain unresolved at this point. Even if the mechanical analysis of a movement is essential for the question of what is the most economic tempo, i.e., identifying the efficient or inefficient cooperation of active and passive forces, the significance of physiological factors cannot be disregarded. It is very well possible that another tempo is more economical in which the cooperation of active and passive forces is not optimal but instead the relation of contraction and relaxation of muscles, or excitation and inactivity of the nervous centers, is most favorable for the maintainance of function.

On the other hand, we regard it as an essential result of the present study that the activity of the nervous centers is not the only necessary basis for the generation of voluntary as well as reflexive movements but that also passive forces, such as inertia and elasticity, are shown to play an important role. These are hypotheses which have been pursued by Rieger[14] and Pfahl[15] for quite some time but their attempt to infer the existence of passive forces from the characteristics of the displacement profile has not yet been generally recognized. We hope that the present investigations have given sufficient empirical support to these hypotheses, but simultaneously also detailed the relative proportion of active and passive forces contributing to movements performed at different speeds.

Summary

Focusing on continuous forth and back movements of the elbow, wrist and finger joints, we examined the action currents of agonists and antagonists in their mutual relations as well as in their relation to the phases of the displacement profile. We conclude from the results that such movements are not only generated by muscle activity but also to a significant degree by inertial and elastic forces.

The kind of interrelations of active and passive forces changes with the speed of the movement. For slow movements the reversal is brought about solely by elastic forces from the stretched tissues (muscles), but a constant activity of the agonists is required to decelerate these elastic forces so that the reversal happens sufficiently slowly. For fast movements strong inertial forces have to be opposed by a contraction of the antagonists in order to bring about the required fast change of direction. At a certain intermediate speed, on the other hand, inertial and elastic forces are exploited to initiate the reversal of direction and only a repeated impulse of muscle activity is needed to sustain the movement. This apparently optimal economical tempo is at approximately one cycle per second for the forearm, at approximately two cycles per second for the wrist, and at just below three cycles per second for the finger.

Wachholder's Legacy

This paper, the ninth in the series, is a good example of Wachholder and Altenburger's style of addressing research questions: The experiments were carefully controlled and technically sound, the interpretation of the data was conservative, and the arguments were presented in a circumspect fashion. In comparison with more recent studies, one shortcoming, though, may be that Wachholder and Altenburger described their findings mostly in verbal detail without the extensive quantification that is customary and expected nowadays: Measures on the exact timing between kinematic and EMG events, and inferential statistical analyses of data from more than a few selected subjects, are missing. And yet the scientific value of Wachholder's papers cannot be overestimated.

It appears strange that Wachholder's work disappeared almost entirely into obscurity. One reason surely is that Wachholder and Altenburger's joint work on movement coordination lasted only five years. While Wachholder turned to other issues, Altenburger moved to Foerster's laboratory and introduced the EMG techniques into the electroencephalogram studies of Foerster. This could have been potentially important continuation if he had not died only a few years later at a very young age. Another major reason obviously was the devastating political circumstances in Germany that began to develop soon after the publication of their work. The war and the subsequent separation of Germany, with Wachholder working in Rostock, East Germany, allowed only severely restricted scientific activity; and there was next to no scientific exchange between the eastern and the western parts of Germany.

The German language surely was an obstacle to a wider appreciation in the Anglo-American community, but even in the German academic world Wachholder's name is no longer widely known. In fact, it was in France that his contemporaries first recognized the significance of his research. In 1926, Fessard in Paris dedicated a paper to Wachholder's work: "Le Movement Voluntaire d'apres K. Wachholder" (Fessard, 1926). Later, Paillard, who started as Fessard's research assistant, incorporated Wachholder's concepts on movement coordination in his own work, *The Patterning of Skilled Movements,* with due mention of the pioneering work of Wachholder and Altenburger (Paillard, 1960). In 1967, Wiesendanger in Zürich published a paper in which he reported the triphasic burst pattern in simple ballistic movements with reference to Wachholder's primary contribution (Wiesendanger, Schneider, & Villoz, 1967). However, this work also remained largely overlooked, as it was published in a Swiss medical journal in the German language. It was only in the 1970s—40 years later and after Wachholder's death—that an article by Angel (1974) on EMG activity in discrete movements resulted in a whole series of studies on the triphasic burst pattern, leading to hypotheses about single-joint movement control such as pulse-height control (Ghez & Gordon, 1987) and the dual-strategy hypothesis (Gottlieb, Corcos, & Agarwal, 1989). In these publications, references to Wachholder's name resurfaced. However, aside from the few tributes to his work on discrete movements, details of Wachholder's experimental results, as well as the broader scope of his efforts, remained largely unknown.

Relevance and Influence on Current Issues in Motor Control

The selected paper on rhythmic movements contains a number of observations that have direct relevance to more contemporary work on rhythmic movements.

Elastic Tempo, Natural Frequency, and Nonlinear Oscillations

One prominent topic in Wachholder and Altenburger's paper was the notion of elastic tempo and the role of active and passive forces involved in movement generation. On the basis of the complementary analysis of EMG and kinematic profiles, Wachholder and Altenburger inferred, using physical and physiological arguments, that the most economical frequency of oscillation was at an intermediate level where "the inertial and elastic forces are exploited for the execution and the deceleration of the movement, and the only function of active forces is to sustain the movement by repeated impulses of similar magnitude" (Wachholder and Altenburger, 1926, p. 639). In other words, the only role proposed for the nervous system was to provide an impulse at the right phase of the cycle to sustain the oscillation and to offset the energy loss. The authors showed that these types of movements displayed the smoothest trajectories with least activity in the involved muscles.

This definition of elastic tempo dovetails with that of the natural frequency, or "comfort mode," in rhythmic movements, as proposed by Turvey, Kelso, and colleagues in their development of a dynamic systems perspective on movement coordination (Kelso, 1995; Kugler & Turvey, 1987). Consistent with Wachholder and Altenburger's concepts, rhythmic activity performed at this preferred frequency plays a central role in the theorizing of the dynamic systems perspective because it is interpreted as one major stable expression, that is, a periodic attractor of a nonlinear dynamic system. In different strands of their work, Turvey and colleagues demonstrated that subjects, when asked to swing a handheld pendulum rhythmically at their most comfortable tempo, reliably and repeatedly chose one frequency closely matching the eigenfrequency of the moving limb. In detailed empirical studies on single-joint wrist, finger, and hand pendulum movements, amplitude and frequency relationships of oscillations performed at different frequencies were shown to have features of limit cycle attractors of nonlinear oscillators (Beek et al., 1995; Beek, Rikkert, & van Wieringen, 1996; Kay, Saltzman, & Kelso, 1991; Turvey et al., 1988; Kay et al., 1987; Kugler & Turvey, 1987).

Rhythmic activity was a central topic for Wachholder also in a more fundamental way: In conjunction with his results on the alternation of agonist and antagonist activity in discrete movements (observed in the triphasic pattern as well as in the corrective adjustments after over- and undershoot at movement termination), he argued that rhythmic movements were the "natural" expression of activity of the nervous system. On the basis of further detailed EMG analyses in his 1928 monograph, he presented a classification of movements in which the categorical distinction between rhythmic and discrete movements was pivotal. He applied these findings to ergonomic designs and recommended that working movements should be repetitive and should be performed at these most economical intermediate frequencies (Wachholder, 1928). While hypotheses about the most "natural" movements always have a touch of speculation, Wachholder and Altenburger's insights into the details of muscular activity in relation to the corresponding kinematics and their arguments for the economy of intermediate frequencies remain an important contribution.

Relation Between Electromyographic Activity and Kinematic Phases As Underlying "Mechanism" of Phase Transitions

Another central result from Wachholder and Altenburger's contribution was the asymmetry of the flexion and extension phases, especially under voluntary accentuation. It was noted that the accentuated part of the movement cycle, typically flexion, was preceded by a flexor burst that was relatively advanced, such that the unaccentuated extensor burst was closely followed by the accentuated flexor burst. In contrast, the interval between the flexor burst and the following extensor burst was relatively longer. This asymmetry in the phasing was reported to be more pronounced for faster frequencies and accompanied by a progressively more irregular electrical pattern.

This observation holds some interest with respect to the interpretation of phase transitions in rhythmical movements. Kelso and colleagues pursued a strategy that identified phase transitions from a less stable to a more stable coordination pattern as a phenomenon typifying the movement system as a nonlinear dynamical system of coupled oscillations (Kelso, 1984). The generic nature of phase transitions in rhythmic movements, specifically from anti-phase to in-phase behavior, has been underscored when similar transitions have been found not only in various interlimb movements but also in between-person situations, and—important in this context—in single-finger oscillations where they were synchronized with a metronome beat. Recently, Carson and Riek (1998) pointed out that many of the transition phenomena could be better understood when the underlying neuromuscular and biomechanical properties were considered. An experiment originally performed by Kelso, Delcolle, & Schöner (1990) and replicated by Carson (1996) showed that when subjects were asked to oscillate their index finger to a metronome beat, the coordination pattern in which flexion was synchronized with the beat (i.e., accentuated) was more stable than when extension was synchronized (i.e., accentuated) with the beat. Phase transitions from extensions to flexions with the beat were obtained in the typical experiment in which one initial coordination pattern was performed at increasingly higher frequencies. Carson showed that this phenomenon was dependent on the forearm position, such that phase transitions occurred earlier and more frequently when the forearm was in a pronated orientation. Additionally, he offered a set of physiological explanations for the preference of flexion, such as the fact that flexors have more monosynaptic cortical projections. While this is substantiation of the differential stability, it does not explain the actual mechanism for the switching process. With a view to Wachholder and Altenburger's results, the accentuation to the beat is accompanied by an asymmetry in the EMG pattern with respect to the kinematic trace, and this asymmetry is accentuated at higher frequencies. As the movement frequency is increased, the temporal adjacency between flexion burst and extension burst also increases, eventually leading to co-contraction. This cramplike state is avoided by reorientation of the anchoring to the next metronome beat, which results in a switching of patterns. Evidently, this extrapolation from Wachholder and Altenburger's results still has a hypothetical character, but the type of reasoning may provide another level of understanding for the transient breakdown and switching of coordination patterns.

"Blocking"—Limitations in Temporal Accuracy of Agonist and Antagonist Activity During Fast Rhythmic Tapping

Heuer (1998) developed a very similar argument to reevaluate the phenomenon of *blocking* in rapid single-finger tapping, a study in which he explicitly recognized the classic work of Wachholder on rhythmic movements. *Blocking* refers to the occasional occurrence of intertap intervals of about twice the duration of the normal interval. While its origin had been unclear, this phenomenon had been interpreted as a sign of fatigue and the exceeding of attentional demands. Heuer (1998) recorded EMG and kinematic data in single-finger tapping executed at a maximal rate. In replicating Wachholder and Altenburger's results, he reported that the flexion and extension bursts were significantly shifted with respect to the kinematic "flexion" and "extension" phases, to such a degree that the EMG bursts were almost entirely anti-phase with the kinematic trace. In detailed analyses, Heuer quantified the temporal relations between EMG bursts and the kinematic landmarks and found that a blocking event was associated with a deviant temporal organization such that the flexor burst occurred too early in the cycle, in close succession to the extensor burst, leading to an omission of a tap. Heuer concluded that rapid rhythmic movements were not limited by contraction rates, but rather by the temporal accuracy at which antagonistic muscles of the oscillating limb were coordinated. With increasing frequency the time window for the precise onset became smaller, allowing small timing errors to effect a disruption of the rhythmic sequence.

These are only three examples suggesting that Wachholder's work holds more than historical interest. Many of his results and insights are remarkably fresh and modern and can be directly related to more current issues. One hope is that these three examples and some of the speculations offered may renew interest in and respect for old and forgotten work.

Acknowledgments

This research was supported by NSF Research Grant SBR 97-10312. I would like to thank Greg Anson for long discussions and a careful reading of the manuscript.

Endnotes

[1] Wachholder distinguished among agonists, antagonists, and synergists. Synergists are all the muscles that contribute to the function of the prime mover.

[2] Translation: Wachholder never uses the term "rhythmic" movements but rather "forth and back" movements. While the translation uses "rhythmic" in the title in order to better relate the contents of the paper to current terminology, Wachholder's own coining will be maintained throughout the text.

[3] The nowadays unusual term "action current" *(Aktionsströme)* refers to the electromyographic activity of muscle fibers.

[4] *Fulton*, Proc. of the Roy. Soc. of London, Ser. B **97**, 424. 1925.

[5] *Haas*, Pflügers Arch. F. d. ges. Physiol. **212**, 651. 1926.

[6] *Wagner*, Mitteilung. Pflügers Arch. f. d. ges. Physiol. **212**, 666. 1926.

[7] VIII. Mitteilung. Pflügers Arch. f. d. ges. Physiol. **212**, 666. 1926.

[8] *R. Wagner*. See footnote 6.

[9] *Pfahl*, Zeitschr. F. Biol. **82**, 377. 1925.

[10] *Isserlin*, Kräpelins Psychol. Arb. **6**, 1. 1914.

[11] Larger differences in the duration and magnitude of the two muscle action currents can also be found independent of accentuation, when the forth and back movements are not performed at the central range of motion but at the joint's extreme ranges of motion. (Note that, for all reported results, the movements were performed at an intermediate range of motion.) In this case one finds that the muscle which moves the limb away from the extreme joint position is less active than the one moving in the opposite direction. If the movement is nevertheless executed with the same speed and extent in both directions, then this is only possible if additional passive forces act in support of the one direction. These passive forces are most likely the very strong elastic forces which are generated by the stretched tissue of the opposite muscles (see below).

[12] In agreement with these results, *Atzler* and colleagues recently found in measurements of oxygen consumption that turning a crank at intermediate speeds is most economical (Pflügers Archive f. d. ges. Physiol., **208**, 184, 1925).

[13] *Pfahl*, Zeitschr. F. Biol. **82**, 378, 1925 see p. 383.

[14] *Rieger*, Zeitschr. f. Psychol. u. Physiol. d. Sinnesorg. **31**, 1 and **32**, 1903.

[15] *Pfahl*, see footnote 13.

References

Angel, R.W. (1974). Electromyography during voluntary movement: The two-burst pattern. *Electroencephalography, Clinical Neurophysiology, 36*, 493-498.

Beek, P.J., Rikkert, W.E.I., & Wieringen van, P.C.W. (1996). Limit cycle properties of rhythmic forearm movements. *Journal of Experimental Psychology, 22*(5), 1077-1093.

Beek, P.J., Schmidt, R.C., Morris, A.W., Sim, M.-Y., & Turvey, M.T. (1995). Linear and nonlinear stiffness and friction in biological rhythmic movements. *Biological Cybernetics, 73*, 499-507.

Berger, H. (1929). Über das Elektroencephalogramm des Menschen. *Archiv für Psychiatrie und Nervenkrankeiten, 87*, 527-570.

Bethe, A. (1931). Plastizität und Zentrenlehre. In A. Bethe, G. von Bergmann, G. Embden, A. Ellinger (Eds.), *Handbuch der normalen und pathologischen Physiologie. Arbeitsphysiologie II: Orientierung, Plastizität, Stimme und Sprache* (pp. 1045-1129). Berlin: Springer.

Carson, R.G. (1996). Neuromuscular-skeletal constraints upon the dynamics of perception-action coupling. *Experimental Brain Research, 110*, 99-110.

Carson, R.G., & Riek, S. (1998). Moving beyond phenomenology: Neuromuscular-skeletal constraints upon coordination dynamics. In J.P. Piek, (Ed.), *Motor behavior and human skill: A multidisciplinary approach.* Champaign, IL: Human Kinetics.

Fessard, A. (1926). Le mouvement volontaire d'apres K. Wachholder. *Chachine*, 1-69.

Foerster, O. (1902). Die Physiologie und Pathologie der Koordination. *Monatsschrift der Psychiatrie, 5.*

Ghez, C., & Gordon, J. (1987). Trajectory control in targeted force impulses: I. Role of opposing muscles. *Experimental Brain Research, 67*, 225-240.

Gottlieb, G.L., Corcos, D.M., & Agarwal, G.C. (1989). Strategies for the control of voluntary movements with one mechanical degree of freedom. *Behavioral and Brain Sciences, 12*, 189-250.

Hering, H.E. (1865). Beitrag zur Frage der gleichzeitigen Tätigkeit antagonistisch wirkender Muskeln. *Zeitschrift für Heilkunde, 16*, 129.

Heuer, H. (1998). Blocking in rapid finger tapping: The role of variability in proximodistal coordination. *Journal of Motor Behavior, 30*(2), 130-143.

Hoffmann, P. (1910). Beiträge zur Kenntnis der menschlichen Reflexe mit besonderer Berücksichtigung der elektrischen Erscheinungen. *Archiv für Anatomie und Physiologie/ Physiologische Abteilung, 1*, 223-246.

Holst von, E. (1939/73). Relative coordination as a phenomenon and as a method of nervous system function. In R. Martin (Ed. and Trans.), *The collected papers of Erich von Host: Vol I. The behavioral physiology of animal and man* (pp. 3-135). Coral Gables, FL: University of Miami Press.

Jung, R. (1973). Some European scientists: A personal tribute. In F.G. Worden, J.P. Swazey, & G. Adelman (Eds.), *The neurosciences: Paths of discovery* (pp. 477-517). Cambridge, MA: MIT Press.

Kay, B.A., Kelso, J.A.S., Saltzman, E.L., & Schöner, G. (1987). Space-time behavior of single and bimanual rhythmical movements: Data and limit cycle model. *Journal of Experimental Psychology: Human Perception and Performance, 13*(2), 178-192.

Kay, B.A., Saltzman, E.L., & Kelso, J.A.S. (1991). Steady-state and perturbated rhythmical movements: A dynamic analysis. *Journal of Experimental Psychology: Human Perception and Performance, 17*(1), 183-197.

Kelso, J.A.S. (1984). Phase transitions and critical behavior in human bimanual coordination. *American Journal of Physiology: Regulatory, Integrative, and Comparative, 246*, R1000-R1004.

Kelso, J.A.S. (1995). *Dynamic patterns: The self-organization of brain and behavior.* Cambridge, MA: MIT Press.

Kelso, J.A.S., Delcolle, J.D., & Schöner, G. (1990). Action-perception as a pattern formation process. In M. Jeannerod (Ed.), *Attention and performance XIII*. Hillsdale, NJ: Erlbaum.

Kohnstamm, O. (1901). Über Koordination, Tonus und Hemmung. *Zeitschrift fürDiät und Physikalische Therapie, 4*, 112-122.

Kugler, P.N., & Turvey, M.T. (1987). *Information, natural law, and the self-assembly of rhythmic movement.* Hillsdale, NJ: Erlbaum.

Paillard, J. (Ed.). (1960). The patterning of skilled movement. *Neurophysiology*, Vol. II. Washington, DC: American Physiological Society.

Piper (1913). Die Aktionsströme menschlicher Muskeln. *Zeitschrift für biologische Technik und Methoden, 3*, 3-52.

Sherrington, C.S. (1906). *The integrative action of the nervous system.* London.

Turvey, M.T., Schmidt, R.C., Rosenblum, L., & Kugler, P.N. (1988). On the time allometry of co-ordinated rhythmic movements. *Theoretical Biology, 130*, 285-325.

Wachholder, K. (1922). Über den Wischreflex des Frosches. Ein Beitrag zur Analyse der Reflexfunktionen des Rückenmarks. *Zeitschrift für allgemeine Physiologie, 19*, 91-118.

Wachholder, K. (1923a). Über rhythmisch alternierende Reflexbewegungen. *Zeitschrift für allgemeine Physiologie, 20*, 161-184.

Wachholder, K. (1923b). Untersuchungen über die Innervation und Koordination der Bewegungen mit Hilfe der Aktionsströme. I. Die Aktionsströme menschlicher Muskeln bei willkürlicher Innervation. *Pflüger's Archive, 199*, 595-624.

Wachholder, K. (1923c). Untersuchungen über die Innervation und Koordination der Bewegungen mit Hilfe der Aktionsströme. II. Die Kooridnation der Agonisten und ANtagonisten bei den menschlichen Bewegungen. *Pflüger's Archive, 199*, 625-650.

Wachholder, K. (1923d). Beiträge zur Physiologie der willkürlichen Bewegungen. III. Über die Form der Muskeltätigkeiten bei der Ausführung einfacher willkürlicher Einzelbewegungen. 2. Die Antagonisten. *Pflüger's Archive, 200*, 266-285.

Wachholder, K. (1928). Willkürliche Haltung und Bewegung. *Ergebnisse der Physiologie, 26,* 568-775.

Wachholder, K. (1937). Allgemeine Muskelphysiologie. In J. Buhmke & O. Foerster (Eds.), *Handbuch der Neurologie.*

Wachholder, K., & Altenburger, H. (1925a). Beiträge zur Physiologie der willkürlichen Bewegungen. IV. Über die Form der Muskeltätigkeiten bei der Ausführung einfacher willkürlicher Einzelbewegungen. 3. Die Synergisten. *Pflüger's Archive, 209,* 286-300.

Wachholder, K., & Altenburger, H. (1925b). Beiträge zur Physiologie der willkürlichen Bewegungen. V. Vergleich der Tätigkeit verschiedener Faserbündel eines Muskels bei Willkürinnervation. *Pflüger's Archive, 210,* 644-660.

Wachholder, K., & Altenburger, H. (1925c). Beiträge zur Physiologie der willkürlichen Bewegungen. VI. Über die Beziehungen der Agonisten und Synergisten und über die Genese der Synergistentätigkeit. *Pflüger's Archive, 210,* 661-671.

Wachholder, K., & Altenburger, H. (1926a). Beiträge zur Physiologie der willkürlichen Bewegungen. VII. Willkürliche Haltungen. *Pflüger's Archive, 212,* 657-665.

Wachholder, K., & Altenburger, H. (1926b). Beiträge zur Physiologie der willkürlichen Bewegungen. VIII. Über die Beziehungen verschiedener synergisch arbeitender Muskeln bei willkürlichen Bewegungen. *Pflüger's Archive, 212,* 665-675.

Wachholder, K., & Altenburger, H. (1926c). Beiträge zur Physiologie der willkürlichen Bewegungen. X. Einzelbewegungen. *Pflüger's Archive, 214,* 642-661.

Wachholder, K., & Altenburger, H. (1927a). Beiträge zur Physiologie der willkürlichen Bewegungen. XI. Über die Genese der Antagonistentätigkeit. *Pflüger's Archive, 215,* 622-627.

Wiesendanger, M. (1997). Paths of discovery in human motor control. A short historical perspective. In M.C. Hepp-Reymond & G. Marini (Eds.), *Perspectives of motor behavior and its neural basis* (pp. 103-134). Basel: Karger.

Wiesendanger, M., Schneider, P., & Villoz, J.P. (1967). Electromyographische Analyse der raschen Willkürbewegung. *Schweizerisches Archiv für Neurologie, Neurochirurgie und Psychiatrie, 100,* 88-99.

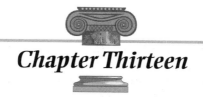

Chapter Thirteen

Woodworth (1899): Movement Variability and Theories of Motor Control

Karl M. Newell and David E. Vaillancourt
The Pennsylvania State University

Revisiting the work of
Robert Woodworth

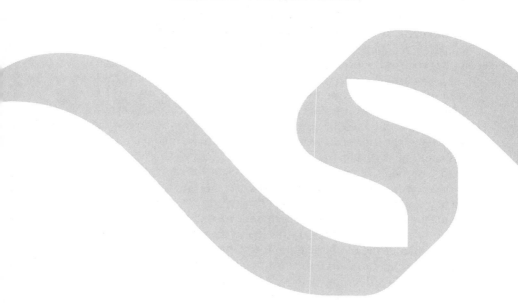

The publication of this collection of classic papers is most timely because it allows us to capture a centennial view of Woodworth (1899). By any standards and, moreover, in relation to a variety of criteria, it is clear that Woodworth has had a profound and lasting influence on the emerging and expanding field of motor control. Here we reproduce selected pages suggesting most important themes of one of Woodworth's papers and provide notes and comments to link these themes to work that has been conducted during the last 100 years. Thus, several segments of text from Woodworth (1899) are reproduced here verbatim. There is no substitute, however, for reading the original Woodworth (1899) paper in its entirety, together with many of the other ground-breaking papers that were written during his era.

We have selected for emphasis four major themes from Woodworth's (1899) paper. The first theme captures some of Woodworth's background theoretical ideas about the psychology and physiology of motor control. Second, we outline key methodological and analysis techniques that Woodworth helped establish for the operational study of limb movement. Third, we turn to his analysis of the relation between movement speed and accuracy. Finally, we emphasize Woodworth's theoretical concept of initial impulse control and subsequent corrections. These four sections are preceded by a few words on Woodworth's academic background and career, and it is to this biographical sketch that we now turn.

Brief of Woodworth's Career

Robert Sessions Woodworth (1869-1962) had a long life and a productive career as a psychologist.[1] Throughout his distinguished career at Columbia University he worked with many well-known psychologists including Wundt, Royce, James, Hall, Thorndike, and Ebbinghaus, and with physiologists such as Bowditch, Sherrington, and Canon. Woodworth was president of the American Psychological Association in 1914 and became a member of the National Academy of Sciences.

The paper included in this chapter, "The Accuracy of Voluntary Movement," is one of the earliest in Woodworth's academic career and formed the basis of the award of his PhD degree in psychology from Columbia University in 1899. His mentor was James McKeen Cattell, who had published a monograph on the psychophysics of movement production[2] that was clearly the background to Woodworth's (1899) effort and that should also be required reading. The late 19th century was the period of the general development of psychophysics in America and Europe, and Woodworth was in essence trying to develop a psychophysics of movement to balance the then-current interest in a psychophysics of perception. Like many scholars, Woodworth shifted the scholarly focus of his research on receiving his doctoral degree, and he published very few additional papers on the topic of movement and accuracy.

The breadth of Woodworth's scholarly contribution is essentially defined and contained in his highly successful book *Experimental Psychology*.[3] He is well recognized for helping to foster experimental psychology as a legitimate and vital subcomponent of psychology. It is noteworthy that Woodworth included aspects of motor learning and skilled performance within this subfield of psychology.

Theme 1: Woodworth's Psychology and Physiology of Movement

Woodworth had training and interests in both psychology and physiology, and his dissertation subject matter, movement accuracy, afforded him an opportunity to integrate these views. Woodworth later published a broader and more fully developed view on this topic in *Dynamics of Behavior*.[4] In the following section we reproduce from Woodworth's paper some introductory comments on these general background issues.

Excerpts From Introduction of Woodworth (1899, pp. 1-7)

In view of all this interest, it is somewhat surprising that the subject of movement has received so little attention from one of the great departments of psychological research. We have as yet no psychophysics of the voluntary movements. By this I mean that we have no large mass of detailed study into the normal relations of voluntary movement to consciousness.

We have nothing in this line that can compare with the immense amount of work done on the relation of perception to the stimulus perceived; or, to widen our view, we have nothing in the general subject of voluntary movement that can compare in completeness with the work done and still doing in all departments of sensation.

It is further noticeable that when the topic of voluntary movement is treated, it is nearly always from the point of view of the *perception* of movement. It is not the movement as produced, but as perceived, that has been the object of study. Much has been written on the sensations or perception or memory of movement, but scarcely anything on the production of movement.

The observation may here suggest itself that this neglect of the mere production of movement is quite fitting in psychology, inasmuch as movement enters into consciousness only as perceived. The objection is, however, not well taken. Movement enters consciousness not only as perceived, but as intended. And the relation of the movement executed to the movement intended is just as important in the study of conscious life as is the relation of the perception to the stimulus perceived. It is quite true that the anatomical and physiological details of the process by which a muscular movement is carried out have no direct bearing on the consciousness that is concerned with the movement. But it is no less true, on the side of sensation, that the anatomy and physiology of the sense organs have nothing directly to do with the consciousness of sensation. Consciousness knows no more of the physiological process by which its sensations reach it than of that by which its intentions are executed. Particular interest attaches to the details of the incoming process, because they condition the details of consciousness. Yet, on the other side, the details of the outgoing process are conditioned by consciousness; and consciousness, like other things, should be studied by its effects as well as by its causes. In short, there is no theoretical reason why the outgoing process should not be studied equally with the incoming, by those who are trying to come to an adequate conception of the conscious life of the human organism. We regard this conscious life as built up on the basis of the reflex arc. We have, so far, studied the afferent portion of this arc. We must advance to the study of the efferent portion. And especially we must endeavor to study the arc as a unit, to trace cause and effect from sense stimulus to muscular response. And we should do this not simply in cases of involuntary response, but in cases of voluntary action. We should, namely, trace the effect upon voluntary actions of varied conditions of sensation. A striking instance of what I mean is afforded by the old observation of Duchenne and of Sir Charles Bell, that a patient whose muscular sense was abolished could execute voluntary movements like extending the hand, when his eyes were open, but either very imperfectly or not at all when his eyes were closed. The outgoing current was apparently impossible when both incoming currents were checked.

The present study is concerned partly with the relations of incoming and outgoing currents in normal individuals. The question raised is not as to the possibility of any movement at all, but as to the relative accuracy of the movement under the control of different senses. A thorough and detailed study of this whole field would be a useful addition to psychology. At present the study of psychological elements is concerned almost wholly with sensation. We see programs of courses written in these terms— "Beginning with a study of sensation, the course proceeds to the higher mental processes—memory, reasoning, emotions, and finally will." This assumes that the elementary study of consciousness must start exclusively from the side of sensation, as if the will were exclusively a 'higher' process. It ignores the fact that movements begin as early in life and as far down in life as any sensation. It fails to see that there is a development of voluntary acts from lower to higher just as truly as there is a development of intellectual life from sensation to abstract thought. And it further overlooks the close dependence of intellectual development on the elementary reactive and voluntary processes. We need, alongside of our elementary study of sensation, a study of the elements of the active side. And since the primary action, the primary volition, consists in bodily movements, that elementary study will devote itself to an analysis of voluntary movements as related to the consciousness that intended them and to the perceptions by which they are governed. Just as we base our conception of sensation on a study of sensations, and our theory of association on a study of associations, so we should base our conception of the will on a study of volitions, and primarily of voluntary movements.

This has, indeed, been the basis on which the best modern discussions of the will have been founded. They have used the material at hand, largely of a clinical character. And this is, of course, a valuable kind of material. But as in the study of the functions of the brain clinical and physiological material supplement and correct each other, so we may reasonably expect that a detailed study of the elements of voluntary action would cooperate to a fuller understanding of the will and of the relation of consciousness to its acts.

In an extended study such as is here conceived, the present paper aims, of course, to fill but a very modest place. Just as the study of sensation has consisted largely in an examination of the accuracy of sensations, so a study of movement will be largely an examination into the accuracy of movement. This side of the subject has hitherto received less attention than has the maximum of movement (dynamogenesis, fatigue experiments, etc.). Practically, however, the accuracy of movement is the more important of the two. It is the accuracy of a movement that makes it useful and purposive. While some few movements require only brute force of a comparatively ungoverned sort, in most cases there must be a considerable degree of control and adaptation to a particular end. The movement must have a particular direction, a definite extent or goal, a definite force, a definite duration, a definite relation to other movements, contemporaneous, preceding and following. Even in comparatively unskilled movements it is remarkable how many groups of muscles must cooperate, and with what accuracy each must do just so much and no more.

And later Woodworth (1899, p. 27):

Some doubt may arise whether my work is really psychological or physiological. The field of voluntary movement undoubtedly lies, like the field of sensation, in the borderland between the two sciences. On which side of the border the present studies lie, I have not thought it worth while to attempt to decide.

Notes and Comments on Theme 1

The preceding segment clearly reveals that Woodworth had identified at least three key issues that remain cornerstones of theoretical psychology and motor control today. First, he pointed up the disparity of research effort at that time with regard to the study of the perception as opposed to the production of movement. This unevenness of inquiry has remained with us through the subsequent 100 years of psychology in spite of the heightened interest currently in the study of movement and action. Second, Woodworth recognized the significance of intention to the link between consciousness and perception. In essence, he endorsed the importance of studying action in perception and perception in action. Furthermore, reflexes were to be understood in the context of voluntary movement and not as isolated segments of intentional behavior. In short, he was clearly against the standard view of the senses as the *beginning* of consciousness and purposeful activity. This position seems a given today for most scholars of motor control, but 100 years ago it was far from the received position. Third, Woodworth emphasized the importance of studying the accuracy of movement as opposed to maximal-effort tasks. He saw accuracy tasks as emphasizing the purposefulness of movement in action and the particular organizational properties of the movement kinematics and kinetics. Accuracy tasks have developed a very significant place in motor control research during the 20th century, and they may well be the most frequently studied category of motor tasks.

One of the most intriguing issues in this opening segment, though, comes by way of the comment that explicitly finesses the distinction between the psychological and the physiological. Given that during this time psychology was striving to establish itself as a separate discipline from philosophy and physiology, this comment would have run the risk of being seen as antiestablishment. Nevertheless, this was a general perspective that Woodworth fostered throughout his career.[4] Today, the disciplinary boundaries to contemporary motor control are being strongly challenged by the notions of interdisciplinary study and modeling attempts of movement and action that are scale independent. One wonders if Woodworth would see the current interdisciplinary array of poster topics at the Society for Neuroscience and other venues of motor control research as a sign of progress.

Theme 2: Methods and Analysis of Motor Control

Woodworth's dissertation, when considered along with the monograph of Fullerton and Cattell (1892),[2] instituted a number of experimental methods and analysis approaches toward a psychophysics of movement that are still central to motor control research some 100 years later. In this section we emphasize portions of Woodworth's methodology and highlight these four main contributions: "Woodworth's Introspection," "Experimental Devices," "Measures of Error," and "Experimental Procedures."

Woodworth's Introspection: Excerpt Taken From Woodworth (1899, pp. 4-7)

An Italian day-laborer breaking stones in the street or hammering on a hand drill, is not classed as a skilled laborer, and yet the movement of swinging the large hammer—requiring as it does the concerted action of muscles of all the limbs and of the trunk, each of which must contract in proper time and force—is executed with such precision that the hammer hits the drill every time.

It is not difficult, by use of the theory of the probable distribution of cases about their average, a theory which undoubtedly holds with approximate correctness for all ways of hitting at a target, and hence for all movements directed to a definite end, to calculate the degree of accuracy of any movement. We have only to determine within what limits the movement must remain in order to escape a 'miss,' and then to count the number of misses in a large number of trials. It is clear that a movement so accurate that though often repeated it seldom misses its mark must, in the great majority of trials, fall far within the limits of a miss. If a marksman can put ninety-nine shots out of a hundred within a certain ring of a target, he can put nine out of ten within a ring only a half or third as large. Knowing the percentage of cases in which the error exceeds certain limits, we can determine by means of the probability curve, or by the corresponding table, the value of the average error, the error of mean square, or any of the standards. The reliability of our determination would increase as the square root of the number of cases observed. The only difficulty with this method is that the number of cases counted would generally have to be large. In any movement which was at all well-practised and efficient the proportion of misses would be very small, and hence the number of cases counted must be large in order to get the true proportion of misses. But if this proportion is too small to be accurately determined within a reasonable time of observation, we can still determine an upper limit beyond which the average error does not lie.

The following is an example of the use of this method of computing the accuracy of every-day movements. I stood for an hour watching four Italians pound on two hand drills. As the two couples kept time with each other, it was easy to count the blows and the misses. I counted 4,000 blows in all, and in that number there was but a single miss. Moreover, that one was the first blow after a rest, and was made by a man who seemed less skilled and confident than his companions. So that the average of 1 in 4,000 is too high rather than too low. The radii of the drill and of the hammerhead were each about two centimeters. The deviation from the center sufficient to constitute a miss measured therefore 4 centimeters. If then an error of 4 centimeters occurs in this movement once in 4,000 trials, the *average* error would be, according to the probability curve, about 0.9 cm. This is small in comparison with the whole movement, since the distance traveled by the hammerhead is at least a meter and a half, or over 160 times the average error. In other words, the error in direction—that of extent is not here involved—averages about one-third of a degree. Yet these laborers swing the hammer almost carelessly, using the eyes to guide them only for the last half of the blow.

In smaller movements, such as those of writing, the absolute though probably not the proportionate value of the average error is still smaller. In letters a centimeter in height I have found the error to average about half a millimeter, or one twentieth. Much more accurate and undoubtedly most accurate of all our ordinary movements, are those of the vocal organs. The adjustments of the vocal cords for pitch, of the breath for loudness, and of the cavity of the mouth for the quality of a tone, must be very fine indeed. The accuracy of pitch may be roughly determined by a method similar to that just used in the case of hammer blows. A large share of us are able to strike a given tone time after time without appreciable discord. The error necessary to constitute a miss will be measured by the smallest difference in pitch that can be detected. This is given as 0.2 of a vibration per second; but that is undoubtedly too small for ordinary quick observation. If we multiply it by 25, and take 5 vibrations per second as the measure of a perceptible miss, we shall be sufficiently conservative. Any one who can sing well enough to make a perceptible discord only once in 20 notes would then, according to the probability curve, have an average error of not over 2 vibrations per second. In order to compare this with the errors in other movements, we need to express the 2 vibrations as a fraction of the extent of the whole movement. The denominator of this fraction would, of course, vary with the size of the interval jumped, and also with the absolute pitch. If the pitch be middle C, or let us say a pitch of 250 vibrations per second, and if the jump be an octave, then the interval, measured in vibrations, is 125 when the jump is from the C below, and 250 when from the C above. And the average error of the singer, under the conditions assumed, would be 2/125 for the jump from the C below, and 1/125 for the jump from the C above. In striking the next C higher, since the vibration rate is doubled, the same percentage of misses would mean an average error of half the size, in proportion to the whole movement or jump. When we consider that along with the precision in pitch there must go a precise adjustment of the current of air and of the parts of the mouth, and that the whole combination of movements must be executed with great promptness, we can hardly doubt that the movements employed in singing a high note are the most accurate under our control. This accuracy is largely the result of the extremely delicate sense—that of pitch—that furnishes its guide. And, indeed, when this sense is applied to the movements of the arm and fingers, the latter can by long practice attain an accuracy perhaps equal to that of the vocal cords. Evidently the same line of reasoning that has been applied to the movements of the cords can be applied to the movements of the violinist's hand, and if the violinist is able to strike a given pitch, and jump a given interval, with the same accuracy and speed as the singer, the same fractions as were obtained above would represent his average error. Probably the movements of the violinist's left hand are, in point of extent, the most delicately graded of any rapid manual movements. It is known that the good violinist must begin very early and grow up in art. The movements of the piano player need not be so accurate in extent, as a much greater leeway is allowed by the breadth of the keys. The remarkable feature of the movements of a skilled pianist is rather their combination of speed and accuracy with great variety and extreme complexity.

Experimental Devices: Excerpt Taken From Woodworth (1899, pp. 16-19)

My experiments have been carried on almost exclusively by the use of various forms of the graphic method. The particular advantage of this method was that it allowed the movements to be made at any desired speed and interval. It also allowed the performance of a large number of tests in a short time, leaving the measurements till afterward. In the way, I have been able to accumulate a number of tests (over 125,000 movements have been used in preparing this paper) that would have been quite impossible in any other way. The subsequent measurements took, indeed, a large amount of time; but as they were very simple and mechanical in character, they could be made by an assistant.

In studying the accuracy of the *extent* of a movement, I used a kymograph rotating on a horizontal axis, and carrying a continuous roll of paper 24 centimeters wide, at a rate of 1-5 mm. per second. Over the drum was fitted a desk-like cover. This concealed the paper, except a narrow area, which showed through a slot parallel to the axis of the kymograph. Along the nearer edge of this slot was a brass straight-edge, which could be moved to and for, and so vary the width of the slot. At one end was fixed another piece of brass to serve as a 'stop,' or, better, as a starting-point for the movements. When the desk-top was in position the brass straight-edge lay 2-3 mm. from the surface of the paper beneath. A hard drawing pencil, beveled to a very tapering point, and held by the fingers in the ordinary position, was now inserted through the slot so that its point rested on the paper. The movement consisted in ruling a line along the straight edge in either direction. Then, as the paper moved slowly by, the movement was repeated at regular intervals indicated by a metronome, and the record came out with the appearance represented in Fig. 1 [*figure 13.1 here*].

The principal advantage of this method lies in the quickness with which a large number of movements can be made and recorded. If it is desired to study the relation of the accuracy of movements to the interval between them, or if for any reason it is necessary to have the movements follow each other at a small interval, some automatic registering apparatus is indispensable. Especially is this true in the case of fatigue. In order to induce fatigue the movements must of course follow so quickly as to allow little time for recuperation between them.

An apparent disadvantage of the particular arrangement here adopted is that the movement of the pencil point does not represent exactly the

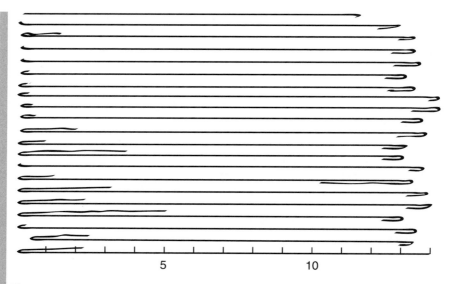

Figure 13.1
Sample tracing of lines ruled on the kymograph, each required to be equal to the preceding. Reduced to 2/3 original size. A centimeter scale is drawn in the last line (reproduction of Woodworth, 1899, Figure 1).

movement of the hand which holds the pencil. As there is a certain amount of free play between the hand and the point of the pencil, and as the resistance to the motion is applied mainly at the point, it is clear that the hand must always move somewhat further than the pencil. This can be observed to be the case, and the more so in proportion to the speed of the movement and to the pressure upon the pencil.

But though this would be a slight source of error if the study were primarily of the *perception* of movement, it is not so when the emphasis is laid on the *production* of movement. In the latter connection the movement must always be studied with respect to some result aimed at. In the present method the result attempted is the drawing of a line of a certain length. This attempt lies nearer common experience, and is more definite and tangible, and so a fairer test of accuracy, than the attempt to make a mere movement of the hand which shall have a certain extent.

The experiment was varied in several ways. Sometimes the normal was seen line, which the subject was to copy time after time. Sometimes the line was reproduced from memory. Sometimes a line was previously drawn on the moving paper, at right angles to the direction of the movements, and movements were required to terminate just on that line. But the most useful method was to require each line to be equal to the one made just before. However much error had been committed in that preceding line, no correction was to be attempted in the new line. The subject was impressed with the idea that his sole duty was, without reference to the errors he had committed in the past, to make the present line equal to that immediately preceding. The width of the slit was so adjusted that the subject saw the line he had just made. The advantage of this method lies, first of all, in the stimulus it gives to the attention. When a large number of repetitions of the same movement are attempted the attention flags and the movement becomes more or less automatic. But by this method the normal is constantly changed, though but slightly. Automatism is excluded. There must be each time a new adjustment to fresh conditions. In the second place, this method is almost necessary if a series of movements is to be made with the eyes closed. If the eyes are closed, and a single normal is required to be repeated time after time, the test is one of memory rather than of accuracy of movement; but when the normal is in each case the line just made, the error of memory is mostly excluded. Another very marked advantage of this method is that each movement is in every way comparable to that which it imitates. In the usual method of psychological experiments one stimulus is presented as a standard and the other as a quantity to be compared with the standard. The attitude of the observer toward the two is different. The one he stores in memory; the other he compares with a memory image. From this difference in attitude arises a constant time-error. In the reproduction of movements this error is specially in evidence, as has been remarked by Delabarre. The normal movement and the reproduction are made at different speeds, and with different innervations of the muscles antagonistic to the movement. As contrasted with this source of error, the method which makes each movement first a reproduction of the preceding, and then a normal to the following, insures that each movement shall receive the same quality of attention and be carried out in the same way.

Measures of Error: Excerpt From Woodworth (1899, p. 20)

Another advantage of this device of making each movement the normal for the following is that the calculation of results, the most tedious part of the use of the graphic method, is much simplified. Instead of measuring the whole lines and computing their average length and average error, we need measure only the difference between the end of each line and the end of the next. These differences give the errors directly. Moreover, if, as often happens, two or more successive errors lie in the same direction, it is not necessary to measure them separately, but only their sum. And still further, if we get the sum of all the errors in one direction, and also the difference between the first and last lines of the series, we can easily compute the sum of the errors that lie in the other direction, and so the total and the average error.

The 'constant error' is also readily obtained by this method, being simply the difference between the first and the last lines divided by the number of lines less one. The curve itself gives a direct demonstration of the direction and amount of the constant error. This may be seen by reference to Fig. 1 [*figure 13.1 here*]. Here, as in most cases, except where the speed is so great as to make it difficult to complete the movement, the constant error is positive (often more strikingly so than here). This figure also illustrates the method indicated above of calculating the average error. The sum of all the positive errors is 62 mm. Now if the sum of the negative errors were equal to that of the positive, the constant error would be 0, and the last line would be of the same length as the first. Since the last line is 17 mm. longer than the first, the sum of the negative errors must be 17 mm. less than that of the positive errors. We may express the calculation in a general formula. If p be the sum of the positive errors and c the last line minus the first, then p-c represents the sum of the negative errors, and 2 p-c represents the total error. On dividing by the number of trials we get the average error. If it is desired to get the pure variable error, the correction can easily be made, first finding the constant error. As, however, the constant error is usually very small, the correction is not worth making.

The average error seems as any rate to be the best general measure of the accuracy of movement, when the normal is *perceived* without much constant error. Evidently the accuracy of a movement cannot be stated wholly in terms of the variable error. Its accuracy must be tested by the closeness with which it attains its goal. The constant error and the variable error may well be isolated and studied separately. But for a complete measure of accuracy the two must somehow be taken in connection with each other, and there seems no better way of connecting them than to leave them combined as nature made them.

There is one source of error in the method of making each line equal to the preceding: since the normal varies in length, the different movements in the same series are not strictly comparable. As the positive constant error is cumulative in its effect, the normal tends to become longer and longer. But this can be practically avoided by making the series short, or by dividing it according to length.

Experimental Procedures: Excerpt Taken From Woodworth (1899, pp. 22-23)

In the first, which may be called the 'coordinate paper experiment,' the movement consisted in hitting with a pencil point at the center of each in turn of the small squares in a sheet of coordinate paper. The coordinate paper used was ruled in square of either one-quarter or one-fifth inch sides (6.4 or 5.1 mm.). The squares within a block of one square inch were aimed at in the order of reading. After a large number of hits had been made the misses were counted. A hit that fell outside of the square or on its sides was counted a miss. A miss would thus measure longer in the corners than in the middle of the sides. But this introduced no error into the calculation, since the accuracy would in any case be proportional to the per cent of misses. The disadvantage of this method is that a large number of hits must be made in order to get a reliable determination of the per cent of errors. Its advantage is that the subsequent calculation of results requires only counting instead of measuring. This is a point of considerable importance in studying fatigue, since, in order to get fatigue, an immense number of hits is necessary, and some device for shortening the calculation is therefore almost indispensable. Besides that, it was desired not to confine the study exclusively to a single sort of movement, but to extend the observations to a reasonable variety of movements. The act of hitting rapidly at a series of targets is quite different from that of ruling a line equal in extent to another. It requires accuracy of direction as well as of extent. And it turned out also to be a more complicated act than that of hitting repeatedly at the same target. The motion is double; besides the vertical striking movements, there is a horizontal motion of the hand along the row of squares. The control of each is to some extent independent of the other. At the faster rates, however, it was not possible to aim each hit separately; the horizontal movement of the hand along a row, and the four of five striking movements for that row, had all to be performed as one act. It is perhaps on account of the complexity of this movement that its accuracy was subject to great variation at different times. For this reason it does not commend itself as a test in individual psychology, or for possible clinical purposes.

Better adapted, because giving much more uniform results, is a device which may be named the 'three target experiment':

Three dots about a millimeter in diameter were made on a sheet of paper at mutual distances of 15 cm., forming thus an equilateral triangle. The sheet was fastened to a table, at a definite position with respect to the subject of the experiment, so, namely, that two dots were about 5 cm. from the nearer edge of the table, and the other dot beyond. One of the two nearer dots—the one on the left when the right hand was to be used, and the one on the right when the left hand was to be used—was brought into the subject's medial plane. A metronome prescribed the speed.

Beginning at the further dot, and going round and round the triangle in a direction opposite to the hands of a watch, the subject aimed in succession of each dot. Exactly 50 hits were made at each dot. Then, to measure the accuracy of the result, the method was simply to find, by trial with compasses, the radius of the circle which would just enclose 34 of the 50 hits, and leave 16 outside. Those counted were, of course, the 16 lying outside. The center of the circle was so chosen that the hits were distributed around it about equally on each side. It represented the center of distribution of the hits. The distance of this center from the dot aimed at gave thus the constant error, which could be determined in direction as well as in extent. The radius of the circle gave the variable error of mean square, which is such that 68% of the cases lie within that distance from the average.

Comments on Theme 2

This extended segment from Woodworth on the analysis of movement error reveals two foundational aspects of his approach to measuring movement accuracy: the importance of linking the measures of movement to both statistical and psychophysical concepts.[2] The section "Woodworth's Introspection" contains an early discussion of the theoretical relevance of the various measures of movement error that arise from the *distribution* of the movement outcome. Woodworth pointed up the important difference between measures of accuracy and measures of variability. This is still an important issue today in the study of movement accuracy and motor control in general,[5] although there is a tendency for modern researchers armed with computers and packaged statistical programs to finesse or even ignore the significance of these fundamental operational issues raised by Woodworth. He also outlined the links between the quantitative technique of measuring performance as an error from a standard and the related qualitative technique of measuring error as merely a miss from a standard (this latter approach, of course, is best known through research that relates to Fitts' [1954] law).[6]

In the next three sections, "Experimental Devices," "Measures of Error," and "Experimental Procedures," Woodworth describes the details of his research methodology. While the theoretical significance of Woodworth's thesis provided a wealth of complex issues, his apparatus and measures of accuracy were simple in their design. Here he used a metronome as the primary tool for controlling the timing of movements and even estimated the minimal visual processing time (400 ms) by this method. In various experiments, he had subjects perform writing, tapping, and aiming movements that remain central issues in motor control research today. Woodworth also introduced important measures of error, namely the constant error, average error, and variable error, in the study of movement accuracy and variability.

This discussion on measurement and movement error is not, however, confined to operational procedures and statistical issues. It also outlines issues pertaining to the relevance of some basic operational protocols that can be studied in movement accuracy tasks, including location versus distance, speed versus no speed requirement, and discrete and sequential movements. Finally, Woodworth links the types of errors measured to theorizing about memory, intention, introspection, perception, and error correction in movement. These are all issues that sit behind research today on movement accuracy, including the related situations in which accuracy tasks are in essence merely used to study some other movement-related construct.

Theme 3: Movement Speed and Accuracy

Woodworth is perhaps best known today in the motor control domain for his early work on the movement speed-accuracy relation. This paper implemented methods to assess issues such as the function of the movement speed-accuracy relation, estimates of minimal visual processing time, and the role of vision in movement limb control. Woodworth's early work in these areas set the theoretical and operational standards that all work since is inevitably and appropriately contrasted against. Indeed, it is useful to keep in mind the question as you read this section: What have we accomplished since Woodworth (1899)?

Excerpts Taken From Woodworth (1899, pp. 27-34)

It is clear that the study of accurate movement must consider at every step the speed of the movement. Two movements are not necessarily the same because they have the same length. If one is more rapid than another, a factor is thus introduced which will very conceivably affect the accuracy. We must, somehow, be able in our experiments to know the speed of the movements. The method here adopted for this purpose is based on the ease with which we can 'keep time.' The *metronome* has been my constant companion during all this work. The subject has been required to make one movement at each stroke of the metronome, which might be set anywhere from 40 to 200 strokes per minute. In case still greater speed was desired the subject was required to make two or three movements to each stroke of the metronome. After a little practice almost everyone can meet these requirements without devoting any attention to keeping time.

Beside the methodological necessity of taking account of the speed of a movement, the relation of accuracy to speed is in itself worthy of study. Common observation teaches us that the accuracy diminishes when the speed becomes excessive, but further than that we shall have to rely on experiment. Will the accuracy diminish regularly, as the speed is increased, or will there be an optimal rate, at which the accuracy surpasses that at either faster or slower rates? How much more accuracy is attainable at low speeds than at high? Is the curve the same for the two hands, and the same with eyes shut as with eyes open? For answers to all such questions we must turn to special experiments.

I have tested the relation of accuracy to speed in several sorts of movements, which may however all be grouped into two classes: the ruling of lines on the drum, and the hitting at targets in different ways. I shall base my discussion of the matter on the results gained in ruled lines, and bring in the other experiments to confirm or to illustrate particular points. The movements of the experiments recorded in Tables I.-IV. [*not reproduced here*] were made by the method, defended above, of requiring each line to be equal to that which immediately preceded. Besides the tables, which give separately the results obtained from the individual subjects, I introduce composite diagrams representing the average results for the four subjects. These diagrams will form the basis of the exposition, and the tables will be directly referred to only in noting individual differences.

The relation of the accuracy of a movement to its speed is presented in Fig. 2 [*figure 13.2 here*]. Since the ordinate is proportional to the average error of the movement, a rise in the curve denotes an increase in the error, and consequently a decrease in accuracy. We see therefore that in a general way the movement loses accuracy as its speed is increased. As the number of movements per minute is increased from 20 to 200—as, therefore, the speed is increased tenfold—the error increases sixfold. We cannot reduce the result of so simple a formula as that the error is proportional. In the left hand, as we shall see, it increases too rapidly to be proportional.

On looking more closely, we see that it is not even true that equal increments of speed produce equal increments of error. The line of ascent is not straight, but steeper in the middle portion than at either end. In fact, at each end there is a portion in which no perceptible increase in error attends the increase in speed. Movements at 40 per minute—that is, at intervals of 1.5 seconds—are on the whole quite as accurate as movements at 20, with intervals of 3 seconds. And movements at 140, 160, 180 and 200 are all about equally accurate. These facts will be studied more in detail in later connections. Here, by way of general explanation, it may simply be suggested that an interval of 1.5 seconds allows time for all the fine adjustments at the end of a movement—all the *groping about,* or adding on of slight additions—that can be done in an interval of 3 seconds. There is, therefore, a lower limit beyond which decrease in speed does not conduce to greater accuracy. And at the upper end there is a limit beyond which increase in speed does not produce much further inaccuracy. The reason is that beyond a speed of 140 to 160 movements per minute it is no longer possible to control the movements separately. Much has to be left to the automatic uniformity of the hand's movements, and this, as we shall see, does not diminish as the speed increases.

In formulating this inverse relation between speed and accuracy we have been limiting our view to movements that were regulated by sight. If we now take into account movements designed to be equal but made without the help of sight, we shall find this inverse relation to hold no longer, at least as a general rule. Figure 3 [*not reproduced here*] shows the relation that obtains when the eyes are closed, and also when the movement is careless or 'automatic.' (For explanation of the 'automatic' movements consult the text to Tables I.-IV. [*not reproduced here*]) We see that the automatic movements gain slightly in uniformity as the speed is increased, while the studied movements made with closed eyes are almost equally accurate (or inaccurate) throughout. The correlation between accuracy and speed is much slighter than when the eyes are used.

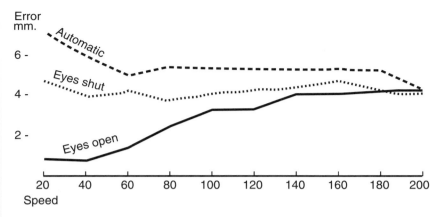

Figure 13.2
Relation of accuracy to speed. Right hand. (Reproduction of Woodworth, 1899, Figure 3.)

As between the three sorts of movement, we notice that that which is governed by the eye is much the most accurate at low speeds, and that the movement with eyes shut, though less accurate than this, is still decidedly better than the careless movement. But though this is true at low speeds, it is less and less true as the speed is increased. The gradual decrease in accuracy when the eyes are used, and the gradual increase in the uniformity of the automatic movements, finally bring all the curves to about the same level. From 140 on, the accuracy is about as great blind as seeing and at 200 no effort avails to improve on the automatic uniformity of the movement. We may put these results in another form as follows: at high speeds the accuracy contributed by voluntary attention, using either the muscle (joint) sense or the eyes, amounts to zero. By decreasing the speed we greatly increase the accuracy due to visual control, but do not increase that due to the muscle sense.

All these inferences have been drawn from movements of the right hand. Figure 4 [*not reproduced here*] shows that the left hand confirms them, with one exception. We do not find at the beginning of the curve for eyes open a flat portion, as in the right hand. An interval of 1.5 seconds is not here as good as one of 3 seconds. The accuracy diminishes rapidly up to the rate of 120 movements per minute, and from there up remains practically constant. The curves for automatic movements and for movements with eyes shut betray no decided tendency, no closer correlation between accuracy and speed than obtains under similar conditions in the right hand. The only general tendency is a sagging of both curves in the middle. The minimum of error—that is, the maximum of accuracy—occurs at intermediate speeds. The point at which attention ceases to add any accuracy to automatic movement comes here at a lower speed than with the right hand. The interweaving of the curves begins as low as 100.

In order to compare more easily the accuracy of right and left hands, and thus to contribute a little to the study of bilateral asymmetry of function, the corresponding curves of figures 3 and 4 are paired off in figures 5, 6, and 7 [*not reproduced here*]. Figure 5 [*not reproduced here*] enables us to compare the accuracy of movements controlled by aid of the eye. At the slowest rate employed, the accuracy attained by the left hand is practically the same as that attained by the right. But as the speed is increased the two curves diverge more and more showing that the left hand is much more quickly and extremely affected by speed than the right. We find in figure 6 [*not reproduced here*] that the superiority of the right hand over the left is marked when the eyes are not used, and in figure 7 [*not reproduced here*] that the same is true even of the uniformity of automatic movements. In both cases the superiority is clearly visible at the lowest rates, but still more so at the high speeds.

These differences between the hands are not peculiar to this one sort of movement, but appear also in target experiments of different kinds, as is shown in Tables XII. and XIV. [*not reproduced here*]

The advantages of the right hand over the left, in point of accuracy, would accordingly seem to be three:

(1) While not capable of greater precision than the left when plenty of time is allowed, it can be controlled much more rapidly. Slow movements can be made as accurately with the left hand, provided the eyes are used—which means, provided a delicate sensory control is used. If plenty of time is allowed, either hand can probably be adjusted as fine as the naked eye can see. But if the speed is increased beyond a certain point—a point which will have different positions for different kinds of movements—the left hand can no longer be controlled as closely as the right. The seat of this superiority of the right hand is probably in the motor centers. The same may be said of the next point of superiority.

(2) Even in automatic movements, the right hand shows a greater uniformity than the left. This is presumably an effect of the greater practice that the right hand has had in making uniform movements. It furnishes a basis of regularity on which the voluntary accuracy of the right hand can build.

(3) In as much as the right hand gives better results also when the eyes are closed, it would seem that the muscle, joint and skin sensations from the right arm are probably more delicate than those from the left. Yet it is possible that (3) is simply an effect of (2).

Comments on Theme 3

The topic of this segment reflects the theme of Woodworth's dissertation and captures the problem for which he has become so well known in the area of motor control. He mapped out the relation between movement speed and accuracy and the influence of vision on this function. This work also represents what may be the earliest attempt to determine the minimal visual processing time in motor control and the influence of bilateral mechanisms on limb control.

The speed-accuracy problem has remained an active research area and has tended through the last 100 years to incorporate the dominant theoretical view of the day.[7] Woodworth's experiments clearly revealed some of the basic features of the speed-accuracy function: first, the concept that movement spatial accuracy tends to decline with increments of movement speed, and second, the concept that the influence of movement speed on accuracy is not linear. This was a confirmation of the earlier findings of Fullerton and Cattell (1892)[2] that Weber's law does not hold for movement accuracy and the psychophysics of movement. Third, there are differences between the error functions for the location and extent of movement. Fourth, there are subtle asymmetrical differences between the influence of handedness on limb control. These basic findings on the speed-accuracy relation all hold today, and they form the empirical backdrop for much current research in motor control.

The other major contribution of Woodworth in the speed-accuracy area relates to the investigation of the influence of vision on movement accuracy. He showed that there are lower and upper velocity bounds to the influence of vision on movement accuracy. In essence he gave an early estimate of the minimal visual processing time in limb control, a topic that has continued to stimulate lively interest.[8] Research since Woodworth's time has tended to show that vision influences limb control in shorter temporal durations than was evident in his work. These differences in the estimates of the temporal limitations of visual control could be due to measurement issues. There is also the postulation that the influence of vision is task specific, thus rendering the search for an absolute minimum less relevant in a general sense than has been periodically proposed through the years.

Theme 4: Initial Adjustment and Current Control

Woodworth introduced the notion of initial impulse control followed by subsequent current control. This is an important theoretical concept that has remained until today, although the labels for the respective phases of the movement have changed some from author to author and theory to theory. In a sense, this two-phase concept of movement control provided the relevant theorizing for the speed-accuracy functions that Woodworth had identified.

Excerpts Taken From Woodworth (1899, pp. 54-62)

The phrases 'initial adjustment,' 'finer adjustments' and 'current control' have been bandied about so freely in the last few pages that the patient reader doubtless hopes they will soon be either given a rest or else made to give an account of themselves. We shall do the latter first.

If one reader desires a demonstration of the existence of the 'later adjustments' which constitute the most evident part of the 'current control,' let him watch the movements made in bringing the point of his pencil to rest on a certain dot. He will notice that after the bulk of the movement has brought the pencil point near its goal, little extra movements are added, serving to bring the point to its mark with any required degree of accuracy. Probably the bulk of the movement is made by the arm as a whole, and the little additions by the fingers. If now the reader will decrease the time allowed for the whole movement, he will find it more difficult, and finally impossible, to make the little additions. Rapid movements have to be made as whole. If similar movements are made with eyes closed it is soon found that the little additions are of no value. They may bring us further from the goal as likely as nearer. We have no extra knowledge of where the goal is, and so cannot use our finer adjustments.

Another demonstration can be had by drawing a free hand line joining two points. The line will record the changes in direction and so give us an insight into the later adjustments as far as they are applied to the direction of the movement. Increasing the speed or shutting the eyes produces the same effects as before. There is, however, one new fact that appears and gives us an insight into the character of the first adjustment. If lines of considerable length, say a foot or two, are made at a rapid rate, the changes in direction will probably be found to be about the same in them all. They all start out at nearly the same angle from the true direction and make about the same sweeping curve around to the goal. This curve is not a simple arc, but bends back on itself. As this curve appears, moreover, when the eyes are closed, the changes in its direction cannot be due to later adjustments. The initial impulse takes the hand along a curve. We aim around a corner; not according to geometrical straight lines, but according to the make-up of our arm. From the geometrical point of view, the simplest movement that we can make—the movement as determined solely by its first impulse, and not complicated with later adjustments—is still a complex affair. The initial adjustment is itself complex. It includes the innervation of different muscles one after another. The coordination adapted to produce a straight line is probably more complex than that to produce certain curves. The first impulse includes also a command to stop after a certain distance. These later effects of the first impulse are probably in some degree reflex. The proper continuation of a movement which has been started seems, from pathological cases, to be dependent on the preservation of the arm's sensibility. Yet the first impulse of a movement contains, in some way, the entire movement. The *intention* certainly applies to the movement as a whole. And the reflex mechanism acts differently according to the difference in intention. We must suppose that the initial adjustment is an adjustment of the movement as a whole.

A graphic demonstration of the later adjustments in the matter of extent of movement is not so easy as in the matter of direction. But by means of a rapidly rotating kymograph it can be accomplished. By this means a curve of the speed of the movement—similar to the curve of muscular contraction—is obtained, and any little additions to the movement can be detected.

As representing the standard curve of a movement governed entirely by its initial adjustment, we take the curve of 'automatic' movements. Since no attention was paid to the extent of these movements, there is no call for later adjustments. With this standard we may compare the curves obtained when each movement was required to imitate the preceding, or to terminate at a given line. We may compare movements also at different speeds, and of the right and left hands. The comparison will reveal the causes of the differences in accuracy between these several movements. See figures 9 and 10.

The most striking difference between these tracings is that between the sharpness of their tops. At the slowest rate the automatic movement gives a sharper top than any other, and the studied movements with eyes open the bluntest. The order of sharpness is: automatic, left hand with eyes shut, right hand with eyes shut, left hand with eyes open, right hand with eyes open. The blunt top is an expression of extreme slowness of movement at the close. To make up for this, the beginning and middle of the movement, and also the return to the staring point, are considerably hastened. This slowness at the end is useful because it allows for the fine adjustments. Evidences of these can be seen in the curves. They are visible as irregularities in direction or as marked differences from the run of the automatic movement. Some of the fine adjustments consist in little *additions* to the movement, carrying it beyond where it would otherwise have gone; and others in a *subtraction* or inhibition of the movement, making it shorter than it would otherwise have been. The latter seem to give the best results; the former seem to be corrections of mistakes. The best type of later adjustment is that which brings the movement so smoothly to a stop that no sharp change in direction is possible. This type is the best, since it is clearly the least awkward. The whole movement runs smoothly to its desired end, without any break or correction.

Turning now to the records of movements at more rapid rates, we see the differences between the different sorts gradually disappear. At 40 the differences are still present; the time allowed is still sufficient for nearly all the later adjustment that can be profitably used. At 80 only the right hand, eyes open, shows any perceptible broadening of the top; at 120 even this is almost gone. Above this the later adjustments are about *nil*, and all movements have to depend on their initial adjustment.

These tracings demonstrate the truth of our previous assumption that the loss of accuracy at high speeds was due to impossibility of later adjustments. Or, as it was expressed, the *bad effect of speed is exerted on the current control of the movement.* A rapid movement does not allow time enough for the later adjustments. The later adjustments are reactions to stimuli set up by the movement, and a rapid movement does not allow for the reaction time. That this is a sufficient explanation of the bad effect of speed, at least up to 120, is seen on comparing the degree of loss of accuracy with the degree of failure of the later adjustments.

The tracings serve also to bring out clearly the differences between the hands. At the slowest rate, the left hand, as well as the right, has plenty of time for its later adjustments, and, therefore, it attains about equal accuracy with the right. The adjustments of the left hand are, however, more awkward. As the speed is increased the left hand loses its fine adjustments much more quickly than the right. We found before that one point of inferiority of the left hand was that, though it could be accurate slowly, it could not combine accuracy with speed. We may now be more explicit, and say that the left hand can make the fine later adjustments of a movement slowly, but not rapidly. Another point of inferiority that was noted was a less delicate tactile sense. This also appears in the tracings. When the eyes are shut and the speed is low the right hand gives a less pointed top than the left. This means that the right hand did more in the way of later adjustment, undoubtedly because it had a keener sense of the normal length.

The presence of later adjustments can be detected in many common movements, as, for instance, in singing. Ordinary singers do not always strike the note accurately at one jump, but must feel around a little after reaching the neighborhood, guiding themselves by the sense of pitch. Probably the ordinary run of violinists, and certainly the beginner, find their notes in this groping way. The path to skill lies in increasing the accuracy of the initial adjustment, so that the later groping need be only within narrow limits; and through increasing the speed of the groping process, so that finally there seems to be no groping at all. The later adjustments are combined with the bulk of the movement in that smooth and graceful way which we picked out from our tracings as the most perfect type. Whether the great virtuosos do away entirely with the later adjustments and achieve their wonderful accuracy by means of the first impulse, would be an interesting thing to find out. The speed and *verve* of their performances make it difficult to suppose there is anything there of the nature of groping. Yet these artists have had to work up through the groping stage, and it is likely that some traces of the process by which they reached perfection should remain in the perfected results. The later adjustment is probably there, but it is made with perfect smoothness, and has by long and efficient practice attained the sureness and the speed of a reflex.

The question, how much of the accuracy of a movement is attained by the initial adjustment, and how much is left to the later adjustments, is difficult of accurate answer. We cannot take the accuracy attained with closed eyes as a measure, for there is some attempt even with eyes closed at later adjustments. And, besides, the accuracy of the initial impulse may increase with the clearness of the normal. Our *aim* is better with eyes open than with eyes closed. A better measure would be the accuracy attained by use of the eyes at high speeds. Since the power of later adjustments is mostly lost at high speeds, the degree of accuracy remaining must be attributed to the initial impulse. But we have found the accuracy of the impulse to be greater at short intervals. So that if we were to take the total accuracy attained at high speeds (and short intervals) as equal to that portion of the accuracy at low speeds which is due to initial adjustment, we should be making the adjustment more accurate than it really is. It would seem proper, however, to take *the accuracy attained at high speeds and long intervals* as approximating to the desired measure. The mere speed, it has been argued, does not interfere with the accuracy of the initial adjustment. What affects it is the interval. If then the interval remains the same, and only the speed is varied, the accuracy of the initial adjustment will remain constant. And if at any speed we can assume the later adjustment to be *nil*, then the accuracy remaining will be that of the initial adjustment at that interval. If then we turn to Tables VII-XI. [*not reproduced here*], and examine the horizontal lines, we shall probably find approximately the measure we are seeking. We have to allow for some chance irregularities, and perhaps can do no better than to take the error at 200 as representing that of initial adjustment when uncorrected by later control. According to this measure we find the final error to be at low speeds very much less than the error of initial adjustment. The final error expressed as a per cent of the error of initial adjustment is as follows:

Table 13.1

	Speed 20	Speed 40	Speed 100
Subject D	9	3	37
Subject W	16	11	74
Subject P	9	–	91
Subject F	6	8	76
Subject F	2	2	86

From these numbers we infer that the initial impulse contributes but a small part of the accuracy of slow movements, but a good share of all the accuracy that remains at 100.

It is quite possible that the numbers in the first two columns are too small. My reason for supposing so is that the initial adjustment, as measured by this method, turns out to be sometimes less accurate than the automatic movements at the same rate. It seems proper to regard the latter as furnishing a zero of accuracy, and anything below this must be due to some disturbance. Perhaps the disturbance consists in the unusual combination of high speed and long interval. At the same time it is quite possible that the initial adjustment of careless movements is fully as accurate as that of careful, when each movement is a repetition of the one before.

The error of initial adjustment can be more readily calculated for the *direction* of movement. In the experiment, described above, of drawing a free-hand line to connect two points, we have a record of the direction in which it started as well as of the point to which it finally came. The direction in which it started is an indication how accurate the first aim was; it represents the initial adjustment. If we produce the line in the direction in which it started, we shall see where the first adjustment alone would have sent it. We can see how far it would have come from the goal, and compare that error of the original adjustment with the error finally made. We can also detect the successive corrections that were made, and see how much accuracy each added. The only difficulty with the method is that not all the changes in direction are real attempts at correction. As stated above, the movement, at least when rapid, proceeds naturally by a curved path. Some of the changes in direction are, therefore, provided for in the initial adjustment. By practice we can distinguish pretty well between such changes and those which record a correction. And this sort of confusion is comparatively absent in slow movements.

I will give the results of one such test. The lines were about 50 cm. in length. They all started at a common center and radiated toward dots which served as goals. They were required to keep time with a metronome beating at a slow rate. When the metronome beat 20 times a minute the average error of the initial adjustment was 23.0 mm. and the final error 2.1 mm. When the beat was 40 a minute the average error of initial adjustment was 38.8 mm., the final error 4.8. The final error was, at the slower rate, 9% of the initial, and at the faster rate 12%. We see here the error in initial impulse increasing as the interval is shortened, contrary to what we observed above. But this need not disconcert us. The movements are here much longer, and not mere repetitions of each other; and the perception of the new target was difficult at short intervals. Hence, the optimal interval is longer than in the simpler movements.

The general conclusion is then fairly clear. The accuracy of the original impulse is slight compared with that added by the later adjustments, when the speed is low and the eyes are used; otherwise, almost as great. In other words, in the situations which permit great accuracy that accuracy is due mostly not to the initial adjustment of the movement as a whole, but to the current control, consisting of finer adjustments.

Comments on Theme 4

Woodworth proposed the important theoretical idea that movements in accuracy tasks are composed of two segments or phases. There is an initial impulse phase that gets the movement going in the right direction. This is followed by a current-control phase that provides adjustments and fine-tunes the movement to realize the desired accuracy in the task. This idea of distinct phases of movement control has persisted through the 100 years subsequent to Woodworth.[9] Furthermore, the notions of current control and successive corrections might in many ways be seen as forerunners of the cybernetically inspired principles of closed-loop control in movement.

Woodworth showed experimentally that it is the current-control phase that fundamentally accounts for the accuracy of movement. He also proposed that the speed of the initial impulse does not influence the accuracy of movement. This latter idea has since been shown to be misplaced through findings emanating from the impulse variability theory of movement accuracy.[10] This difference in experimental findings may be due simply to the limited range of short-duration movements examined in Woodworth's experiments. Nevertheless, one can argue that Woodworth inspired the concept of error correction in current limb control, and this important idea has been shown to be robust over a variety of conditions.[11] This two-phase model of limb control is still seen as central to accounts of the speed-accuracy function for movement control.[5]

Woodworth also identified a problem that still mystifies researchers today: how the fundamental curvilinear motion of limbs is translated to produce linear movements. He did not offer a theoretical account of this empirical issue, but he certainly identified a key problem that theories of limb control need to accommodate.[10,11]

Concluding Comments

One of the features of classic papers in science is that one can continue to distill new ideas and twists on the topic at hand. This is certainly true in the case of Woodworth (1899), and not just because the paper is long and difficult to consume at a single reading. There are several shades of gray to a number of the theoretical and operational points advanced.

The key theoretical contribution to motor control in this paper is undoubtedly the postulate of a two-phase model of limb control, involving an initial impulse and subsequent corrections. Indeed, this idea has a highly contemporary ring. It would be difficult for any scholar of the 20th century to sustain an argument that he or she has made a more fundamental contribution than Woodworth to the study of movement accuracy.

Finally, it is worth noting that Woodworth obtained his experimental findings with what we would view as primitive technology and without a computer. One senses that Woodworth had a strong feel for the phenomena at hand that was enriched by his comprehensive empirical agenda. This was a hallmark of Woodworth's classic approach to experimental psychology and motor control.

Acknowledgment

We would like to thank Howard N. Zelaznik for helpful comments on an earlier version of the paper.

Endnotes

Brief of Woodworth's Career

[1] Key treatments of Woodworth's career including bibliography may be found in the following: Murphy, G. (1963), Robert Sessions Woodworth, *American Psychologist, 18,* 131-133; Poffenberger, A.T. (1962), Robert Sessions Woodworth: 1869-1962, *American Journal of Psychology, 75,* 677-689; Seward, G.S. & Seward, J.P. (Eds.) (1958), *Current psychological issues: Essays in honor of Robert S. Woodworth,* New York: Henry Holt and Company; Woodworth, R.S. (1939), *Psychological issues,* New York: Columbia University Press.

[2] Fullerton, G.S. & Cattell, J. McK. (1892), On the perception of small differences, *The Pennsylvania Philosophical Series, No.2,* Philadelphia: University of Pennsylvania Press.

[3] See texts: Woodworth, R.S. (1938), *Experimental psychology,* New York: Henry Holt and Company; Woodworth, R.S. & Scholsberg, H. (1954), *Experimental psychology,* New York: Henry Holt and Company.

Woodworth's Psychology and Physiology of Movement

[4] See Woodworth's texts elaborating on this issue: *Dynamic psychology* (1918), New York: Columbia University Press; *Dynamics of behavior* (1958), New York: Henry Holt and Company.

Methods and Analysis of Motor Control

[5] See Schutz, R.W. & Roy, E.A. (1973), Absolute error: The devil in disguise, *Journal of Motor Behavior, 5,* 141-153; Newell; K.M. (1976), More on absolute error, etc., *Journal of Motor Behavior, 8,* 139-142; Newell, K.M. & Hancock, P.A. (1984), Forgotten moments: A note on skewness and kurtosis as influential factors in inferences extrapolated from response distributions, *Journal of Motor Behavior, 16,* 320-335.

[6] Fitts, P.M. (1954), The information capacity of the human motor system in controlling the amplitude of movement, *Journal of Experimental Psychology, 47,* 381-391.

Movement Speed and Accuracy

[7] For some contemporary theoretical views on the movement speed-accuracy relation, see Crossman, E.R.F.W. & Goodeve, P.J. (1963), Feedback control of hand movements and Fitts' Law, paper presented at the Experimental Psychology Meeting, Oxford, England, 1963, published in *Quarterly Journal of Experimental Psychology, 35A,* 251-278; Hancock, P.A. & Newell, K.M. (1985), The movement speed-accuracy relationship in space-time, in H. Heuer, U. Kleinbeck, & K.H. Schmidt (Eds.), *Motor behavior: Programming, control and acquisition* (pp. 153-188), Berlin: Springer; Meyer, D.E., Smith, J.E.K., & Wright, C.E. (1982), Models for the speed and accuracy of aimed movements, *Psychological Review, 89,* 449-482; Plamondon, R. & Alimi, A.M. (1997), Speed/accuracy trade-offs in target-directed movements, *Behavioral and Brain Sciences, 20,* 1-31; Schmidt, R.A., Zelaznik, H.H., Hawkins, B., Frank, J.S., & Quinn, J.T., Jr. (1979), Motor output variability: A theory for the accuracy of rapid motor acts, *Psychological Review, 86,* 415-451.

[8] Carlton, L.G. (1981), Processing visual feedback information for movement control, *Journal of Experimental Psychology: Human Perception and Performance, 7,* 1019-1030; L. Proteau & D. Elliott (Eds.), *Vision and motor control,* Amsterdam: North-Holland; Vince, M.A. (1948), Corrective movements in a pursuit task, *Quarterly Journal of Experimental Psychology, 1,* 85-103; Zelaznik, H.N., Hawkins, B., & Kisselburgh, L. (1983), Rapid visual feedback process-

ing in single-aiming movements, *Journal of Motor Behavior, 15,* 217-236; Slifkin, A.B., Vaillancourt, D.E., & Newell K.M. (2000), Intermittency in the control of continuous force production, *Journal of Neurophysiology, 84,* 1708-1718.

Initial Adjustment and Current Control

[9] Crossman, E.R.F.W. & Goodeve, P.J. (1983), Feedback control of hand movement and Fitts' law, paper presented at the meeting of the Experimental Psychology Society, Oxford, July 1963, published in *Quarterly Journal of Experimental Psychology, 35A,* 251-278; Elliott, D. (1992), Intermittent versus continuous control of manual aiming movements, in L. Proteau & D. Elliott (Eds.), *Vision and motor control,* Amsterdam: North-Holland; Jeannerod, M. (1988), The neural and behavioural organization of goal-directed movements, Oxford: Clarendon Press; Keele, S.W. (1968), Movement control in skilled motor performance, *Psychological Bulletin, 70,* 387-403.

[10] Schmidt, R.A., Zelaznik, H.H., Hawkins, B., Frank, J.S., & Quinn, J.T., Jr. (1979), Motor output variability: A theory for the accuracy of rapid motor acts, *Psychological Review, 86,* 415-451; Newell, K.M. & Carlton, L.G. (1988), Force variability in isometric tasks, *Journal of Experimental Psychology: Human Perception and Performance, 14,* 32-44; Carlton, L.G. & Newell, K.M. (1988), Force variability and movement accuracy in space-time, *Journal of Experimental Psychology: Human Perception and Performance, 14,* 24-37.

[11] Polit, A. & Bizzi, E. (1978), Processes controlling arm movements, *Science, 201,* 1235-1237; Morasso, P. (1981), Spatial control of arm movements, *Experimental Brain Research, 42,* 223-227; Flash, T. & Hogan, N. (1985), The coordination of arm movements: An experimentally confirmed mathematical model, *Journal of Neuroscience, 5,* 1688-1703.

Index

Note: The italicized *f* and *t* following page numbers refer to the figures and tables, respectively.

Contributors

Rob Bongaardt, PhD, is an Associate Professor in the Section for Health Science, Faculty of Social Sciences and Technology Management at the Norwegian University of Science and Technology at Trondheim, Norway.

Alan M. Brichta, PhD, is a Senior Lecturer in the Discipline of Anatomy at the University of Newcastle in Australia.

Robert J. Callister, PhD, is a Senior Lecturer and also serves as Head in the Discipline of Anatomy at the University of Newcastle in Australia.

Brian L. Davis, PhD, is a Staff Scientist for the Department of Biomedical Engineering at the Lerner Research Institute of the Cleveland Clinic Foundation in Cleveland, Ohio.

Stan Gielen, PhD, is a Professor and Chairman of the Department of Medical Physics and Biophysics at the University of Nijmegen in The Netherlands.

Sid Gilman, MD, is a Professor in the Department of Neurology at the University of Michigan School of Medicine and also serves as Chairman.

Arthur D. Kuo, PhD, is an Associate Professor for the Department of Mechanical Engineering at the University of Michigan in Ann Arbor.

Ari Levine works for the Department of Biomedical Engineering at the Lerner Research Institute of the Cleveland Clinic Foundation in Cleveland, Ohio.

Jennifer C. McDonagh, PhD, PT, is an Associate Professor of Physical Therapy at the Arizona School of Health Sciences in Phoenix.

Onno G. Meijer, PhD, is on the Faculty of Human Movement Sciences at Vrije Universiteit at Amsterdam, The Netherlands.

Karl M. Newell, PhD, is a Professor for and Head of the Department of Kinesiology at The Pennsylvania State University.

T. Richard Nichols, PhD, is a Professor in the Department of Physiology at Emory University in Atlanta, Georgia.

Patricia A. Pierce, MEd, is a Research Specialist in the Department of Physiology at the University of Arizona College of Medicine in Tucson.

Boris I. Prilutsky, PhD, is the Senior Research Scientist for the Center for Human Movement Studies, at the Georgia Institute of Technology in Atlanta.

Maunak V. Rana, MD, works for the Department of Biomedical Engineering at the Lerner Research Institute of the Cleveland Clinic Foundation in Cleveland, Ohio.

John C. Rothwell, PhD, works for the MRC Human Movement and Balance Unit at the Institute of Neurology in London, UK.

Dagmar Sternad, PhD, is an Assistant Professor for the Department of Kinesiology at The Pennsylvania State University at University Park.

Douglas G. Stuart, PhD, is a Regents' Professor in the Department of Physiology at the University of Arizona College of Medicine in Tucson.

David E. Vaillancourt is an NIA fellow in the Department of Kinesiology and The Gerontology Center at The Pennsylvania State University.

Joel A. Vilensky, PhD, is a Professor in the Department of Anatomy at the Indiana University School of Medicine at Fort Wayne.

Vladimir M. Zatsiorsky, PhD, is a Professor of Kinesiology and Director of the Biomechanics Laboratory at The Pennsylvania State University.

About the Editors

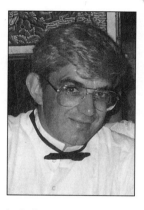

Mark L. Latash, PhD, is a professor of kinesiology at Penn State University. Since the 1970s he has worked extensively in the areas of normal and disordered motor control. He is the author of *Neurophysiological Basis of Movement* and *Control of Human Movement* and the editor of *Progress in Motor Control,* volume 1, and the journal *Motor Control.* He also translated Bernstein's classic *On Dexterity and Its Development* in 1996. He has written more than 100 papers published in refereed journals.

Dr. Latash was an assistant professor and associate professor in the department of physiology and the department of physical medicine and rehabilitation at Rush Medical College in Chicago, Illinois.

He earned a master's degree in physics of living systems from the Moscow Physico-Technical Institute in 1976 and a PhD in physiology from Rush University in 1989. He is a member of the Society for Neuroscience and the American Society of Biomechanics.

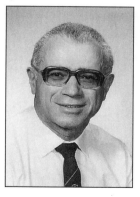

Vladimir M. Zatsiorsky, PhD, is an expert in the biomechanics of human motion. He has been a professor in the department of kinesiology at Penn State University since 1991 and is the director of the university's biomechanics laboratory. Before coming to North America in 1990, Dr. Zatsiorsky served as professor and chair of the department of biomechanics at the Central Institute of Physical Culture in Moscow. He has received several awards for his achievements, including the Geoffrey Dyson Award from the International Society of Biomechanics in Sport (the society's highest honor).

Dr. Zatsiorsky has authored or co-authored more than 250 scientific papers. He has also authored or co-authored 11 books on various aspects of biomechanics that have been published in English, Russian, German, Italian, Spanish, Portuguese, Chinese, Japanese, Polish, Romanian, Czech, Serbo-Croatian, and Bulgarian. His latest books are *Science and Practice of Strength Training* (1995), *Kinematics of Human Motion* (1997), and *Biomechanics in Sport* (2000, editor).

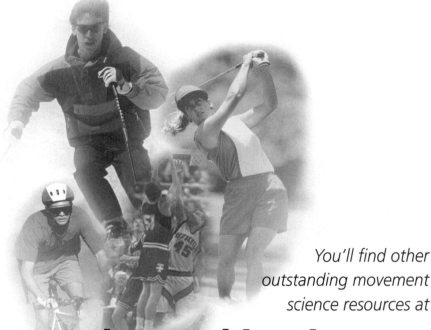

JUN 2 9 2001

DATE DUE
